9225

D1068958

ADVANCES IN NEUROLOGY
VOLUME 8

Advances in Neurology

Advances in Neurology
Volume 8

Neurosurgical Management
of the
Epilepsies

Editors:

Dominick P. Purpura, M. D.
Professor and Chairman
  Department of Anatomy
Director
  Rose F. Kennedy Center
  for Research in Mental
  Retardation and Human
  Development
Albert Einstein College of Medicine
New York City, New York

J. Kiffin Penry, M.D.
Chief, Applied Neurologic
  Research Branch
Head, Section on Epilepsy
Collaborative and Field Research
National Institute of Neuro-
  logical Diseases and Stroke
National Institutes of Health
Bethesda, Maryland

Richard D. Walter, M.D.
Professor, Department of
  Neurology
Center for the Health Sciences
University of California
  School of Medicine
Los Angeles, California

Raven Press, Publishers ■ New York

Made in the United States of America

International Standard Book Number 0–911216–88–x
Library of Congress Catalog Card Number 74–80533

ISBN outside North and South America only: 0–7204–7534–1

Sponsors

NATIONAL INSTITUTE OF NEUROLOGICAL DISEASES AND STROKE

Director
Donald B. Tower

EPILEPSY ADVISORY COMMITTEE

Chairman
Richard D. Walter

Executive Secretary
J. Kiffin Penry

Milton Alter

Lillian R. Elveback

James R. Fouts

Brian B. Gallagher

Richard L. Masland

Dominick P. Purpura

Theodore Rasmussen

Ewart A. Swinyard

Glenn E. Ullyot

Preface

The basic premise that a cortical epileptogenic focus, once identified, should be surgically excised, with proper respect for vital functions, has never been seriously challenged in principle. Neither has it been universally accepted in practice. The reason for this is not a shortage of neurosurgeons possessing the necessary skills and experience for the operative procedures, but rather a lack of consensus as to the role of surgical intervention in the management of the epilepsies. In essence this volume attempts to address this problem, which was identified as a central issue in workshop sessions of the Epilepsy Advisory Committee, National Institute of Neurological Diseases and Stroke, National Institutes of Health. In the planning of this volume, foremost consideration was given to evaluation of the candidate population for surgical intervention, methods and problems of patient selection and study, surgical procedures, and analysis of follow-up. Additionally, it was considered important to review the salient neurophysiological and pathophysiological principles that constitute the rationale for current and some potentially promising neurosurgical approaches to the management of the epilepsies.

If there is one point that emerges from this volume it is that claims to the therapeutic value of any surgical procedure for epilepsy—whether this be cortical resection, temporal lobectomy, or cerebellar stimulation—cannot be evaluated without adequate and prolonged follow-up. Measuring the efficacy of surgical treatment of the epilepsies is even more complicated than measuring the efficacy and toxicity of an antiepileptic drug. For this reason, emphasis was placed on evaluation of the collective experience from several prominent centers with relatively large numbers of cases and with detailed histories of the largest follow-up in several areas of neurosurgical management. Out of this arose another area of concern: the definition of beneficial result over a prolonged period. The goals of any program of epilepsy management are not met solely by statistical documentation of seizure reduction, however salutary such data may be. Psychosocial rehabilitation and integration are equally important determinants of therapeutic success. This calls into examination both purely medical and medico-surgical programs of epilepsy management as necessary components of the inquiry. In this regard it is anticipated that the data presented here will contribute to a continuing examination of the criteria for evaluation of the comprehensive management of the patient with epilepsy.

The surgical treatment of epilepsy was conceived in antiquity, languished for three millennia, and emerged as a modern methodology only forty years ago. The period of growth and development thereafter is highlighted in this volume. But it is not enough that the record be examined without reflection as to the promise for the future. It is hoped that the present volume will reveal additional milestones to assess further development of the opportunities for neurosurgical management of the epilepsies.

The Editors
(September 1974)

Contents

CONTRIBUTORS

Cosimo Ajmone-Marsan, M.D.
Chief, Electroencephalography and Clinical Neurophysiology Branch, National Institute of Neurological Diseases and Stroke, National Institutes of Health, Bethesda, Maryland 20014

Paul H. Crandall, M.D.
Attending Neurosurgeon, Department of Surgery, UCLA Center for the Health Sciences, and Professor of Surgery (Neurological), UCLA School of Medicine, Los Angeles, California 90024

William Feindel, M.D., D.Phil.
Director, Montreal Neurological Institute, and Professor, Department of Neurology and Neurosurgery, McGill University, Montreal, Quebec H3A 2B4, Canada

Pierre Gloor, M.D.
Chief, Laboratory of Electroencephalography and Clinical Neurophysiology, Montreal Neurological Institute and Hospital, and Professor (Clinical Neurophysiology), Department of Neurology and Neurosurgery, McGill University, Montreal, Quebec H3A 2B4, Canada

Gordon Mathieson, M.D., Ch.B., F.R.C.P.(C)
Neuropathologist, Montreal Neurological Institute, and Associate Professor, Department of Neuropathology, McGill University, Montreal, Quebec H3A 2B4, Canada

Francis L. McNaughton, M.D., F.R.C.P.(C)
Neurologist, Department of Neurology, Montreal Neurological Institute and Hospital, and Professor of Neurology, Department of Neurology and Neurosurgery, McGill University, Montreal, Quebec H3A 2B4, Canada

Brenda Milner, Sc.D.
Head, Psychology Department, Montreal Neurological Hospital, and Professor of Psychology, Department of Neurology and Neurosurgery, McGill University, Montreal, Quebec H3A 2B4, Canada

Naomi Mutsuga, M.D., D.Med.Sc.
Visiting Fellow, Surgical Neurology Branch, National Institute of Neurological Diseases and Stroke, National Institutes of Health, Bethesda, Maryland 20014

George A. Ojemann, M.D.
Attending Neurological Surgeon, University Hospital, and Associate Professor of Neurological Surgery, University of Washington School of Medicine, Seattle, Washington 98195

Wilder Penfield, M.D., F.R.S.
Honorary Consultant of the Montreal Neurological Institute, Montreal, Quebec H3A 2B4, Canada

Theodore Rasmussen, M.D.
Senior Neurosurgical Consultant and Former Director, Montreal Neurological Institute and Hospital, and Professor, Department of Neurology and Neurosurgery, McGill University, Montreal, Quebec H3A 2B4, Canada

J. Preston Robb, M.D.
Neurologist-in-Chief, Montreal Neurological Hospital, and Professor of Neurology, McGill University, Montreal, Quebec H3A 2B4, Canada

Doris A. Sadowsky, B.S.
Mathematical Statistician, Office of Biometry, Collaborative and Field Research, National Institute of Neurological Diseases and Stroke, National Institutes of Health, Bethesda, Maryland 20014

E. A. Serafetinides, M.D., Ph.D.
Associate Chief of Staff (Research), Brentwood Veterans Administration Hospital, and Professor of Psychiatry, UCLA School of Medicine, Los Angeles, California 90024

John M. Van Buren, M.D., Ph.D.
Chief, Surgical Neurology Branch, National Institute of Neurological Diseases and Stroke, National Institutes of Health, Bethesda, Maryland 20014

A. Earl Walker, M.D.
Professor Emeritus, Department of Neurological Surgery, Johns Hopkins University School of Medicine, and Clinical Associate, University of New Mexico School of Medicine, Albuquerque, New Mexico 87106

Richard D. Walter, M.D.
Attending Neurologist, UCLA Medical Center, and Professor of Neurology, UCLA School of Medicine, Los Angeles, California 90024

Arthur A. Ward, Jr., M.D.
Chief of Service, Neurological Surgery, University of Washington Affiliated Hospitals, and Professor and Chairman, Department of Neurological Surgery, University of Washington School of Medicine, Seattle, Washington 98195

Advances in Neurology, Vol. 8, edited by D. P. Purpura, J. K. Penry, and R. D. Walter. Raven Press, New York © 1975.

Introduction:
The Physiology of Epilepsy

Wilder Penfield

John Hughlings Jackson, listening to the patients who described to him their epileptic seizures, or watching a fit at the bedside, surmised that this was evidence of brain action caused by unruly discharge in some area of gray matter. He was actually declaring that epilepsy has a neurophysiology of its own. That was one hundred years ago and the entire idea of the localization of semi-separable physiological mechanisms that account for function within the brain was a new and very exciting discovery.

Here was the beginning of neurology as a "science" and the beginning of that part of neurophysiology having to do with brain action and the localization of function. First among the founders of neurology as a science were four men who made very different approaches to the mystery of the brain and the mind.

Paul Broca (1), a French surgeon who was also a pathologist, showed, at autopsy, that speech function has a localization within the brain of man. Fritsch and Hitzig (2), two German physiologists, proved by electrical stimulation that motor function can be localized within the precentral gyrus of a dog. Hughlings Jackson (3), an English neurologist, *primus inter pares,* listened to what epilepsy was saying about the function of the brain.

The authors of the chapters in this book each has special experience and skills that will be of use to anyone who is concerned with the management of the epilepsies. This book deals with the *art* of neurosurgical treatment of "the epilepsies," and includes chapters by neurologists, neuropathologists, neurophysiologists, electrophysiologists, a neurological psychologist, and neurosurgeons whose special experience is varied and vast. Their goal is to see the dawning of the day of perfect practice of the art. Epilepsy is as old as the race, older perhaps. As long as there is brain action, epilepsy will appear from time to time, presenting problems forever difficult and yet revealing.

It is 46 years now since the spring of 1928 when Otfrid Foerster and I completed, in Breslau, Germany, our study of radical cortical excision under local anesthesia as a treatment of focal epilepsy [published in 1930 (4, 5)]. Neurosurgery was far short of being a well-developed art then. But we had seen the microscopic structure of epileptogenic brain lesions and were both excited about the significance of the progressive closures of small blood vessels that were present in all of them. We were sure there were many avenues of access to knowledge and to better therapy in this form of treatment and the use of the electrode.

Montreal Neurological Institute Reprint No. 1164.

The six months that I spent working with Foerster in Breslau were for me an interlude between New York and Montreal. Consequently I sailed with my wife and children from Breslau directly to Montreal. We went with high hopes, realizing that advance in neurology called for special facilities, more varied training, and better medical teamwork.

Six years later, in 1934, two institutes that had been built with the generous financial assistance of the Rockefeller Foundation of New York were opened and "dedicated to the treatment of sickness and pain and to the study of neurology":[1] Foerster Institute in Breslau and the Montreal Neurological Institute.

I have no doubt that Foerster's hopes and dreams, like my own, had had to do, at least in part, with all that might be done for epileptics in such an institute, and all that epilepsy might in turn teach us about the brain and the mind of man, particularly as the techniques for operation under local anesthesia were perfected. Alan Gregg of the Rockefeller Foundation joined us in this dreaming, fortunately for us. In a certain sense, paraphrasing Proverbs, it might be said of both institutes:

> Epilepsy "hath builded her house.
> She hath hewn out her seven pillars."

There is, as I have suggested above, a physiology of epilepsy. This was recognized in the rationalizations of Hughlings Jackson, but that was only a beginning. Today it is not enough to bring to the study of each case electrical stimulation, electrical recording, and other new techniques; we must continue to listen to the patient, with sympathetic insight.

That the epileptic patient had secrets to reveal was discovered long ago by Hippocrates. How delightful is the lecture he gave to Greek physicians and medical students! That was 400 B.C., when no one could have guessed that he would one day be called "Father of Scientific Medicine." The lecture shows the attitude of the man to the art and the practice of Medicine, and to the patient:

I urge you not to be too unkind, nor to consider too carefully your patient's superabundance of means. Sometimes, give your services for nothing . . . For where there is love of man, there is also love of the art. For some patients, though conscious that their condition is perilous, recover their health simply through their contentment with the goodness of the physician.[2]

---

[1] This quoted dedication comes from a tablet on the McGill institute. It would apply equally, no doubt, to the Breslau institute. Unfortunately for Foerster, the Hitler dictatorship paralyzed constructive work in Breslau almost at once, and the World War, which began in 1939, soon put an end to the institute. My dear friend Otfrid Foerster died in Switzerland during the war. In Montreal we were more fortunate. Canadians have supported our enterprise most generously, giving us freedom to contribute to the evolution of neurology in time of peace and even in wartime.

[2] This and other quotations from Hippocrates in this Foreword may be found in Greek and English in Jones, W. H. S., *Hippocrates 1952–1958*. Cambridge, Mass., Harvard University Press; London, Heinemann. The Loeb Classical Library.

This quotation tells us something about the man, but also suggests that he listened to his patients. This may account for the fact that, when other men believed the heart to be the organ of intelligence, he, alone, glimpsed the truth. "To consciousness," he wrote in this same lecture, "the brain is messenger." Then he added, "Men ought to know that from the brain, and from the brain only, arise our pleasures, joys, laughter and jests, as well as our sorrows, pain, griefs and tears. Through it, in particular, we think, see, hear and distinguish the ugly from the beautiful, the bad from the good, the pleasant from the unpleasant."

This amazing statement, which I have quoted many times, is taken from the only one of his preserved lectures that has to do with *Epilepsia,* a malady which, he explained, comes from the brain "when it is not normal." And then his mind leaped beyond the subject of his discussion for a moment, and he made another startling assertion in a brief aside: "Madness, too, comes from the brain when it is not normal."

How could this clinician who knew nothing of the hidden structure of the brain have understood its function so clearly? A clue to the answer is to be found in the excellence of the histories he left behind, written on papyrus. Although brief, they are nonetheless models of critical insight: he loved men. But he listened with attention, as well as compassion, to the many epileptics who must have come to him for help. He pondered their revealing stories and watched each attack that occurred in his presence. Thus he came upon the secrets that *Epilepsia* was ready then, as she is now, to reveal to any physician who comes to her with a prepared mind.

We know something of how Hippocrates had prepared his mind. He had defied the superstitions of that day and denied what he called the "unprovable hypotheses of the philosophers" of his time. He had reached his own conclusion that disease in general was *not* an evidence of sin or of disfavor on Mount Olympus, and that epilepsy in particular was not the curse of any god or devil. Truth, he had concluded, was to be found in nature and in the observation of man in health and in disease. Thus he listened and observed and pondered the nature of man's being.

I can so easily imagine now how it came about that some patient, suffering from temporal lobe seizures, might have given him the first clue. Let us suppose that, as a boy, the patient had fallen from a cliff and Hippocrates could see a depression in the skull. The brain beneath must have been injured. Now, as a man, the patient described to him how, in his recurring small attacks, he relived a past experience. Suddenly then, it might well have dawned on Hippocrates, "the record of consciousness must be in the brain!" From that and other cases he would guess that epilepsy was "produced by the brain when it was not normal." Suddenly, I imagine, a new hypothesis flashed upon him, a provable hypothesis: "To consciousness, the brain is messenger."

But the problem of substantiating this proposition still lies before us. It is our task and our opportunity.

Twenty-three centuries after Hippocrates, another clinician with an enquiring mind took time to observe epileptics. He listened to what *Epilepsia* was still waiting to confide. The clinician was John Hughlings Jackson. As he made his rounds in the Queen's Square Hospital and the ancient London Hospital, he explained each epileptic seizure with reference to the hypothesis that the attack was caused by, and began with, an unruly "discharge" in some area of gray matter. This discharging state, he argued, might spread into neighboring areas. If so, it moved slowly. As the hypothesis was accepted, "spread" came to be called a "Jacksonian march."

In his Hunterian Lecture in 1872, Jackson, whose approach to medicine had been that of one previously interested in philosophy, remarked that "Medical men, since they, only, witness the results of experiments of disease on the nervous system of man, will be looked to more and more for facts bearing on the physiology of the mind."

Today, epilepsy—I like to personify her sometimes by using the Hippocratic name *Epilepsia*—has more secrets to confide to the neurologist or neurosurgeon who can understand the "tongue" she speaks.

A century has passed since Jackson made his illuminating observations and much has been learned about the physiology of the brain and the function of semi-separable mechanisms within the brain. It is clear today that the "unruly discharge"—we recognize it now to be electrical—is the cause of each fit. Jackson was right. It does begin in some local area of gray matter. But there is more to understand, and this is part of the basic physiology of epilepsy.

1. The initial discharge interferes for the moment with the normal use of that area of gray matter. Call it *epileptic interference*.

2. In addition to that interference, the discharge may bring forth a *positive response*. Each positive response can be explained by axon conduction of neuronal potentials along a normally active tract with resultant activation of a distant area of gray matter. This activation is functional rather than explosive.

For example, if the interfering discharge occurs in the motor gyrus, the activation occurs in the functionally related gray matter of the medulla or spinal cord. This is the *secondary cell station*.

If the discharge occurs in a sensory convolution of the cerebral cortex, activation is produced in a functionally related nucleus or cell station of the diencephalon. Thus, the patient is suddenly aware of a feeling or a sight or a sound that is elementary in character. It seems logical to conclude that these sensory nuclei in the higher brainstem activate, in their turn, a brain mechanism more closely related to consciousness.[3]

In the neurosurgeon's hand, the stimulating electrode has the same effects when applied to the cerebral cortex—the same local interference and the same distant

---

[3] Under normal circumstances, afferent impulses pass along this pathway, and sensory perception comes to the level of consciousness unless the impulses are inhibited by lack of the subject's attention. Thus, normally, the sensory message approaching the highest level of integration (the highest level of brain function) is subjected to selection and elimination. This is part of the process of *centrencephalic integration*.

activation. Thus, discharge in, or stimulation of, convolutions in the interpretive areas of the temporal lobe brings back past experience by activation of the record of consciousness. This active response can only be called "psychical" as compared with "sensory" and "motor."

The record of the stream of consciousness seems to be located within the diencephalon, not in the cortex near the stimulating electrode as I once assumed. The record, it would seem, consists of a thread or threads of *facilitation for the passage of a subsequent stream of electrical potentials.*

Figure 1 (which I have used in several recent publications) explains the production of active responses by epileptic discharge and by electrode stimulation.

Jacksonian march is only one method of spread of epileptic seizures. In that method, the unruly discharging state moves from cell to adjacent cells. A seizure may also spread by a second method, *bombardment.*

Neuronal potentials traveling from a focus of discharge over a functional pathway to a second cell station may or may not activate it. But if the activating current becomes too strong and lasts too long, the bombardment produces a second focus of unruly discharge in the gray matter of the secondary station.

In Fig. 1 I have referred to what the editors of this book have called "the epilepsies." They are caused by discharges in various areas of the cerebral cortex and they produce positive responses: (1) movement, (2) sensation, (3) interpretive illusion, and (4) experiential recall. There are, of course, discharges in the so-called "silent areas" of the cortex also and in the speech areas. These do not declare themselves as active responses.

I must refer to two more "epilepsies," both associated with unruly discharges located in the diencephalon (higher brainstem): epileptic automatism and generalized convulsive seizure.

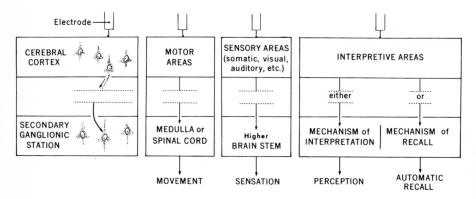

FIG. 1. Positive responses to epileptic discharge or electrical stimulation of cerebral cortex. The mechanisms involved in four types of positive response are suggested here. The stimulus produces interference with the function normally carried out in the cortex near the electrode. When active response results, it is due to axonal activation of a secondary ganglionic station at a distance from the stimulating electrode.

Epileptic Automatism

The unruly discharge takes place within the gray matter of that brain mechanism which makes consciousness possible. This we may call the *highest brain mechanism*. It is localized within the brainstem but not yet charted clearly. Discharge within this gray matter interferes with the action of the mind. When the discharge originates there, clinicians are apt to say the patient is having a petit mal attack. There is a lapse of consciousness while other functions, which depend on brain mechanisms, remain intact. This is epileptic automatism of the brainstem.

But automatism can also be produced secondarily by bombardment from one of two separate areas of gray matter in the cerebral cortex on either side—anterior frontal and antero-inferior temporal.[4]

Anterior Frontal. There may be no clinical evidence of discharge when it begins here unless it is mental confusion.

Periamygdaloid Area. There may be no evidence of the initial discharge here either, unless it comes from neighboring discharge in the deep sylvian cortex.

Except when these initial differences are observed, or when an electroencephalogram shows the difference of origin, the attacks in these three epilepsies (petit mal, temporal automatism, and frontal automatism) seem quite the same.

Consciousness is gone, as it is in deep sleep or in coma. In coma, due to pressure, concussion, or ischemia in the diencephalon, there is similar loss of consciousness but there is also interference in the patient's motor and sensory functions. Not so in automatism, during which interfering discharge is amazingly selective. Only the function of the highest brain mechanism is affected. Consciousness vanishes without interference in the function of the diencephalon's second major mechanism. The man becomes an automaton controlled by this second mechanism.

Call it the *automatic sensory and motor mechanism.* As long as the attack lasts, this mechanism is left alone in the driver's seat, so to speak, with no direction from the mind.

This automatic mechanism is a computer, but it can be programmed only when the man is normally conscious and is paying attention to the subject matter that is being introduced. During automatism, with the highest brain mechanism out of commission, no further guiding program can be given to it.

William Feindel and I (6) found that epileptic automatism could be produced by *electrical stimulation,* using an electrode, insulated except at the tip, thrust deeply into the periamygdaloid area of the cortex in one or other temporal fossa. But the automatism developed *only* when the stimulation was strong enough, and continued long enough, to produce an attack (as proven by the persistence of electrical afterdischarge on withdrawal of the electrode). I surmise, now, that the

---

[4] It is interesting that these are the two areas of brain that are so amazingly enlarged in passing from the brain of the ape to the human brain, a fact that is no doubt related to man's greater intellectual capacity.

long continuance of the stimulation eventually precipitated an unruly discharge in the gray matter of the highest brain mechanism. Thus it interfered instantly with the neuronal action that makes consciousness possible.

Moreover, our clinical experience is in conformity with this. Epileptic automatism is never produced secondarily by bombardment from local discharge in the sensory or motor cortex, although not infrequently it is set off by cortical discharge in the anterior frontal or inferior temporal areas (7).

The function of the automatic sensory and motor mechanism is best understood by a consideration of what the automaton, deprived of the conscious mind, can do during an attack of epileptic automatism. The automaton can carry out all the action that a normal individual in routine life carries out so skillfully while his attention is turned to something else. During such routine behavior, the mind programs the automatic sensory and motor mechanism before turning attention to other considerations. The individual must then reprogram it as often as necessary.

If the automatic mechanism has been previously programmed, then, at the time of the onset of an attack of automatism, the automaton will continue to behave as expected. Otherwise the automaton either follows an habitual pattern such as walking home, or is quite purposeless, unpredictable, and potentially dangerous.

The automatic sensory and motor mechanism may be defined as the mechanism capable of controlling the automaton and receiving direction from the highest brain mechanism. But, under normal circumstances, the automatic mechanism does more: it receives sensory input and selects from it whatever part of that input is to be presented to the highest mechanism in accordance with the momentary focusing of the mind's attention. It must be this same automatic mechanism that, almost simultaneously, recalls appropriate information from the record of past experience, introducing what is appropriate into the stream of consciousness. And certainly it is the automatic mechanism that normally executes coordinated action whether it is voluntary or involuntary, thus using the acquired and inborn reflexes as it has been conditioned to do in the past when the individual was paying conscious attention to the matter.

The evidence derived from a study of epilepsy, then, shows that the automatic sensory and motor mechanism has neuronal circuits, in the diencephalon and the cerebral cortex, that control behavior when the individual's attention is diverted and when local epileptic discharge interferes with the action of the highest brain mechanism. Thus, the integration of (1) sensory and motor mechanisms, (2) conditioned and inborn reflex mechanisms, and (3) mechanisms that can recall memory, as preserved in the record of the stream of consciousness, is carried out in a coordinated fashion by this amazing "computer."

This regulatory activity I have in the past called centrencephalic integration. Its detailed anatomy has still to be worked out, yet the evidence derived from a study of epilepsy and from cortical stimulation suggests that the central gray matter related to this mechanism (like the central gray matter for the highest brain mechanism) is localized in the diencephalon.

Between the incoming stream of sensory information and the highest brain mechanism stands the automatic sensory and motor mechanism. It stands, too, between the highest brain mechanism and the final patterning of the voluntary motor output.

The highest brain mechanism, as indicated by what I have said of the ways in which bombardment occurs, must have a direct relationship with the anterior frontal areas of cortex and the non-sensory areas of the temporal lobes. And, to repeat, it would seem to have no relationship with the motor and sensory cortex except the indirect connection through the automatic sensory and motor mechanism, man's portable computer.

The direct functional interchanges between the two great mechanisms of the diencephalon must normally be voluminous and very active. This is one part of the centrencephalic neuronal interchange which serves the purposes of final functional integration in the brain.

These are some of the hypotheses that come to us from a consideration of the physiology of epilepsy. In the future, let those who work in the exciting field of the neurosciences use them with discretion as they move into the century of work on the neurophysiology and neuroanatomy of the brain that lies before them.

Generalized Convulsion or Grand Mal

This type of seizure is produced by an unruly discharge in the gray matter that forms the central area of the automatic sensory and motor mechanism. This too may be considered an "epilepsy" like the others I have mentioned. The exact localization of this cellular station is yet to be charted, but it is certainly in the diencephalon. The discharge interferes with the mechanism's normal function and, at the same time, it activates, by bombardment, all the distant motor cell stations. The central controlling gray matter is apparently connected with them all. It bombards them all producing many simultaneously active responses from them. That does not mean, necessarily, that these peripheral motor cell stations, which are scattered through the cerebral cortex, lower brainstem, and spinal cord are themselves involved in epileptic discharge.

They are activated simultaneously and, so to speak, often pitted against each other. This results in tonic, clonic tensing movements, unconscious groaning with salivation, and opening of the sphincters. No wonder the ancients called this major seizure the "curse of the gods"!

If the attack continues long enough, some of the secondary stations may eventually explode in epileptic activity as the result of the continued bombardment.

Consciousness is invariably lost in generalized convulsive seizures, and one may surmise that the automatic sensory and motor mechanism has functional tracts (normally, no doubt, carrying selected sensory information) that lead into the mind's mechanism and provide a pathway for bombardment that would instantly interfere with the function of the highest brain mechanism.

Epileptic seizures, like electrical stimulation of the human cerebral cortex, may be reviewed as though they were functional experiments on the human brain, which of course they are not. Clinicians can ask revealing questions and they should learn to record meaningful answers. It is our urgent duty to report to Science, and it is obvious that in discharging that duty we shall become better clinicians.

In this Introduction, I have presented hypotheses and proven facts drawn from a study of epilepsy and a long experience with cortical stimulation. Indeed, in the past year I have reconsidered, as best I could, the neurophysiology that is related to consciousness (8). I began my professional career in the laboratory of Sir Charles Sherrington and entered neurosurgery in the hope of becoming a physiologist in this field as well as neurosurgeon.

The hypotheses presented here that have to do with brain function and the physiology of epilepsy will, I hope, be tested, criticized, and used by those who are responsible for the management of the epilepsies. I am delighted that so many with whom I have discussed these interpretations through the years are today numbered among the very able authors of this book.

There is so much for basic scientist and clinician alike to learn from epilepsy! So much, too, for the psychologist and the philosopher who can turn to it with an open mind.

Doth not Wisdom cry?
And understanding put forth her voice?

REFERENCES

1. Broca, P., *Arch. Anat. Physiol. Swiss. Med.,* 37:300–382 (1870).
2. Fritsch, G., and Hitzig, E., *Bull. Soc. Anat. (Paris),* 2 Série, 6:355 (1861).
3. Jackson, H., *Trans. St. Andrews Med. Grad. Assoc.,* Vol. III (1970).
4. Foerster, O., and Penfield, W., *Brain,* 53:99–120 (1930).
5. Foerster, O., and Penfield, W., *Ztschr. Ges. Neurol. Psychiat.,* 125:475–572 (1930).
6. Feindel, W., and Penfield, W., *Arch. Neurol. Psychiat. (Chi.)* 72:605, 1954.
7. *Epileptic Seizure Patterns.* Penfield, W., and Kristiansen, K. Charles C Thomas, Springfield, Ill., 104 pp., 1951.
8. Penfield, W., *The Mystery of the Mind—A Study of the Physiology of Consciousness.* Princeton University Press, Princeton, New Jersey, 1975 *(in press).*

Advances in Neurology, Vol. 8, edited by D. P. Purpura, J. K. Penry, and R. D. Walter. Raven Press, New York © 1975.

1
Focal Epilepsy: The Problem, Prevalence, and Contributing Factors

Preston Robb

James was 20 months old when he had his first attack, a severe convulsion lasting 3 hr. The second attack a year later differed from the first in that no convulsive movements occurred but there was rolling of the eyes and a period of absence. He was well then until the age of 10 when he started having attacks of absence lasting 5 to 10 sec, followed by a period of confusion for a few minutes. He continued having absence attacks about once a week followed by a period of automatism and pallor. Four months after the onset of these seizures he was admitted to the Montreal Neurological Institute. There the EEG demonstrated a diffuse dysrhythmia with maximum abnormality over the right Sylvian and temporal regions. He was put on medication and followed at regular intervals. He continued to have irregular minor attacks, particularly under pressure. Some were associated with automatic behavior.

At the age of 17 he started work for a large insurance company in the accounting department, and attended night school. He was able to complete his training as a certified public accountant, but advance in the company was limited because of the frequent seizures and the toxic effects of heavy medication. Many attacks were accompanied by automatic behavior such as undressing, and were a frequent source of embarrassment. In 1967, at the age of 22, he was readmitted to the Montreal Neurological Institute. After complete investigation, Dr. Charles Branch did a right anterior temporal lobectomy and removal of epileptogenic brain tissue from the orbital surface of the frontal lobe (Figs. 1 and 2). Pathological examination revealed neuronal loss and gliosis of the right hippocampus. A year later, an EEG showed a minimal residual abnormality over the right temporal region. Since then he has continued on small doses of anticonvulsants. Seven years later, he is seizure-free, doing well in the business world, married, and completely independent.

This is the type of success story that makes the surgical treatment of epilepsy worthwhile. Today, it is well established that in selected patients with seizures of focal cortical origin, excision of the cicatrix, whatever the cause, is an effective and safe form of therapy. Patients with uncontrolled seizures of cortico-reticular origin continue to be a problem. Whether stereotactic destructive lesions or electrical stimulations are the answer is yet to be resolved.

In ancient times the methods used to fight epilepsy were rational and supersti-

---

Montreal Neurological Institute Reprint No. 1165.

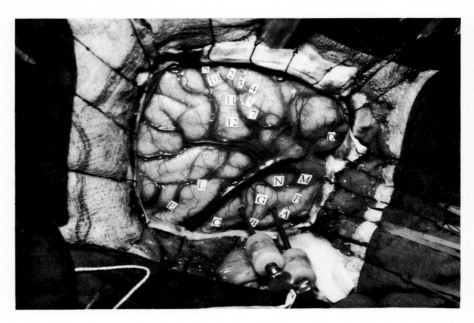

FIG. 1. Patient J. operated on by Dr. Charles Branch. Pre-excision, showing depth electrodes and marker for cortical response to stimulation.

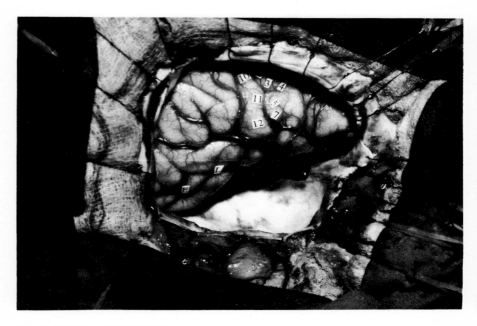

FIG. 2. Patient J., post-excision.

tious on the one hand and magic and religious on the other. In his delightful history, *The Falling Sickness,* Temkin (1945) records some treatments of the past. The rational cure made use of diet and drugs, however inadequate. A weird treatment of a convulsion is suggested by Guainerius (early 15th century) as a form of superstitious prescription: "to give a frog's liver, to smear the patient's mouth with blood, to kill a dog and let the patient have its bile and let the person who first saw him fall, urinate in his own shoe, stir the urine, and give it as a drink to the patient, afterwards, the patient will be entirely delivered." Thomas Willis in the 17th century took exception to this type of treatment: "I say this kind of practice is often too roughly instituted or ordained, because after this manner is double-trouble put on nature to wit one from the disease, and the other not lighter from the standers by, and helpers, when it were much better, for the fit to be suffered to pass over and after its own manner, and the sick endure but one trouble only."

Attention was paid in the past to head injuries as a cause of epilepsy and some were cured with surgery. "In the 14th century Valescus de Tharanta had described the case of a man with a head-wound penetrating to the pia mater. A fetid ichor had reached the brain and had caused epileptic attacks seven or eight times a day till the patient died. Some 150 years later, Berengarius da Carpi treated a severe wound of the head where the epileptic paroxysm had supervened about sixty days after the injury 'because of the matter contained in the brain.' Berengarius had the man placed feet up and head down, he opened the wound, evacuated a large quantity of watery substance of the color of milk, whereupon the epilepsy ceased immediately. It was, moreover, realized that epileptic seizures might appear many years after the injury to the head. This is proved by the following observation told by Duretus (1527–86). 'A bone of the skull of a twelve-year old youth had been broken and depressed by a fall and had by negligence not been restored. The brain was therefore hindered in its growth, since the injured bone itself could not grow so as to become able to hold a larger brain. Consequently in his eighteenth year the youth suffered from epilepsy because of the oppression of the brain. He was, however, cured by the perforation of the depressed bone, for thus the oppression of the brain was removed.' This observation is classical in its brevity and clarity and sounds so rational and modern in the treatment reported."[1]

It was not until the mid-19th century that significant progress was made in the understanding of epilepsy. Delasiauve in his *Traité de l'Epilepsie* (1854) pointed out that in some instances the cause was known, in others it was obscure. He classified epilepsy as follows:

"1. Essential or idiopathic epilepsy manifesting itself merely in functional deviations without lesion, corresponding to simple nervous afflictions and in a word constituting a veritable neurosis.

"2. Symptomatic epilepsy, belonging to a more or less appreciable cerebral lesion, the convulsive spasm being here the symptom and not the disease.

---

[1] From Temkin (1945).

"3. Finally a third epilepsy called sympathetic, produced by the irradiation of abnormal impressions which can have their seat in all parts of the body except the brain or its appendages."

However, it was the monumental works of John Hughlings Jackson that initiated the modern era for epilepsy. Knowledge was developing on localization of cerebral function, to which Jackson was a major contributor. Based on his knowledge and experience, he developed a rational approach to the understanding of the epileptic process. He defined epilepsy as "the name for occasional, sudden, excessive, rapid and localized discharges of grey matter." It was clear to him that there were degrees of epilepsy. "A fit which is limited to the hand is not a fit of a different *kind,* from one which begins in the hand, and then *spreads* all over the body, and is after a certain stage, 'attended by' loss of consciousness. The latter seizure is but the result of a much stronger discharge." He stressed the importance and difficulties in determining the site of origin of an epileptogenic focus. "Surely it is as important to localize 'discharging lesions' as it is to localize the 'destroying lesions.' "

On the basis of his study he urged Mr. Victor Horsley to surgically explore patients. At first he recommended that operation on patients with epileptiform seizures due to a brain tumor only be done where "optic neuritis" exists. He subsequently modified his opinion when in a footnote to the Bowman Lecture of 1886 he wrote, "I have advised operation in the case of a man who had epileptiform seizures beginning in his left thumb, but who had no optic neuritis and no severe headache; there were no signs of injury. Mr. Victor Horsley removed a tumor from the right cerebral hemisphere, and at my suggestion, cut out part of the thumb centre. Mr. Horsley showed the patient at the Brighton Meeting of the British Medical Association on August 13, 1886. The man was quite well except for some weakness of the left hand; the fundi were normal."

Initially "epileptic surgery" was done in the hope of being able to remove a tumor or remove fragments of bone pressing on the brain as a result of trauma. The prognosis must have been very grim indeed when one considers the lack of facilities at that time. The important thing was that with careful inquiry, examination, and observation of attacks, the site of origin of the excessive discharge could frequently be determined and provide a basis for surgical therapy.

The advent of antisepsis, and later asepsis, the discovery of anesthesia, and the knowledge of cerebral localization enabled the surgical treatment of epilepsy to move ahead. The terrible mortality rate that had accompanied previous attempts to treat posttraumatic epilepsy was reduced and gratifying results were obtained. A brief history of the surgical treatment of epilepsy following the initial efforts of Sir Victor Horsley is given by Penfield and Erickson in their volume *Epilepsy and Cerebral Localization* (1941). For obvious reasons the surgical treatment of epilepsy in the first quarter of the 20th century continued to be unsatisfactory and to depend on the clinical findings, as contrast studies were not available and the electroencephalogram still had not been discovered. At the same time, one must remember that anticonvulsants were not readily available and the medical treatment of epilepsy was virtually nil. Phenobarbital was not discovered until 1912 and did not become popular in this country until after World War I. Diphenylhydantoin was not discovered until 1937. As a result there were many epileptics, who today would be controlled with medication, demanding that something be done to alleviate the severe and recurring attacks.

Penfield became convinced, based on his pathological studies of posttraumatic cerebral cicatrix, that cortical excision could benefit the patient with focal cerebral seizures. Following work with Otfrid Foerster in Germany, he came to Montreal in 1928 when he abundantly proved this hypothesis. He developed new techniques, introduced the EEG into the operating room, and, more important, trained many surgeons in the skills required for cortical excision.

Today the use of anticonvulsants enables most epileptics to lead a normal life; there remains, however, a hard core of at least 10% of patients with a focal epileptogenic abnormality who do not respond to medication. It is this group of uncontrolled patients that challenges the neurologists and neurosurgeons today.

PREVALENCE

In a given epilepsy population, a certain percent fail to respond to medication, have focal cerebral lesions, and are candidates for cortical excision. The question is, how many are there?

The National Institute of Neurological Diseases and Stroke recently published Monograph No. 14, *The Epidemiology of Epilepsy.* Here the many problems of studying incidence and prevalence within the disorder of multifactorial origin and multiple symptomatology of the epilepsies are presented (Robb, 1973). The prevalence of epilepsy tends to fall with advancing age and maturation of the brain. Rose et al. (1973) found a prevalence rate of 18.6 to 20.1 per 1,000 based on a questionnaire survey of third-grade students in Washington County, Maryland. This is a much higher prevalence rate than generally reported (5 per 1,000) and adds further proof that epilepsy is much more common in younger age groups.

The optimum time for operation on a patient with active focal epilepsy should be at an age when the chances of spontaneous arrest of attacks due to maturation of the brain are at a minimum and before there is serious interference with educational and career plans. The majority of patients are in their late teens or early twenties, an age when they can cooperate with the surgeon during the procedure. In a series of 720 patients with seizures originating in the temporal lobe at the Montreal Neurological Institute, Rasmussen found that 67.8% were between the ages of 21 and 35.

In 1959 Kurland and his colleagues reported the incidence and prevalence of convulsive disorders in a small community (Rochester, Minnesota). Although they believed that a large majority, if not all, of the local residents with diagnosed convulsive disorders were included in the survey, the computed rates were considered as minimal values. The prevalence rates for all types of epilepsy, age adjusted to the U.S. population, was 3.7 per 1,000 population. A review of the literature on the prevalence of epilepsy would suggest that the figure is definitely low. Pond and his associates (1960) in a study in England found a prevalence rate of 6.2 per 1,000 persons. Brewis and associates (1966) in another study in England found a prevalence rate of 5.5 per 1,000 persons.

The fact that there is no universally accepted classification of epilepsy has contributed to the lack of accepted uniform standards for epidemiologic studies. The result is that the prevalence rate reported by one group of investigators cannot be compared with those of another. Nevertheless, if one is to talk in round figures, a conservative estimate, considering the present available knowledge, is a prevalence rate of 5 per 1,000 persons; i.e., one person in 200 has epilepsy.

FOCAL EPILEPSY

In a search for information on the incidence of focal epilepsy, one naturally looks at the literature on head injuries as a cause of epilepsy. Caveness, Walker, and Ascroft (1962) point out that not every individual who has a severe head injury develops epilepsy. The incidence of posttraumatic epilepsy in such cases is 50%. Patients with depressed skull fractures in the frontal region have an incidence of epilepsy that does not exceed 60%. As long as there are automobiles, wars, and children playing in the streets, head trauma is going to be a major cause of epilepsy. Patients with posttraumatic epilepsy, followed over a number of years, have a decreasing tendency to have seizures (Walker and Erculei, 1969). In the early period up to 4 years following a head injury, the epileptic phenomena are usually severe and often frequent. After this time there is a tendency for the epileptic phenomena to manifest only focal characteristics. Patients who experienced generalized manifestations simply experience the initial phenomena or aura of their attacks. After a period of 5 years, 50% of the individuals who experienced generalized seizures will have stopped having attacks and in the next 25 years have no further attacks. Occasional attacks may occur and these are usually attributed to a stoppage of medication or excessive use of alcohol. An interesting observation made by Caveness (1963) is that there is no relationship between the severity of injury and the intensity or duration of the seizures. This may support the concept that there is a genetic factor in posttraumatic epilepsy.

Temporal lobe epilepsy is common in children. Chao and her associates (1962) found that 15% of their epileptic children had seizures originating in the temporal lobe. Our own experience would support the concept that many children with diffuse or migrating EEG abnormalities frequently end up with clear-cut temporal lobe abnormalities. It may be that the severe convulsions of infants and children are the cause of the hippocampal sclerosis. Certainly, Falconer thinks so (1970).

THE PRESENT PROBLEM

The population of the United States in 1973 was over 209 million. Based on the prevalence rate of 5 per 1,000, there were approximately 1,048,585 patients with epilepsy. A conservative estimate would be that 20% of these patients are not controlled with medical therapy and 10% would benefit from surgical excision. In other words, there are roughly 105,000 patients in the U.S. who should be considered for surgical treatment of their epilepsy.

FACTORS CONTRIBUTING TO THE SURGICALLY TREATABLE EPILEPTIC DISORDERS

There are several factors which contribute to the development of an epileptogenic focus: (1) the degree of cerebral maturation; (2) genetic factors; and (3) cerebral pathology. As far as importance is concerned, there is a fluctuating interplay. What may be important in one patient may be negligible in another.

Cerebral Maturation

An epileptic seizure is a herald of pathology most frequently found in the maturing brain. As man advances from birth to old age, the tendency toward seizures decreases.

Recently, Merlis (1973) reviewed the literature on the age of onset of seizures in populations of epileptics. Averaging the results of five most recent authors, 67% had onset of seizures between birth and 19. In the Lennox and Lennox (1960) group of 4,000, 77% had onset in this age range. Their figures are reasonably representative.

Age of onset	Percent	
0–19	77.0	A large number
20–29	12.7	of children
30–39	6.1	
40–49	2.7	
50+	1.7	

The figures of Bicard, Gastaut, and Roger (1955) are probably the most representative of all of those papers reviewed by Merlis.

Age of onset	Percent	
0–20	67	Private non-
21–30	11.8	hospital patients
31–40	8.5	
41+	12.7	

Regardless of selection factors, between 65 and 75% of patients had onset of seizures before the age of 20.

Breaking down the early age group, Kurland (1959) showed that there was a continuous drop in incidence of epilepsy from birth to age 29.

Age group (yr)	Rate/1,000
0–4	1.52
5–9	0.25
10–14	0.25
15–19	0.19
20–29	0.04

Although the incidence was a little higher in Crombie's series (Crombie et al., 1960), due to different criteria for selection, the rate of fall-off was about the same.

Age group (yr)	Rate/1,000
0–4	3.46
5–9	0.58
10–14	0.58
15–24	0.84
25–34	0.23

It is clear that as man ages and his brain matures, the tendency to have seizures decreases. It would decrease even more if alcohol and tobacco could be avoided.

Epilepsy is a disorder of neurons made hypersensitive by changing conditions, either physiological or pathological. Insults to groups of neurons as they develop make them hypersensitive. The brain responds to similar insults in different ways depending on the degree of maturation, or, conversely, different insults or lesions may cause identical clinical response depending on the degree of cerebral maturation. For example, infantile massive spasms in two children may appear to be identical, but postmortem examinations reveal a completely different type of pathology. Absence seizures were identical in two of our children, yet time revealed a cerebral lipoidosis in one, and in the other no cause was ever found other than a positive family history. Purpura (1964) points out that developing cell systems of the brain do not mature at the same rate or at the same time. Consequently, functional disturbances resulting from insult to the immature brain will depend not only on the nature and severity of the insult but also on the ontogenetic phase of development of the brain. For example, similar degrees of anoxia in a 7-month premature child and a child at term produce different results: in the first, spastic diplegia; in the second, athetosis.

Purpura's data (1959) on the time course of cerebral and cerebellar cortical development indicate that the fundamentally different patterns of neuronal morphogenesis in these structures satisfactorily account for the different electrographic characteristics of evoked potentials observed in immature cerebral and cerebellar cortex.

We are concerned with the maturing brain, its growth and development, the production of new and continually maturing cells. It should also be remembered that, at the same time, death of isolated units or entire cell populations is a normal occurrence in morphogenesis. The onset and pace of degenerative changes during development are ultimately under genetic control (Saunders et al., 1962). It is intriguing to speculate as to the role of the genetically controlled "death clock" in the production of membrane instability and epilepsy.

Genetic Factors

What are the genetic factors in the production of focal epilepsy? It has long been known that heredity plays an important role in the etiology of the epilepsies.

Investigations conducted over the past 20 years, particularly by Metrakos and Metrakos (1973), have done much to substantiate this. It was William Lennox who revived the interest in the genetics of epilepsy when in 1951 he published the results of a study of 4,231 epileptics and 20,000 near relatives. He showed that there was a significantly higher incidence of seizures in families of patients with "essential" epilepsy than in families of patients with "symptomatic" epilepsy. This was really the first significant work on the subject since it was suggested by Hippocrates centuries before.

The work of Metrakos and Metrakos clearly indicates that there is an autosomal dominant gene responsible for the centrencephalic EEG abnormality. They also suggested that genetic factors are partly responsible for "symptomatic" or "acquired" epilepsy. Later studies by Metrakos and Andermann strongly support the concept that there are underlying genetic factors in focal epilepsy. The results of most of their studies were consistent with a unified concept of epilepsy as proposed by Ajmone-Marsan (1961), Bray and Wiser (1965), and Gloor (1968). Metrakos concluded that "no clear line of demarcation exists between localized and nonlocalized forms of epilepsy." Based on their studies, they suggested that spike-and-wave epilepsy, focal epilepsy, and febrile convulsions have at least one common genetically controlled predisposing factor. One can appreciate this when one is confronted with a patient with a focal type of seizure that on repeated EEGs shows a picture of focal abnormalities and cortico-reticular bilaterally synchronous abnormalities.

Bray (1973) expressed the opinion that focal epilepsy and petit mal epilepsy were often hereditary, the two disorders may have the same genetic basis, and the condition appears to be transmitted as an autosomal dominant trait with age-dependent penetrance. The disorder persists into adult life often in a fashion not clearly recognized because the EEG abnormality is lost in many cases in a maturational process. It was Bray's impression that patients with focal disorders are easier to control, perhaps indicating that the focal form of the disorder is a milder form of the disease.

Cerebral Pathology

The oldest and most familiar lesion seen in epilepsy is sclerosis of Ammon's horn. It was observed not only in cases of "idiopathic" but also of "symptomatic" epilepsy. Spielmeyer (1927) and later Scholz (1951) confirmed and expanded the earlier findings. They provided clear evidence that the sclerosis was due to vascular disturbances and/or anoxia. Earle, Baldwin, and Penfield (1953) claimed that "incisural sclerosis" was the most common cause of temporal lobe epilepsy. The lesion was presumed to be the result of herniation of the temporal lobe, or more strictly its most mesial and inferior parts, into the tentorial openings during the head-molding phase of parturition. The concept that incisural sclerosis is a result of molding the head at birth is at variance with the hypothesis that Ammon's horn sclerosis is caused by seizures and related to vascular spasm and anoxia.

Meyer studied the patients who had had an anterior temporal lobectomy by Mr. Murray Falconer. The incidence of sclerosis of Ammon's horn in their cases was just over 70%, followed closely by lesions of the uncus (64%) and to a lesser degree by lesions of the amygdaloid complex (Meyer et al., 1954). Falconer and his colleagues (1964) were of the opinion that hypoxic episodes in infancy and early childhood played a more important role than birth trauma. As well as insular sclerosis, they had 21 patients with small cryptic tumors in their series of 100. Some had dual pathology. There were 18 small glial formations or tumors, three small capillary angiomas, one dermoid cyst, one parasitic cyst, and one lesion suggesting tuberous sclerosis.

Although the pathological lesions seen in many conditions which cause convulsions are known, the exact pathophysiological lesion at the site of the origin of the attack is obscure. Whether at a neuronal level there is ischemia with a shift in the sodium ration and depolarization or whether extracellular potassium is the chief offender is a question yet to be decided.

As the child matures, there are a variety of pathological lesions of the brain that serve as potential causes of focal epilepsy. Some of these may be apparent at birth, such as a Sturge-Weber syndrome or other congenital malformations. Other lesions may be present then but do not become apparent until later, for example, tuberous sclerosis. A traumatic birth may be the cause of small or large cerebral hemorrhages with secondary cicatrix formation and subsequent seizures.

During childhood there are many potential causes such as meningitis, trauma, and postvaccinal cerebrovascular occlusions. Focal encephalitis has been a cause of epilepsia partialis continua. An important cause, as mentioned above, is the mesial temporal lobe sclerosis following the anoxia of a severe febrile convulsion. Children with infantile hemiplegia have a high incidence of seizures. Sometimes the seizures are so uncontrollable, in spite of toxic levels of anticonvulsants, that hemispherectomy is indicated. Very slow-growing astrocytomas may cause seizures. They may be associated with a dilated temporal horn and may go undiscovered until operation. The EMI scanner may prove to be a boon in identifying such masses. Trauma as a cause of focal epilepsy has already been discussed.

These pathological lesions of the brain are mentioned, not to list all of the disorders that cause focal epilepsy, but rather to emphasize the many different sources of patients with uncontrollable focal seizures.

SUMMARY

The prevalence of epilepsy in the United States is 5 per 1,000, and there are an estimated 1,048,585 patients with epilepsy. Conservative estimates indicate there are 105,000 patients with focal epilepsy in the U.S. who would benefit from surgical therapy. Investigation and treatment of focal epilepsy is expensive and very time-consuming, the result being that there are relatively few centers in the U.S. with a comprehensive program for the surgical treatment of epilepsy. During the maturation period, the brain is particularly prone to insult and subsequent development of focal seizures. There is an autosomal dominant gene that contributes to both generalized and focal epilepsy. There are a great variety of pathological lesions of congenital, traumatic, anoxic, inflammatory, neoplastic, or unknown origin that cause focal seizures that do not respond adequately to anticonvulsant drugs and that are amenable to surgical therapy.

REFERENCES

Ajmone Marsan, C. (1961): Changing concepts in focal epilepsy. Clinical-E.E.G. considerations. *Epilepsia,* 2:217–228.

Bicard, N., Gastaut, H., and Roger, J. (1955): Statistical studies of the different electrical varieties of epilepsy. *Epilepsia,* 4:73–79.

Bray, P. (1973): Inheritance of focal and petit mal seizures. In: *The Epidemiology of Epilepsy. A Workshop.* N.I.N.D.S., Monograph No. 14, D.H.E.W. Public No. (N.I.H.) 73–390, pp. 109–114.

Bray, P. F., and Wiser, W. C. (1965): The relation of focal to diffuse epileptiform E.E.G. discharge in genetic epilepsy. *Arch. Neurol.,* 13:233–237.

Brewis, M., Poskanzer, D. C., Rolland, C., and Miller, H. (1966): Neurological disease in an English city. *Acta Neurol. Scand. Suppl.,* 24:42–89.

Caveness, W. F. (1963): Onset and cessation of fits following craniocerebral trauma. *J. Neurosurg.,* 20:570–583.

Caveness, W. F., Walker, A. E., and Ascroft, P. B. (1962): Incidence of post-traumatic epilepsy in Korean Veterans as compared with those of World War I and World War II. *J. Neurosurg.,* 19:122–129.

Chao, D., Sexton, J. A., and Pardo, L. S. S. (1962): Temporal lobe epilepsy in children. *J. Pediat.,* 2:416–422.

Crombie, D. L., Cross, K. W., Fry, J., Pinsent, R. J. F. H., and Watts, C. A. H. (1960): A survey of the epilepsies in general practice. A report of the research committee of the College of General Practitioners. *Brit. Med. J.,* 2:416–422.

Delasiauve, L. J. F. (1854): *Traité de l'Epilepsie.* Paris, p. 37.

Earle, K. M., Baldwin, M., and Penfield, W. (1953): Incisural sclerosis and temporal lobe seizures produced by hippocampal herniation at birth. *Arch. Neurol. Psychiat.,* 69:27.

Falconer, M. A. (1970): Significance of surgery for temporal lobe epilepsy in childhood and adolescence. *J. Neurosurg.,* 33:233–252.

Falconer, M. A., Serafetinides, E. A., and Corsellis, J. A. (1964): The etiology and pathogenesis of temporal lobe epilepsy. *Arch. Neurol.,* 10:233.

Gloor, P. (1968): Generalized cortico-reticular epilepsies, some considerations on the pathophysiology of generalized bilaterally synchronous spike and wave discharge. *Epilepsia,* 9:249–263.

Horsley, V. (1886): Brain surgery. *Brit. Med. J.,* 2:670–675.

Jackson, J. H. (1932): From J. Taylor, *Selected Writings of John Hughlings Jackson.* Hodder and Stoughton, London.

Kurland, L. (1959–1960): The incidence and prevalence of convulsive disorders in a small urban community. *Epilepsia,* 1:143–161.

Lennox, W. G. (1951): The heredity of epilepsy, as told by relatives and twins. *JAMA,* 146:529.

Lennox, W. G., and Lennox, M. A. (1960): *Epilepsy and Related Disorders.* Little, Brown and Co., Boston.

Merlis, J. K. (1973): Epilepsy in different age groups. In: *The Epidemiology of Epilepsy. A Workshop.* N.I.N.D.S. Monograph No. 14. D.H.E.W. Publication No. (N.I.H.) 73–390, pp. 83–86.

Metrakos, J. D., and Metrakos, K. (1973): Genetic factors in the epilepsies. In: *The Epidemiology of Epilepsy. A Workshop.* N.I.N.D.S. Monograph No. 14. D.H.E.W. Publication No. (N.I.H.) 73–390, pp. 97–102.

Meyer, A., Falconer, M. A., and Beck, E. (1954): Pathological findings in temporal lobe epilepsy. *J. Neurol. Neurosurg. Psychiat.,* 17:276.

Penfield, W. G., and Erickson, T. (1941): *Epilepsy and Cerebral Localization.* Charles C Thomas, Springfield, Ill.

Pond, D. A., Bidwell, B. H., and Stein, L. (1960): A survey of epilepsy in 14 general practices. I: Demographic and medical data. *Psychiat. Neurol. Neurochir.,* 63:217–236.

Purpura, D. P. (1959): Nature of electrocortical potentials and synaptic organizations in cerebral and cerebellar cortex. In: *International Review of Neurobiology*, Vol. 1, edited by C. C. Pfeiffer and J. R. Smythies. Academic Press, New York.

Purpura, D. P. (1962): Synaptic organization of immature cerebral cortex. *Wld. Neurol.*, 3:275–298.

Purpura, D. P. (1964): Relationship of seizure susceptibility to morphologic and physiologic of normal and abnormal immature cortex. In: *Neurological and Electroencephalographic Correlative studies in Infancy*, edited by P. Kellaway and I. Petersen. Grune & Stratton Inc., New York.

Robb, J. P. (1973): A review of epidemiologic concepts of epilepsy. In: *The Epidemiology of Epilepsy. A Workshop.* N.I.N.D.S. Monograph No. 14. D.H.E.W. Publication No. (N.I.H.) 73–390, pp. 13–20.

Rose, S. W., Penry, J. K., Markush, R. E., Raoloff, L. A., and Putnam, P. L. (1973): Prevalence of epilepsy in children. *Epilepsia*, 14:133–152.

Saunders, J. W., Jr., Gasseling, M. T., and Saunders, L. C. (1962): Cellular death in morphogenesis of the avian wing. *Develop. Biol.*, 5:147–178.

Scholz, W. (1951): *Die Krampfschadigungen des Gehirns.* Springer-Verlag, Berlin.

Spielmeyer, W. (1927): Der Pathogenese des epileptischen krampfes. *Z. Ges. Neurol. Psychiat.*, 109: 501.

Temkin, O. (1945): *The Falling Sickness.* The Johns Hopkins Press, Baltimore.

Walker, A. E., and Erculei, F. (1969): Head injured men fifteen years later. Charles C Thomas, Springfield, Ill., pp. 106–118.

Advances in Neurology, Vol. 8, edited by D. P.
Purpura, J. K. Penry, and R. D. Walter. Raven
Press, New York © 1975.

2
Theoretical Basis for Surgical Therapy of Epilepsy

Arthur A. Ward, Jr.

Although research in recent years has provided a growing body of knowledge dealing with the physiologic, morphologic, and chemical substrates that are associated with the epileptic process, our fundamental concepts are solidly based on those presented by Hughlings Jackson in the Lumleian Lectures delivered in 1890 (Jackson, 1931). He proposed that epilepsy of cortical origin arises in a "discharging lesion." He went on to point out that "the highly 'explosive' cells of a discharging lesion will, on their fulminating discharge, overcome the resistance of, and thus produce excessive discharge of, collateral stable nervous elements." Thus we have the concepts of an epileptogenic focus, the development of the local seizure which then spreads to the rest of the brain involving, in the words of Jackson, the "compelled excessive discharges of stable cells," i.e., secondary activation of normal neuronal circuits.

This is a very modern statement of the underlying mechanisms in epilepsy and, in fact, is the basis for the various types of surgical therapy which have been developed in the intervening three quarters of a century. Based even on this crude model of the epileptic process, one would predict that surgical excision of the focus containing a mass of "highly explosive" cells should be therapeutically beneficial. In addition, any technique (pharmacologic or surgical) which blocks the pathways of spread to the rest of the brain should be beneficial.

THE FOCUS

Current knowledge now makes it possible to propose a model of the epileptic process in some detail. In focal cortical epilepsy, the essential feature is the epileptogenic focus since, in its absence, a propagating clinical seizure does not arise. The data indicate that the focus is composed of pathologically hyperactive neurons. The critical mass of such epileptic neurons necessary for spontaneous seizures is unknown at the present time although it is clearly more than one. In dramatic contrast to the firing patterns of normal neurons in cortex, the interictal firing pattern of neurons in the focus is characterized by recurrent, high-frequency bursts of action potentials (Calvin, Sypert, and Ward, 1968; Wyler, Fetz, and Ward, 1973). Firing rates in a burst may vary from 200 to 900/sec; the burst usually starts at high frequency, and there is no decrement in frequency during the burst. In those cells thought to be "pacemaker" epileptic neurons, there are few or no single action potentials between bursts; the bursts repeat 5 to 15 times/sec. These interictal bursts are usually stereotyped, showing little fluctuation in the first few spikes of the burst. An exception is a special type of burst with a structured timing pattern that has been observed only within the area of major EEG spike activity in the focus. The pattern of firing within these unique bursts is characterized by a long first interval between the first and subsequent spikes in the burst, and these have been called long-first-interval bursts (Calvin et al., 1968). They have been recorded with microelectrodes from foci in monkeys with chronic epilepsy as well as from human foci. In the monkey with sensorimotor foci, such long-first-interval burst firing is recorded only from pyramidal tract neurons. In the human, confirmation of cell type is obviously not possible, but such patterns of firing have been recorded from foci in cortex which do not contribute to the pyramidal tract. One can therefore speculate that this unique firing pattern occurs only in epileptic cells whose morphology is pyramidal. In recording the activity of single cells in the focus of the awake, undrugged monkey with chronic epilepsy, only 15% of cells demonstrated such long-first-interval burst firing. In addition, pacemaker or group I (Wyler and Fetz, 1974) cells are encountered intermixed with cells demonstrating either normal firing patterns or shifting between normal tonic firing and epileptic firing in bursts.

We have been undertaking microelectrode recording of the activity of single neurons in the human cortex during the course of operations for epilepsy for the past 20 years. Not only do such data provide an opportunity to confirm, in the human, key observations from more extensive experimental data, but they have also been of some assistance in making surgical judgments in the operating room. The cortical focus is customarily delimited by electrocorticography in which the presence of epileptic spikes in the EEG are the hallmark of the epileptic process. Such spikes can also be propagated, however, and, at times, it may be unclear whether the recorded spikes are arising locally in the vicinity of the pial electrode or whether they are propagated from a more distant focus. Microelectrode recording of the activity of cortical neurons can help resolve this ambiguity. The demonstration that neurons in the suspected focus are generating burst discharges characteristic of epileptic neurons has, for us, provided additional security for this surgical judgment.

Calvin (1972) has pointed out that the synaptic consequences of the high-frequency burst output of epileptic neurons can be appreciably different from those ordinarily considered in our models of the transmission of signals in the central nervous system. Normal neurons tend to fire at a nominal rate of about 20/sec. Such a train of spikes in a presynaptic pathway generates postsynaptic potentials in the postsynaptic neuron which will begin to sum. However, this sum does not keep building up indefinitely because the membrane potential depolarization decays. Thus 200 synapses on a cell (firing asynchronously at 20/sec) can modify the firing of a postsynaptic cell. It is, therefore, not surprising that 2% of a spinal motoneuron's 10,000 synapses firing asynchronously can either elicit rhythmic firing from a silent cell or markedly increase a preexisting firing rate.

Since group 1 a afferents account for only 2% of the synaptic inputs on a spinal motoneuron, the fact that the knee jerk can be elicited with ease indicates that this small number of synapses can be most effective. Epileptic neurons, on the other hand, instead of firing at 20/sec, often fire at rates of 200 to 900/sec during their bursts, which may last from 10 to 40 msec or longer. Assuming 200/sec rates within an epileptic burst, only 20 synapses with overlapping bursts would be capable of significantly disrupting the normal activities of the postsynaptic neuron. Furthermore, by Calvin's computation, a mere 80 bursting input boutons would be sufficient to cause high-frequency firing in the postsynaptic cell. Thus only 0.13% of the 60,000 synapses of a normal cortical neuron need to be bursting to convert this cell into another bursting cell.

Thus it is apparent that the epileptic burst is a very efficient "packaging" of synaptic input compared with the firing patterns of normal cortical neurons. A group of pacemaker neurons or primary epileptic bursting neurons in an epileptic focus might be expected to have an appreciable density of synaptic connections to adjacent normal neurons, allowing recruitment of normal neurons to widen the extent of the apparent "focus." Background synaptic activity should bias such recruitment. On this basis, the size of the epileptic focus should expand and shrink depending on background synaptic activity and synchronizing factors. The data of Wyler and Fetz (1974) obtained in the awake epileptic monkey would be consistent with such a formulation. They have shown that, in the chronic focus, autonomous, pacemaker neurons are intermixed with other neurons whose firing patterns may fluctuate between varying degrees of epileptic burst firing and normal patterns of firing. Under conditions of operant conditioning, the activity of the apparent pacemaker cells could not be modified while the firing patterns of the others could be synaptically modified. Thus the critical mass of bursting neurons in the focus does appear to enlarge or shrink depending on the characteristics of synaptic drive upon these secondary cells. Although anatomic studies of the focus in the monkey model of chronic epilepsy or in man with the Golgi technique clearly indicate that many cells have lost much of their dendritic synaptic input (and physiologic studies indicate that partial deafferentation results in spontaneous hyperactivity), the behavioral data indicate that many cells in the focus (particularly those that are not "pacemaker" neurons) must have some synaptic input; otherwise their activity could not be manipulated at all by such maneuvers as operant conditioning or sleep.

These concepts have obvious practical consequences in designing therapy for clinical seizures. It is assumed that, for a mass of epileptic neurons to produce a clinical seizure, they must recruit surrounding neuronal activity into sychronous firing until a "critical mass" is reached, at which point clinical manifestations and/or propagation of the pathologic cellular activity is apparent. When a population of epileptic neurons is segregated to a single, circumscribed area of cortex, we have an epileptogenic focus. When this is destroyed, the source of the seizures is missing and the patient is "cured." This is the goal of subpial resection. Clearly the first criterion is that the population of epileptic neurons

be segregated to a circumscribed area. This is accomplished by the clinical requirements that the clinical seizures be of focal onset and that this cortical focus
be confirmed by localized EEG epileptic abnormalities. If the pathology inducing
the cellular changes which produce epilepsy is more widespread, a complete
surgical removal may not be possible. Thus it would be predicted that the ideal
surgical candidate would be one in whom localized injury has produced a restricted epileptogenic focus which can be identified and confirmed using clinical,
EEG, and radiographic techniques and that this focus is in dispensable cortex.
If the pathologic insult (such as vascular ischemia) induces a widespread and
poorly defined distribution of hyperactive cellular pathology, the surgical attack
obviously becomes more difficult and may even require the surgical extirpation
of the entire hemisphere. A final condition of successful therapy by surgery is
that the surgical extirpation of a localized focus must be undertaken in such a
fashion that the surgical trauma is minimal and does not itself induce a new
margin of cellular pathology around the margins of the excision which can
continue to cause seizures. Thus far subpial resection has proven to be the surgical
technique of choice and its effectiveness is well established.

Obviously an optimal technique would be one which differentially destroys the
epileptic cells in the cortical region of the focus but preserves those cells whose
activity is normal. No such technique exists, but current data do provide some
clues which may have therapeutic potential in the future. It has been shown
(Moseley, Ojemann, and Ward, 1972) that epileptic neurons in the chronic cortical focus in the monkey respond differently to focal cortical hypothermia than
do normal cortical neurons (or neurons excited into epileptic activity by topical
convulsants). The data suggest that hypothermia influences different membrane
mechanisms in epileptic neurons than in other neurons. Furthermore, more
recent data suggest that prolonged local cooling at critical temperatures might
result in neuronal death of epileptic neurons with survival of normal neurons.
This may provide an opportunity to achieve the same results as those following
subpial resection without some of the drawbacks of a direct surgical attack. The
clinical effectiveness of local hypothermia in the treatment of epilepsy is reviewed
in Chapter 12.

In addition, there are clues that it may be possible to modify behaviorally the
activity of neurons in the epileptic focus. The data in the monkey model of
epilepsy indicate that, of all cells within the focus (defined by precise electrocorticography), about one-half exhibit physiologic behavior that cannot be distinguished from that of normal cortical neurons. The remaining neurons in the focus
could be called "epileptic" but their spontaneous activity exhibits a spectrum of
abnormal, hyperactive, burst activity. At one end of the spectrum are group 1
(Wyler and Fetz, 1974) or "pacemaker" epileptic neurons which fire in structured
bursts with high, invariant burst indices and whose activity cannot be modified
either by operant conditioning or other behavioral manipulations such as sleep.
Between this end of the spectrum and normal neuronal activity at the other end
lie a continuous spectrum of abnormal neurons characterized by lower and more

variant burst indices which Wyler and Fetz have called group 2 epileptic cells. Often their spontaneous activity could vary from periods of normal appearing patterns of firing to high-frequency burst firing and, in all, their activity could be as easily conditioned as normal cells.

We have postulated that these group 2 epileptic neurons, because of their inherent lability in burst firing, and because of the proclivity for bursts to be synchronized by massive synaptic influences, might represent the potential "critical mass" available for rapid enlargement of a focus necessary to induce a propagating, clinical seizure. It is precisely this group of neurons that may have their pathologic activity diminished during operant conditioning. Daily periods of single neuron operant conditioning were carried out in a small series of epileptic monkeys after stable seizure frequencies were documented. After some days to several weeks, there was a decrease in clinically apparent seizures and a much more striking decline in the number of abnormal neurons encountered with the microelectrode which was not secondary to the possible cortical damage from repeated electrode penetrations. Thus it appears that single cell operant conditioning is associated with a decrease in single cell interictal epileptic activity and a decrease in spontaneous clinical seizures in epileptic monkeys (Wyler, Fetz, and Ward, 1974). Monkeys who continued to have fits during the weeks of operant conditioning did so only on the weekends when no operant conditioning was undertaken. Such experimental data raise the possibility that, with appropriate biofeedback, operant conditioning in human epileptics might have therapeutic potential. Furthermore, Sterman and Friar (1972) have demonstrated that reinforcement of sensory-motor rhythms in cats increased the threshold to monomethylhydrazine-induced seizures. But the clinical application of operant conditioning techniques has not yet generated controlled data in adequate series of patients to determine the therapeutic potential of this approach.

There is an additional potential therapeutic approach based on known properties of the epileptic focus. There is strong morphologic evidence pointing to partial deafferentation of neurons in the focus of the epileptic monkey and of man. It is also clear that experimental deafferentation of sensory relay cells in spinal cord of the lateral cuneate nucleus and of the nucleus caudalis of the trigeminal system results in dramatic spontaneous hyperactivity of the deafferented neurons (Ward, 1969). This hyperactivity appears some 3 weeks after loss of input and tends to increase with time. In the cerebral cortex, partial or total neuronal isolation of a block of cortex leads to dramatic changes in excitability as well (Sharpless and Halpern, 1962). Threshold decreases and duration of afterdischarges increase over weeks and months following partial or complete isolation of cortex. This phenomenon has been called supersensitivity. Rutledge, Ranck, and Duncan (1967) have shown that chronic electrical stimulation of such an isolated cortical slab in the cat prevents the development of such supersensitivity and, once supersensitivity has developed, chronic stimulation will reverse the process. Such chronic stimulation was undertaken at current strengths subthreshold for afterdischarge. Information is not yet available as to whether chronic electrical stimulation of a cortical epileptic focus in the human would modify seizure frequency, but clearly the surgical and electronic technology currently exist where this technique could be easily undertaken. Thus, experimental research has yielded clues that may lead to therapeutic advances in the treatment of epilepsy. Additional animal research is needed, however, to clarify the problems before there can be any consideration of therapeutic trials in human patients.

The physiological data which has been presented dealing with the properties of group 2 epileptic neurons in the focus may provide a basis for the therapeutic effectiveness of modalities of surgical therapy other than a direct surgical attack on the focus. It is clear that synaptic modulation of the group 2 epileptic neurons can augment or decrease their pathological activity. It may be that either the facilitatory drive on such cortical cells (or an increase in the inhibitory synaptic bias on them) can be achieved by lesions or manipulation of distant circuits. This may be the basis for the observations (Chapter 12) that stereotactic lesions in upper brainstem or in the nonspecific thalamic system reduce seizure frequency in certain patients with seizures. Unfortunately the clinical data available at present do not permit precise delimitation of which cortical foci are best suppressed—nor are the responsible stereotactic lesions precisely delimited from an anatomic standpoint. It has been shown in the experimental animal that lesions in the caudate nucleus may facilitate the spread of acutely induced cortical seizures. Lesions in the anterior thalamic nuclei and inferior thalamic peduncle inhibited the spread of cortical afterdischarge and reduced the frequency of clinical seizures in the chronic monkey model (Kusske, Ojemann, and Ward, 1972). Whether similar stereotactic lesions in the human epileptic will be effective is not yet known.

It is known that modification of input from cerebellum can profoundly modify the precipitation and propagation of seizures arising in cortical foci. Cooke and Snider (1955) clearly showed that cerebellar stimulation usually resulted in either abrupt or gradual termination of afterdischarge in the cerebral cortex induced by electrical stimulation. This inhibitory effect on electrically induced cortical seizures was obtained following stimulation of cerebellar cortex, fastigial nucleus, inferior olive, brachium pontis, and cerebellar peduncle (Cooke and Snider, 1953; Snider and Cooke, 1953). Facilitation of cortical seizure activity was also occasionally seen (Snider and Cooke, 1953). Dow, Fernandez-Guardiola, and Manni (1962) demonstrated that cerebellar stimulation usually inhibited seizure activity induced in cortex by cobalt implantation. This inhibition was often followed by facilitatory rebound. Furthermore, the removal of the cerebellum in rats seemed to enhance the chronic epileptic manifestations provoked by application of cobalt powder on the frontal lobe. Therefore Dow concluded that the cerebellar influence on the development of the epileptic process is mainly of an inhibitory character and is demonstrated by electrical stimulation, ablation, and cooling of the cerebellum.

The role of the cerebellum is further documented by the role it appears to play in the mechanism of action of diphenylhydantoin (DPH). Julien and Halpern (1972) have shown that intravenous DPH induces a dramatic increase in the firing rates of the Purkinje cells in cerebellum. High-frequency sustained discharges reached a maximum 90 min after DPH and persisted for several hours thereafter. Furthermore, similar high-frequency tonic firing of Purkinje cells was recorded in animals chronically pretreated with DPH. Finally, administration of DPH after cerebellectomy was much less effective in reducing seizures than in intact animals.

Thus there is experimental evidence to indicate that activation of cerebellum (Purkinje cells) by electrical stimulation or drugs (DPH, phenobarbital) will reduce many aspects of epileptic phenomena in acute experimental animals. Certainly DPH is an excellent anticonvulsant drug for human epilepsy, and one might anticipate that appropriate electrical stimulation of the same neuronal elements in cerebellum by chronic electrical stimulation should also demonstrate an anticonvulsant effect as Cooper, Amin, and Gilman (1973) have shown. It remains to be seen whether long-term chronic activation of Purkinje cells is best accomplished by electrical stimulation via implanted electrodes which can activate only a limited number of Purkinje cells, or whether tonic inhibition of seizures is more effectively maintained for long periods by activation of Purkinje cells rather generally by the anticonvulsant drug DPH. There is evidence that prolonged, intense activation of Purkinje cells by toxic doses of DPH can induce Purkinje cell death. The consequences of prolonged, intense electrical stimulation are, however, not known.

The mechanisms by which cerebellar activation (by either stimulation or drugs) inhibits the epileptic process is unknown. If the essential feature is activity in Purkinje cells, their efferent fibers go mainly to the deep cerebellar nuclei. However, a few leave the cerebellum without relaying in those nuclei, and such fibers arise from the flocculonodular lobe and from portions of the vermis and mainly the anterior lobe. Electrical stimulation of the latter structure is said to be particularly effective in inhibiting seizures in experimental animals. Thus it is not even established that the effect is mediated via the roof nuclei. In fact, were it not for the observations of Julien and Halpern (1972) which strongly implicate activity in Purkinje cells, the data from electrical stimulation are ambiguous since the distribution of current fields and the neural structures activated are unknown. In fact, the effect may not be a specific inhibitory effect on epileptic processes in cortex. It has long been known (Cooke and Snider, 1953) that stimulation of the cerebellum induces activation of the cortical EEG similar to that following stimulation of the reticular formation. There are clues from both clinical experience and specific physiologic data in the epileptic monkey which indicate that activation, behavioral attention, and desynchronized EEG rhythms depress epileptic neuronal activity in the focus. Cerebellar stimulation may act in this indirect fashion as well.

THE PRECIPITATION OF SEIZURES

The current model of the epileptic process proposes that the epileptic focus is composed of autonomous epileptic cells (group 1) as well as a much larger number of group 2 epileptic neurons whose activity, however, varies between normal activity and high-frequency burst activity. Under certain circumstances, appropriate synaptic input to the latter cells drives them to the upper limits of their range of pathologic activity and their activity now becomes indistinguishable from that of the pacemaker cells. As this group of cells reaches a critical mass, their propagating burst activity can now recruit normal cells to fire also in a bursting mode and the seizure starts to propagate. Alterations of local extracellular K^+ may also be involved in this process.

Although the details of the mechanisms responsible for generating the appropriate synaptic input to precipitate this sequence of events are not known, some general properties can be identified.

One of these is the state of behavioral arousal. Sleep has profound influences upon the natural history of most epilepsies as evidenced by the increased frequency of ictal events during early stages of non-rapid eye movement (n-REM) sleep. Sleep deprivation lowers seizure thresholds. Most of the data have been obtained in humans but the same phenomena appear to be manifested by the epileptic monkey model. Furthermore, studies of the activity of single epileptic neurons in the monkey provide additional insight into the role of sleep in producing changes in activity at the epileptic focus. Wyler (1974) has shown that group 1 (pacemaker) neurons in the focus of monkey which were grossly epileptic during wakefulness did not change firing patterns significantly during spontaneous sleep, whereas group 2 neurons (mildly epileptic during wakefulness) changed drastically during sleep, becoming indistinguishable from group 1 neurons in burst structure. From the vantage point of single cell recording, it is surprising that sleep does not routinely precipitate clinical seizures. Although there is a modest body of knowledge dealing with the neural circuits subserving sleep and wakefulness, there are no clues to indicate that stereotactic surgical lesions in these circuits, either currently or at any time in the foreseeable future, will be beneficial without major morbidity in human patients.

A second well-documented variable that plays a role in precipitation of seizures is behavioral stress. There are narrative data in clinical experience and controlled data in the experimental monkey model to support this conclusion. In the latter instance, Lockard, Wilson, and Uhlir (1972) have shown that emotional stress induced by avoidance conditioning increases seizure frequency in monkeys continuously housed in a behavioral laboratory where all seizures can be recorded. Surgical therapy specifically directed at this factor in the epileptic process has not been explicitly undertaken. However, the reports of benefit in seizure frequency after cingulumotomy in human patients may well be a consequence of alterations in the response to environmental stress rather than a direct effect on seizure mechanisms. Also, there is ambiguity regarding the reported beneficial results after amygdalotomy where Narabayashi and Mizutani (1970) note that the best improvement in seizure frequency is obtained in patients with the best behavioral improvement. But, again, this factor does not appear to be one with significant potential for surgical manipulation at the present time.

Other variables which appear to play a role in the precipitation of spontaneous epileptic seizures have even less potential for surgical manipulation.

PATHWAYS OF SPREAD

Once a critical mass of neurons is firing in high-frequency bursts at the focus, their propagating burst activity can now recruit normal cells to fire in a bursting mode—and this regenerative process leads to propagation of the seizure widely throughout the central nervous system. The circuits of spread obviously depend on the cells of origin. With a focus in motor cortex, the axonal propagation of the seizure will obviously be rapidly manifested by appropriate motor movements. From foci in temporal lobe, there are preferential pathways of spread within the limbic system, and, in fact, the discharge may commonly remain restricted to limbic circuits.

If the anatomic projections from the neurons in and adjacent to the focus are well localized into a projection bundle which can be surgically divided in its entirety, the clinical result should be a complete suppression of clinical seizures. The EEG abnormalities at the focus should be largely unchanged, but the ablation of pathways for propagation should prevent this localized abnormality from influencing normal brain function. Unfortunately, this optimal set of circumstances rarely presents itself spontaneously in nature. However, there is every reason to believe that there are clinical circumstances where it is surgically possible to destroy stereotactically a major projection pathway from the focus and thereby produce significant clinical improvement. This may well be the basis for the improvement reported to follow lesions of the fornix and other structures in the efferent pathways from temporal lobe as is discussed in Chapter 12.

Consideration of pathways from a focus may also be important for reasons other than the propagation of the occasional clinical seizure. The continuous interictal firing of neurons in the focus is providing abnormal input to those distant cells to which their axons project. It can be proposed that such abnormal input will, in varying degrees, modify the otherwise normal functioning of these circuits. Such functional deficits may be difficult to document clinically because of the well-known redundancy of circuitry in the central nervous system. Certainly such abnormal input will inject an appreciable amount of "noise" into normal circuits and the resultant modification of efficient information processing may only make itself evident by subtle functional changes. Circuits subserving the more complex functions may be the most susceptible to modification by such "noise." Thus interictal neuronal burst firing in critical neuronal pathways might result in a variety of behavioral and cognitive deficits. If so, the goal of therapy should be directed at reduction of interictal as well as ictal epileptic events since interictal firing may not be functionally innocuous.

In addition to such functional (and reversible) changes, this hyperactivity may, in time, induce other, more lasting changes. In the experimental setting, it has been shown that chronic, electrical stimulation of a locus in the cortex over a period of weeks can, particularly in lower mammalian forms, induce changes in threshold such that propagating afterdischarge and actual clinical seizures appear in time. After this process is well established, cessation of electrical stimulation can be followed by continuation of spontaneous EEG spiking and other evidences of alterations of spontaneous excitability. This process has been given the name "kindling" (Goddard, McIntyre, and Leech, 1969). The phenomenon is of interest to experimental psychologists since it may form a neurophysiologic model for learning or memory. It is obviously of interest to an understanding of epilepsy. Although little is known of the detailed mechanisms involved at this time, the phenomenon may be related to several observations in clinical epilepsy.

Obviously the phenomenon of "kindling" has certain similarities to those observations dealing with what has been termed the "mirror focus." The mirror focus is usually considered to be an area (commonly the homotopic area of cortex in the opposite hemisphere) receiving projections from an acute, epileptic focus. After a period of time, the EEG spiking at the mirror focus becomes "independent" from that recorded at the primary focus; i.e., the spikes at the mirror focus are no longer synchronous with those at the distant primary focus. However, there is still ambiguity regarding the true "independence" of the mirror focus since there have been relatively few controlled studies to show that such "independent" spiking continues after removal of the primary focus. The phenomenon is most easily demonstrated in lower animal species (especially those with lissenencephalic brains), and, although of interest, there is no clear evidence to indicate that this phenomenon is of clinical importance in man.

In the surgical therapy of epilepsy, it has been noted that, following subpial resection of the cortical focus, continuing spiking in cortex adjacent to the area of resection is not always associated with a poor surgical result. Rather, the patient may be seizure-free and the EEG spiking may spontaneously resolve—as has been described in the kindling phenomenon after cessation of stimulation.

There is another more speculative but potentially more important consequence of involving the kindling phenomenon in the natural history of epilepsy. One might propose the following sequence of events after the production of a focal, traumatic lesion to cortex which is highly epileptogenic (such as sensorimotor) in man. As a consequence of the neuronal destruction, gliosis, and partial deafferentation, a complex sequence of pathologic events sequentially develops. In the dynamic production of an epileptogenic focus, neurons in the scarred area become hyperactive. They provide a continuous bombardment of adjacent neurons which, in turn, "kindles" hyperactivity in them and the focus matures to the point where the first clinical seizure occurs. One might postulate that, if the developing neuronal hyperactivity could be blocked by the prophylactic adminis-tration of anticonvulsant drugs, this sequence could be blocked. In fact, if the hyperactivity can be suppressed for a sufficiently long period of time (perhaps 1 to 2 years), possibly many otherwise clinically evident foci would be aborted. There is clinical evidence that this may be possible and the evidence has recently been summarized by Rapport and Penry (1972). Experimental evidence has demonstrated the efficacy of prophylactic anticonvulsants in animal models of epilepsy (Servit, 1960). Of the clinical reports, there are three controlled series reported since 1947: in these, between 20 and 50% of the patients not receiving anticonvulsant drugs after head injury developed epilepsy. Of those patients receiving only the anticonvulsant drug DPH in modest doses, 4 to 6% developed epilepsy. In the series where the treated patients received prophylactic DPH and phenobarbital, none developed epilepsy in contrast to untreated controls, 20% of whom developed epilepsy.

Thus it may well be that the brain "learns" how to have a seizure—and that the most effective point for blocking the process may be at the beginning with prophylactic anticonvulsant therapy. This matter is clearly of major importance in surgical therapy, since prophylactic anticonvulsant therapy during the postop-erative period would now appear to be essential. Although such postoperative anticonvulsant therapy has been customary in most centers, it has been estab-lished in part through custom and intelligent intuition; now a more firm basis and rationale are available.

Before leaving the complex of pathophysiologic events which constitute the epileptic process, there is one final observation which is clinically relevant to the design of an appropriate therapeutic strategy. Histologic studies in the chronic epileptic monkey by Harris (1972) indicate that continuing clinical seizures are associated with continuing neuronal damage. In monkeys having chronic, sponta-neous seizures for periods of 1 to 5-½ years after the production of the epilepto-genic focus by the intracortical injection of alumina, both axonal and terminal degeneration is continuously occurring as demonstrated by the Nauta-Gygax and Fink-Heimer reduced silver methods. There are also some data which indicate that the continuing neuronal degeneration is related to the continuing seizures and their frequency and severity rather than to other variables. Thus the original clues reported by Westrum, White, and Ward (1964) indicating that an active epileptogenic focus continues to undergo active pathologic changes has now been confirmed in the monkey model. More importantly, it has also been confirmed in human (Scheibel and Scheibel, 1973). Brown (1973) has also reported that electron microscopic studies of temporal lobe removed at operation show evi-dence of ongoing degeneration of boutons, spines, and axons in these cortices.

Thus it may be that the occurrence of clinical seizures is not innocuous. This has a bearing on clinical decisions regarding surgical therapy for intractable seizures. Based on these data, the prudent strategy would appear to consist of aggressive medical therapy in the attempt to achieve complete control of clinical seizures as quickly as possible. The attempt should then be continued only for that period of time necessary to make the judgment in that patient that a spontaneous remission is not likely to occur. To delay surgical therapy for long periods of time appears to carry the inevitable price of continuing neuronal damage in the vicinity of the focus. This may be undesirable, not only in its own right, but also because the continuing neuronal degeneration may add to the pathophysiologic alterations and augment the total epileptic process, thereby making future seizure control more difficult by any means. Of course, this conclusion is yet to be proven by hard, clinical data.

An increasing body of knowledge has been generated by all disciplines of neuroscience that bear on the process called epilepsy. This discussion has concentrated almost exclusively on selected concepts supported by recent evidence largely from the discipline of electrophysiology with supporting data from neuromorphology. It should be remembered, however, that there is now a significant body of data in the fields of neurochemistry and neuropharmacology which is essential to any comprehensive modern view of epileptic mechanisms. However, much of the development of surgical therapy and its rationale rest on physiologic concepts, which accounts for the current emphasis. As the disciplines of neuroscience increase our understanding of the basic mechanisms involved in epilepsy, there is every reason to believe that new avenues for therapy will be developed in the future.

REFERENCES

Brown, W. J. (1973): Structural substrates of seizure foci in the human temporal lobe. In: *Epilepsy: Its Phenomena in Man,* edited by M. A. B. Brazier. Academic Press, New York.

Calvin, W. H. (1972): Synaptic potential summation and repetitive firing mechanisms: Input-output theory for the recruitment of neurons into epileptic bursting firing patterns. *Brain Res.,* 39:71–94.

Calvin, W. H., Sypert, G. W., and Ward, A. A., Jr. (1968): Structured timing patterns within bursts from epileptic neurons in undrugged monkey cortex. *Exp. Neurol.,* 21:535–549.

Cooke, P. M., and Snider, R. D. (1953): Some cerebellar effects on the electro-corticogram. *Electroenceph. Clin. Neurophysiol.,* 5:563–569.

Cooke, P. M., and Snider, R. S. (1955): Some cerebellar influences on electrically induced cerebral seizures. *Epilepsia,* 4:19–28.

Cooper, I. S., Amin, I., and Gilman, S. (1973): The effect of chronic cerebellar stimulation upon epilepsy in man. *Trans. Amer. Neurol. Assoc.,* 98:192–196.

Dow, R. S., Fernandez-Guardiola, A., and Manni, E. (1962): The influence of the cerebellum on experimental epilepsy. *Electroenceph. Clin. Neurophysiol.,* 14:383–398.

Fetz, E. E., and Wyler, A. R. (1973): Operantly conditioned firing patterns of epileptic neurons in motor cortex of chronic monkey. *Exp. Neurol.,* 40:586–607.

Goddard, G. V., McIntyre, D. C., and Leech, C. K. (1969): A permanent change in brain function resulting from daily brain stimulation. *Exp. Neurol.,* 25:295–330.

Harris, A. B. (1972): Degeneration in experimental epileptic foci. *Arch. Neurol.,* 26:434–449.

Jackson, J. H. (1931): *Selected Writings of John Hughlings Jackson.* Vol. 1. *On Epilepsy and Epileptiform Convulsions,* edited by J. Taylor. Hodder and Stoughton, London.

Julien, R. M., and Halpern, L. M. (1972): Effects of diphenylhydantoin and other antiepileptic drugs on epileptiform activity and Purkinje cell discharge rates. *Epilepsia,* 13:387–400.

Narabayashi, H., and Mizutani, T. (1970): Epileptic seizures and the stereotaxic amygdalotomy. *Confin. Neurol.,* 32:289–297.

Kusske, J. A., Ojemann, G. A., and Ward, A. A., Jr. (1972): Effects of lesions in ventral anterior thalamus on experimental focal epilepsy. *Exp. Neurol.,* 34:279–290.

Lockard, J. S., Wilson, W. L., and Uhlir, V. (1972): Spontaneous seizure frequency and avoidance conditioning in monkeys. *Epilepsia,* 13:437–444.

Moseley, J. I., Ojemann, G. A., and Ward, A. A., Jr. (1972): Unit activity in experimental epileptic foci during focal cortical hypothermia. *Exp. Neurol.,* 37:164–178.

Rapport, R. L., II, and Penry, J. K. (1972): Pharmacologic prophylaxis of posttraumatic epilepsy. *Epilepsia,* 13:295–304.

Rutledge, L. T., Ranck, J. B., Jr., and Duncan, J. A. (1967): Prevention of supersensitivity in partially isolated cortex. *Electroenceph. Clin. Neurophysiol.,* 23:256–262.

Scheibel, M. E., and Scheibel, A. B. (1973): Hippocampal pathology in temporal lobe epilepsy, a Golgi survey. In: *Epilepsy: Its Phenomena in Man,* edited by M. A. B. Brazier. Academic Press, New York.

Servit, Z. (1960): Prophylactic treatment of posttraumatic audiogenic epilepsy. *Nature,* 188:669–670.

Sharpless, S. K., and Halpern, L. M. (1962): The electrical excitability of chronically isolated cortex studied by means of permanently implanted electrodes. *Electroenceph. Clin. Neurophysiol.,* 14: 244–255.

Snider, R. S., and Cooke, P. M. (1953): Cerebellar activity in relation to the electrocorticogram before, during and after seizure states. *Electroenceph. Clin. Neurophysiol.,* 5:Suppl. 3:78.

Sterman, M. B., and Friar, L. (1972): Suppression of seizures in an epileptic following sensorimotor EEG feedback training. *Electroenceph. Clin. Neurophysiol.,* 33:89–95.

Ward, A. A., Jr. (1969): The epileptic neuron: Chronic foci in animals and man. In: *Basic Mechanisms of the Epilepsies,* edited by H. H. Jasper, A. A. Ward, Jr., and A. Pope. Little, Brown, Boston.

Westrum, L. E., White, L. E., and Ward, A. A., Jr. (1964): Morphology of the experimental epileptic focus. *J. Neurosurg.,* 21:1033–1046.

Wyler, A. R. (1974): Epileptic neurons during sleep and wakefulness. *Exp. Neurol.,* 42:593–608.

Wyler, A. R., and Fetz, E. E. (1974): Behavioral control of firing patterns of normal and abnormal neurons in chronic epileptic cortex. *Exp. Neurol.,* 42:448–464.

Wyler, A. R., Fetz, E. E., and Ward, A. A., Jr. (1973): Spontaneous firing patterns of epileptic neurons in motor cortex of chronic monkey. *Exp. Neurol.,* 40:567–585.

Wyler, A. R., Fetz, E. E., and Ward, A. A., Jr. (1974): Effects of operantly conditioning epileptic unit activity on seizure frequencies and electrophysiology of neocortical experimental foci. *Exp. Neurol.,* 44:113–125.

Advances in Neurology, Vol. 8, edited by D. P. Purpura, J. K. Penry, and R. D. Walter. Raven Press, New York © 1975.

3
Criteria for Selection of Patients for Neurosurgical Treatment

Francis L. McNaughton and Theodore Rasmussen

HISTORICAL INTRODUCTION

Epilepsy is the name for occasional, sudden, excessive, rapid and local discharges of gray matter of some part of the brain. . . .

The mode of onset is the most important matter in the anatomical investigation of any case of epilepsy. . . .

No one can admit more fully than I do the difficulties in the localization of "discharging lesions" . . . I still urge that we should go on trying to localize; and we should, as far as is practicable, work in the same realistic manner as we do in cases of paralysis.

The reader will immediately recognize these as quotations from John Hughlings Jackson. They are taken from his paper "On the Anatomical, Physiological and Pathological Investigation of Epilepsies" published in 1873, and provide a fitting text for this volume on neurosurgical management of the epilepsies. His words have a distinctly modern ring and they remind us, as Temkin (1971) has pointed out, that we are still living in the Jacksonian or modern period in the long history of the Falling Sickness.

Without Jackson's ideas and the approach which he initiated, there might be no modern surgery of epilepsy. The first craniotomy for removal of a brain tumor was performed successfully by a London surgeon, Mr. Rickman Godlee, in 1884. The patient was a young Scotsman with a 3-year history of focal motor seizures involving the left face, arm, and leg. It is of interest that among those present at the operation were Hughlings Jackson and David Ferrier, two men "without whose work it would never have been thought of" (Trotter, 1934). Horsley's brilliant work on the surgery of focal epilepsy followed soon after.

FOCAL AND GENERALIZED FORMS OF EPILEPSY

Throughout his writings, Hughlings Jackson emphasized that epilepsy is a symptom having many varied causes, and is not in itself a disease. He always referred to "the Epilepsies" (in the plural). He stressed the paramount importance of "trying to localize the epileptic process in every patient with seizures" and thereby firmly established the concept of focal epilepsy which we still refer to,

---

Montreal Neurological Institute Reprint No. 1163.

in broad terms, as "Jacksonian" epilepsy, an expression coined by J-M. Charcot in 1887 (Temkin, 1971).

With the development of modern methods of clinical investigation, and electroencephalography in particular, our understanding of focal and generalized epilepsy has been considerably broadened.

This distinction between focal and generalized seizures has been formulated in the International Classification of the Epilepsies (Merlis, 1970). The epilepsies are divided into (1) the partial (or focal) forms, of varied etiology, and (2) the generalized forms, on the basis of clinical and EEG findings. The generalized forms of epilepsy are subdivided into those caused by diffuse or multifocal cerebral lesions ("secondary generalized epilepsies") and those of unknown cause ("primary generalized epilepsies") with a third subgroup of "undetermined generalized epilepsies." Unfortunately, it is often impossible to distinguish between the primary and secondary types.

The large group of the "primary generalized epilepsies," in which genetic factors appear to be of particular importance, has often been labeled in the past by the unsatisfactory term "idiopathic," and more recently by special descriptive terms such as "centrencephalic epilepsy" (Penfield and Jasper, 1954) or "generalized corticoreticular epilepsy" (Gloor, 1968).

Although these broad subdivisions in the International Classification are of practical use, our understanding of the epileptic process is still very limited, and any classification should not be interpreted too rigidly. We feel that epilepsy as we meet it in our patients is a *continuum,* with focal forms at one end of the scale and generalized forms at the other end, but with no boundary line between them. Genetic factors may be important in any form of epilepsy, focal or generalized. Focal seizures often spread rapidly to become generalized without recognizable aura, and may easily be mistaken for one of the generalized types. On the other hand, in so-called primary generalized epilepsy there may be fleeting focal manifestations (Howell, 1955).

If this open relationship between the focal and generalized manifestations is kept in mind, it may lead to earlier recognition and more effective treatment of some hidden forms of focal epilepsy.

BASIC CRITERIA FOR SELECTION OF PATIENTS

The modern surgical management of epilepsy is based on the principle of surgical removal of chronic and reasonably well-restricted focal epileptogenic lesions from the brain in order to reduce the patient's seizure tendency. It is applicable only in patients in whom the clinical and EEG evidence indicates that the attacks are focal in origin and are arising in an area of brain that can be excised without producing significant neurological deficits or without increasing one already present. The principles of clinical investigation involved in establishing a diagnosis of focal epilepsy will be outlined later.

One basic criterion for selection as a possible candidate for surgical treatment is failure of an adequate trial of antiseizure medical treatment to keep the attacks under control to a point where the patient can live a reasonably normal life. When the focal seizures may be caused by a potentially lethal lesion such as a slowly growing glioma, surgical management requires consideration of preservation of life and neurological function as well as alleviation of the seizure tendency, which then usually has a lower priority.

Without doubt, the proper evaluation and selection of patients for surgical management of the symptom, epilepsy, is the most important single factor in determining the success or failure of this form of treatment in reducing the seizure tendency.

Next in importance is the quality of the neurosurgical management. All those with experience in the surgery of epilepsy agree that it requires a team effort which involves not only the collaboration of neurosurgeons, neurologists, and electroencephalographers with a broad experience in every aspect of epilepsy (both clinical and experimental), but also the assistance of specially trained staff nurses and the guidance of the neuroradiologists and the neuropsychologist. The social worker, psychiatrist, and rehabilitation staff may also have an important role. Without such an organized group this type of neurosurgical treatment is frequently unsuccessful.

CLINICAL EVALUATION OF PATIENTS WITH SUSPECTED FOCAL EPILEPSY

The first consideration in the selection of patients for surgical treatment is to gather all the evidence available which will establish the focal nature of the epileptic process. With some patients this may be an easy task, but with others it is a complicated and tedious process.

Epilepsy usually makes its first appearance during infancy or childhood, and onset after the age of 20 is relatively uncommon. The first appearance of epileptic seizures is usually the proper time to undertake a thorough clinical study to determine, if possible, the localization and cause of the attacks and to have available a baseline for future reevaluation.

History

A family history of epilepsy may be important. History of birth trauma, asphyxia, postnatal trauma, febrile illnesses, or contagious diseases may be of etiological significance and should be recorded in full detail. The same will be true of a history of febrile convulsions, "breath-holding spells," or "fainting" episodes earlier in life.

Observation of Attacks

An accurate and detailed description of the seizure pattern (or patterns) is of critical importance in studying localization. The patient or members of the family may be able to describe the true onset of an attack, but often this can be determined with certainty only by direct observation and documentation of the patient's attacks by trained observers in the hospital. The same is true of postictal phenomena such as transient aphasia or one-sided weakness, which may be of critical localizing value.

When a patient is being followed over a period of months or years, it is important to watch for changes in the attack pattern; these changes may occur as the brain of a young patient matures or when a slowly growing cerebral tumor begins to reveal itself. Some of the focal attack patterns commonly recognized in patients are described in Chapters 8–11.

When a patient is under observation in hospital, it is usually necessary to reduce the antiseizure medication and sometimes to withdraw it completely, in order to observe attacks and to obtain satisfactory EEG recordings. Because of the danger of inducing status epilepticus, medication should always be reduced gradually over a period of days, with phenobarbital or primidone the last drug to be withdrawn. When there has been a history of status in the past, or when frequent attacks occur as the medication is reduced, complete withdrawal of medication may be unwise or may need to be of short duration.

Neurological Findings

Findings on routine neurological examination which may aid in localizing an epileptogenic brain lesion include growth asymmetry (e.g., smallness of one hand or foot), subtle motor and reflex changes, a mild cortical sensory deficit, or a hemianopic visual field defect of which the patient is unaware. A history of the patient's handedness and speech development is also important. Psychological assessment and IQ determination should be an integral part of the examination, and in some cases the neuropsychologist may be able to add lateralizing and localizing data of great value (see Chapter 15). The neuropsychological test profile may alert one to the presence of an unusual lateralization of the cerebral speech mechanisms.

EEG Studies

Of equal importance in the evaluation of a patient with epilepsy is the EEG study, which should include recordings on and off medication, sleep recordings when necessary, and, where indicated, more specialized techniques to determine the site of origin of the epileptogenic discharge (see Chapter 5). In attempting to correlate the patient's seizure pattern with the EEG findings, we should remember that the clinical attack pattern observed points to the area of *lowest* seizure threshold, while the EEG record gives better evidence as to the *total extent* of the epileptogenic area.

We would point out that the finding of a bilaterally synchronous 3/sec spike-wave pattern does not absolutely rule out a focal form of epilepsy. Further EEG study will sometimes demonstrate that this is a form of secondary bilateral synchrony produced by a focal unilateral cerebral lesion (Tükel and Jasper, 1952; Madsen and Bray, 1966; Stewart and Dreifuss, 1967). A focal epileptogenic lesion causing secondary bilateral synchrony is apt to be located in the mesial part of the frontal lobe, although lesions elsewhere in the brain may produce a similar pattern (see Chapter 10).

Radiological Studies

Radiological techniques provide valuable evidence of a focal brain lesion or lesions. Plain skull films may demonstrate growth asymmetries (as, for example, a small middle fossa associated with an atrophic temporal lobe), local changes in bone texture and vascular markings, or abnormal intracranial calcifications. In our opinion a pneumogram should be an essential part of the clinical evaluation. In addition, the air study provides a baseline for follow-up studies, if needed later. Angiography is mainly of value in excluding vascular malformations and in the investigation of cerebral neoplasms.

Although cerebral angiography seldom gives as valuable evidence as the pneumogram in the ordinary patient with epilepsy due to a static lesion, it is an essential and usually the first contrast radiological examination to be carried out when there is any suggestion from the age of onset of seizures, neurological examination, ordinary skull X-rays, or EEG that a tumor or vascular lesion may be present.

It is also wise to carry out angiography in a patient with a well-localized seizure pattern whose pneumogram does *not* show definite evidence of an atrophic lesion in the expected location since, occasionally, a small neoplasm or vascular malformation may be found in such patients. It must be emphasized, however, that a negative angiogram does not necessarily rule out a neoplasm (see Chapter 13).

In interpreting radiological findings in patients with epilepsy, we should keep in mind that structural changes may be demonstrated in areas of the brain other than the epileptogenic region.

The computerized tomographic EMI scanner is likely to prove helpful in the early detection of small intracranial neoplasms, particularly an indolent astrocytoma. These may occur in children, as in adults, and can cause focal seizures for a number of years before they are recognized as expanding lesions by standard radiological contrast studies (see Chapter 11).

Radioisotopic Brain Scanning

Brain scanning is useful in detecting vascular malformations and certain types of brain tumor but it rarely detects indolent astrocytomas or other slowly growing gliomas, which not infrequently present as seizures for long periods. It is less helpful in the investigation of focal epilepsy than other diagnostic procedures because it does not show up focal atrophic lesions or areas of gliosis.

Problems in Diagnosis

Once the significance of the symptom (epilepsy) has been established and it is clear that the causative lesion does not itself need treatment, then treatment of the symptoms is in order.

Even after thorough investigation has been carried out along these lines, the focal nature of a seizure problem often remains unsettled or the findings may not be altogether consistent. Real difficulties arise when there is clinical and laboratory evidence of bilateral focal EEG abnormalities (as, for example, bilateral temporal foci), changing foci, or both focal and generalized EEG changes (Chapter 5).

In some patients, a relatively inactive EEG may interfere with a proper study. As mentioned in Chapter 10, focal EEG abnormalities may be singularly absent when the epileptogenic lesion is localized in or near the sensorimotor cortical region.

In the sorting-out process of difficult cases, the most helpful information usually comes from more accurate observation of the patient's attack patterns (particularly when an attack can be observed from its onset) and repetition of EEG examinations after some months or longer, when the seizure activity may have become more clearly defined.

MEDICAL TREATMENT AND ITS LIMITATIONS

The aim of medical treatment of both focal and nonfocal epilepsy is to achieve complete control of all seizures and therefore allow the patient to live a normal life. As yet, there is no perfect drug for the control of epileptic seizures, but without any doubt the drugs available today have enormously improved the outlook for all patients with epilepsy. As more effective anticonvulsant agents appear, the percentage of medically refractory cases in which neurosurgical therapy needs to be considered will decrease.

Although drug therapy is the most important element in medical treatment, the seizure patient often has other problems which require the help of the psychologist, the psychiatrist, the social worker, and other rehabilitation specialists if he or she is to become integrated in society. Social maladjustments may constitute a major obstacle to the patient's ability to function satisfactorily in society and may actually increase the frequency and severity of the seizures themselves.

What constitutes an adequate trial of medical treatment? Before the introduction of diphenylhydantoin (DPH; Dilantin®) in 1938, one could have stated that maximum doses of phenobarbital and bromide, maintained over a period of years, would be considered an adequate trial, because these were the only two effective drugs for the control of epileptic seizures. In 1974, even after extensive trial of many newer drugs, the most dependable drugs available for the control of focal and generalized seizures are probably DPH, phenobarbital, and primidone (Mysoline®). Each of these three drugs may be effective in some patients when used alone. In other patients, a combination of DPH and phenobarbital, DPH and primidone, or all three together may prove to be more satisfactory (McNaughton, 1954; McNaughton and Lloyd-Smith, 1965).

Drug management in epilepsy is still an empirical procedure, and the variations in patient response to treatment are often difficult to explain. The aim of treatment is to bring about complete control of seizures with the minimum dosage of medication and without side effects, so that one starts with a minimal drug dosage, usually related to the age and weight of the patient.

The introduction of reliable routine laboratory methods for measuring blood levels of the common antiseizure drugs has been of distinct help to the clinician. By testing drug levels, one can determine that the patient is actually taking the prescribed medication and absorbing it. (This can be very important.) Because the broad therapeutic range of drug levels is known for each drug, this is also helpful in adjusting the drug dosage to obtain maximum therapeutic effect and at the same time to avoid toxic levels. However, in the long run, it is the patient's clinical response to treatment which is most important. This is still an individual matter, determined by trial and error. Unfortunately, the EEG is not a reliable guide in measuring the effectiveness of drug therapy.

Drug dosage should be managed in a systematic way, with detailed records of the daily dose of each drug used, side effects (if any), and the number of attacks in each period between visits. It is usual to start treatment with a moderate dose of phenobarbital or DPH which can be taken twice daily (morning and night). For example, administration of phenobarbital, 30 mg bid, or DPH, 100 mg bid, might be a beginning dose for a 10-year-old. If laboratory control of blood levels is available, these may be checked after a period of a few weeks, and the dosage increased if levels are low. Primidone may be added at a later date or substituted for phenobarbital, depending on the response to treatment.

If the "first line" drugs fail to bring control even when given in maximal doses tolerated, some of the "second line" drugs may be tried, usually adding one new drug to DPH and phenobarbital or replacing DPH with the new drug; the patient is then followed for a reasonable trial period. Mephenytoin (Mesantoin®) has sometimes been used effectively in place of DPH, but is more likely to have toxic side effects. Carbamazepine (Tegretol®) has recently shown some promise. Other drugs which were designed primarily for the treatment of "absence" attacks (usually considered to be a generalized type of seizure) are ethosuximide (Zarontin®), Trimethadione (Tridione®), and methsuximide (Celontin®). On rare occasions, one of these drugs will prove helpful in controlling focal attacks when combined with DPH and phenobarbital, but they are not effective in focal epilepsy when used alone.

Medical treatment in any patient should not be considered adequate unless the antiseizure drugs have been used in the maximal doses that can be tolerated.

Very accurate figures on the results of medical treatment are not available, since much depends on the selection of patients attending a seizure clinic. However, in clinics where all modern antiseizure drugs are available, treatment usually results in complete control in nearly 50% of patients and greatly reduced incidence of attacks in another 20 to 25%.

Patients without clinical and laboratory evidence of focal or generalized brain damage, and with normal or near normal intelligence levels, usually show the most favorable response to treatment; those with focal forms of epilepsy are more resistant to control, particularly if they belong to the temporal lobe group. Younger patients and those with temporal lobe seizures are more prone to develop behavioral difficulties as a side effect of their medication, or if behavioral problems already exist, these problems may be aggravated by it. In such cases, tranquilizing drugs may be needed in combination with the antiseizure drugs.

GENERAL CONSIDERATIONS IN THE SELECTION OF PATIENTS

Admittedly, drug therapy has many drawbacks. It is a tedious and troublesome form of treatment which usually must be continued for an indefinite period; it can have unpleasant side effects; and it is a form of control, *not* a cure. Apart from drug idiosyncrasies (such as rashes and hematological changes), side effects such as drowsiness and irritability may be bothersome. When contrasted with the possibility of a "cure" by surgical management, it is no wonder that patients and their parents turn eagerly to the neurosurgeon for help.

The possibility of neurosurgical treatment arises whenever adequate medical treatment in a patient with focal epilepsy has failed to give satisfactory control of the attacks, which interfere significantly with the patient's ability to lead a normal or near normal life. When attacks are severe or frequent and particularly if associated with automatism or other overt behavioral disturbances, they constitute a more urgent reason for considering surgical treatment.

When presenting the case for surgical treatment to the patient or to members of the family, one should emphasize that the main purpose of operation is to decrease the seizure tendency rather than to "cure" the epilepsy. In a certain percentage, the reduction in seizure tendency results in the patient becoming completely free of attacks. In others, a marked but incomplete reduction of attacks occurs; in less successful cases, a moderate or slight reduction occurs. In each case, antiseizure medication is continued postoperatively with only gradual reduction in dosage as time proves that the tendency has been satisfactorily reduced.

The majority of patients coming to operation are in the younger age groups, but the duration of the seizures does not reduce the likelihood of a successful result. While only a small percentage of patients present as possible candidates for surgical therapy after the age of 40 to 45, successful results may be obtained with patients in the fifties. Some of the older patients are found to have indolent tumors which have escaped detection by radiological and other investigations (see Chapter 11). The more severe and disabling the seizure problem, as far as a child's intellectual and social development are concerned, the earlier is it worthwhile considering surgical therapy. This must be weighed against the advantages of further delay to increase the likelihood that all epileptogenic areas have become symptomatic and sometimes to permit the operation to be carried out under local anesthesia (see Chapter 7).

In addition, a small percentage of patients with focal cerebral seizures of all types do undergo a gradual spontaneous reduction of seizure tendency in the late teens and early twenties, and can then be well controlled by medication.

Moderate mental retardation is not a contraindication to surgery, providing that the patient's family clearly appreciates the fact that operation will not restore normal intellectual function.

Episodic abnormal, sometimes aggressive, behavior, if closely related to a patient's actual epileptic seizures, may be an important additional factor in recommending surgery. Nonepisodic, continuing aggressive behavior in general is rarely helped by removal of areas of epileptogenic cortex. Patients with stable schizophrenia and paranoid abnormalities of behavior in addition to epilepsy rarely show improvement in psychiatric status as a result of stopping their attacks either medically or surgically, and surgery is usually contraindicated in such patients.

In patients with long-standing seizure problems, eradication of the seizures occasionally may be psychologically disturbing, and psychological and psychiatric support may be particularly important during the early postoperative months or years.

In some patients, relatively mild seizure tendencies are unusually disabling because of intolerance to medication, and early operation is often worthwhile for this reason.

Adequate motivation on the part of the patient beyond middle childhood is essential, because the investigation and surgical procedure require the patient's complete and enthusiastic cooperation. It is also essential that the parents have a clear understanding of the potential risks as well as the potential gains of the surgical procedure. When it seems that the primary motivation toward surgery is that of the parents or the referring physician, it is wise to consider the investigation as a preliminary affair and to postpone serious consideration of operation until the patient himself or herself is thoroughly motivated toward surgery.

Lack of motivation is rarely a problem when the seizure tendency is severe, however, and the patient is old enough to realize the handicaps that result from it.

SPECIAL TYPES OF FOCAL EPILEPSY

Temporal Lobe Epilepsy

This type is worthy of special mention because it is the form of focal epilepsy encountered most frequently, and because it is also very apt to be resistant to medical treatment.

When medical control is clearly inadequate, early operation is advisable to permit as normal schooling and social development as possible. However, the seizure tendency sometimes changes as the brain matures, or multiple epileptogenic areas mature clinically at different rates, so that it is important to be sure that the seizure tendency is a fairly stable one before considering operation. This may mean several complete investigations over a period of years, before recommending operation in a child, even though he initially seems to be a suitable candidate.

The more devastating the social and intellectual effects of the seizures, the earlier the operation should be performed, ideally. If the patient lives well with the seizures, delay until the age of 15 to 16 may be wise, when local anesthesia can be used and when one can be more certain that all epileptogenic areas have declared themselves.

A certain percentage (5 to 10%) of patients in the age range 10 to 15 years with temporal lobe epilepsy experience a definite regression of seizure tendency in the decade following completion of brain maturation. The percentage of patients is small, however, and the degree of regression is often inadequate, so that this is a slender reed to lean on if the patient's attacks are causing a significant handicap during this important period of intellectual and social development.

Posttraumatic Epilepsy

Since epileptogenic areas mature at different rates after brain injury, operation should not be considered until a long enough period of time has elapsed for one to be reasonably sure that all or most of the potentially epileptogenic areas have matured and become symptomatic. Operation is rarely recommended earlier than 3 to 4 years after onset of seizures unless the tendency is unusually severe or becoming progressively worse. Eighty percent of those who develop seizures have done so by 5 years after injury, 60% in the first 2 years.

Since about half of all patients with posttraumatic epilepsy show a spontaneous regression of the tendency with time, operation is not recommended as a rule until the attacks have been present for at least 3 to 4 years. The seizure status is stable in most patients by 5 years after injury (Evans, 1962; Caveness, 1963, 1966; Rasmussen, 1969; Walker and Erculei, 1970; Weiss and Caveness, 1972).

Epilepsy Associated with Infantile Hemiplegia
See Chapter 10.

"Chronic Encephalitis"

A peculiar form of chronic encephalitis sometimes produces focal seizures associated with a very slowly progressive neurological deficit of some sort. The seizures sometimes take the form of epilepsia partialis continua. Sometimes the frequency of the seizures makes early operation necessary even though the presence of a diffuse process is known and there is no possibility of completely stopping the attacks. Operation neither aggravates nor lessens the underlying infectious process which smolders on for several years as a rule before it "burns itself out" after destroying a variable amount of brain tissue. Late operation, when the progression has stopped and the seizure tendency has stabilized, often produces satisfactory reduction of the seizure tendency, but of course cannot reverse the destructive effects of this unusually indolent "chronic encephalitis" (Rasmussen, Olszewski, and Lloyd-Smith, 1958; Rasmussen and McCann, 1968).

Other Syndromes

Other relatively uncommon neurological syndromes deserve mention because of the frequency with which seizures constitute a major problem.

Tuberous Sclerosis

Occasionally, the seizure tendency is well localized despite the fact that this is a diffuse abnormality of the brain. If adequately focal, operation may be indicated in such patients (Perot, Weir, and Rasmussen, 1966). Rarely, "formes frustes" occur in which the cutaneous adenoma sebaceum and mental retardation are absent but the brain lesions are present and epileptogenic. This is usually an operative finding, however, and it is rarely possible to make this diagnosis preoperatively.

Sturge-Weber Syndrome

Sturge-Weber pial angiomatosis is associated with seizures in 90% of cases. The seizures, perhaps because of the abnormal circulation, seem unduly prone to damage the brain in comparison with seizures due to other causes, so early operation in the hope of preventing severe progressive neurological deficits is often wise. "Formes frustes" occur with typical pial lesions but without skin lesions. Maximal removals of the epileptogenic areas and, so far as possible, of the angiomatous area, is necessary in patients with the complete syndrome. In those with pial angiomatosis only, it seems less important to remove all the angiomatous area if a sufficiently complete removal of the epileptogenic area can be achieved. (Alexander and Norman, 1960; Rasmussen, Mathieson, and Leblanc, 1972).

REFERENCES

Alexander, G. L., and Norman, R. M. (1960): *The Sturge-Weber syndrome.* J. Wright and Sons, Bristol.

Caveness, W. F. (1963): Onset and cessation of fits following cranio-cerebral trauma. *J. Neurosurg.,* 20:570–583.

Caveness, W. F. (1966): Variable clinical features of chronic post-traumatic seizure disorders. *Trans. Am. Neurol. Assoc.,* 91:204–205.

Evans, J. H. (1962): Post-traumatic epilepsy. *Neurology,* 12:665–674.
Gloor, P. (1968): Generalized cortico-reticular epilepsies. *Epilepsia,* 9:249–263.
Howell, D. A. (1955): Unusual centrencephalic seizure patterns. *Brain,* 78:199–208.
Jackson, J. H. (1873): *On the Anatomical, Physiological, and Pathological Investigation of Epilepsies.* West Riding Lunatic Asylum Medical Reports, 3:315. Reprinted in: *Selected Writings of John Hughlings Jackson,* edited by J. Taylor, Hodder and Stoughton, London, 1:90–111, 1931.
Madsen, J. A., and Bray, P. F. (1966): The coincidence of diffuse electroencephalographic spike-wave paroxysms and brain tumors. *Neurology,* 16:546–555.
McNaughton, F. L. (1954): Observations on diagnosis and medical treatment. In: *Epilepsy and the Functional Anatomy of the Human Brain,* edited by W. Penfield and H. Jasper. Little, Brown, Boston, pp. 540–568.
McNaughton, F. L., and Lloyd-Smith, D. (1965): Drugs for major epileptic seizures. *Can. Med. Assoc. J.,* 93:607–608.
Merlis, J. K. (1970): Proposal for an international classification of epilepsies. *Epilepsia,* 11:114–119.
Penfield, W., and Jasper, H. (1954): *Epilepsy and the Functional Anatomy of the Human Brain.* Little, Brown, Boston, pp. 622–648.
Perot, P., Weir, B., and Rasmussen, T. (1966): Tuberous sclerosis: Surgical therapy for seizures. *Arch. Neurol.,* 15:498–506.
Rasmussen, T. (1969): Surgical therapy of post-traumatic epilepsy. In: *The Late Effects of Head Injury,* edited by A. E. Walker, W. F. Caveness, and M. Critchley. Charles C Thomas, Springfield, Ill., pp. 277–305.
Rasmussen, T., Mathieson, G., and Leblanc, F. (1972): Surgical therapy of typical and a forme fruste variety of the Sturge-Weber syndrome. *Arch. Suisses Neurol. Neurochir. Psychiat.,* 111:393–409.
Rasmussen, T., and McCann, W. (1968): Clinical studies of patients with focal epilepsy due to "chronic encephalitis." *Trans. Am. Neurol. Assoc.,* 93:89–94.
Rasmussen, T., Olszewski, J., and Lloyd-Smith, D. (1958): Focal seizures due to chronic localized encephalitis. *Neurology,* 8:435–445.
Stewart, L. F., and Dreifuss, F. E. (1967): Centrencephalic seizure discharges in focal hemispherical lesions. *Arch. Neurol.,* 17:60–68.
Temkin, O. (1971): *The Falling Sickness,* second edition. Johns Hopkins Press, Baltimore.
Trotter, W. (1934): A landmark in modern neurology. *Lancet,* 2:1207–1210.
Tükel, K., and Jasper, H. (1952): The electroencephalogram in parasagittal lesions. *EEG Clin. Neurophysiol.,* 4:481–494.
Walker, A. E., and Erculei, F. (1970): Post-traumatic epilepsy 15 years later. *Epilepsia,* 11:17–26.
Weiss, G. H., and Caveness, W. F. (1972): Prognostic factors in the persistence of post-traumatic epilepsy. *J. Neurosurg.,* 37:164–169.

Advances in Neurology, Vol. 8, edited by D. P. Purpura, J. K. Penry, and R. D. Walter. Raven Press, New York © 1975.

4
Principles of Clinical Investigation of Surgical Candidates

Richard D. Walter

The majority of patients treated by surgical means for epilepsy are referred by private physicians to specialized centers or large institutions. In practice, then, this referral process frequently involves a double screening or evaluation—the first on the part of the referring physician who sends the patient to the center having determined that surgical treatment might be considered. The criteria used in making this decision are outlined in the preceding chapter. A second evaluation of the patient, which occurs at the surgical center, is a much more elaborate and detailed study, using techniques and personnel generally not available to the referring physician; this chapter is largely concerned with the principles of this second evaluation.

There is a general agreement among individuals and centers conducting the surgical treatment for epilepsy about the indications for surgery. Some idiosyncrasies in these indications may appear, however, depending on the specific interests and past experience of the group. Since the clinical investigation of the potential surgical candidate is designed to determine if the individual patient meets the indications for surgical treatment, it is appropriate to again review the areas of general agreement for surgical therapy.

HAS MEDICAL TREATMENT BEEN UNSUCCESSFUL?

The determination of medical failure becomes more difficult as new anticonvulsant agents and accurate blood level determinations become available. A recent volume edited by Woodbury, Penry, and Schmidt (1973) is of great assistance in this regard, presenting the current indications, pharmacology, and blood level ranges of most of the available antiepileptic drugs.

Most patients who are referred for surgical consideration to a center have had a long trial on various agents, and it becomes a difficult but important task to review their medication history in regard to the agents used, dosages, drug combinations, and adverse side effects. Such a history will often bring to light an obvious omission, such as an inadequate amount of diphenylhydantoin, a premature discontinuation of primidone because of an initial side effect, or a failure to try one of the more uncommonly used agents because of a concern over serious toxicity.

There are two less easily answered questions that are frequently raised in this area of evaluation. Because the patient has not been controlled with an adequate amount of a specific anticonvulsant in the past, does this mean that a retrial will be unsuccessful? An answer to this question is not in the literature, but every neurologist can cite instances where the reinstitution of a previously unsuccessful drug has provided seizure control. Admittedly the probability is small, yet the variables that make this possible include the ongoing maturation of the patient and possibly the changing aspects of the pathophysiology of the seizure disorder. In general, it has been our policy at UCLA not to defer further surgical consideration on the basis that a previously unsuccessful, adequately administered anticonvulsant might now provide control.

The second question of great difficulty involves a trial of less commonly used or experimental and investigational anticonvulsants. This list of drugs changes with time; examples in 1974 would include considerations of carbamazepine, clonazepam, and clorazepate dipotassium. Putting aside the issue of availability and FDA approval, should surgical treatment be delayed until an adequate trial has been made using these agents? Again, only a clinical and somewhat arbitrary decision can be made, based on the low probability that such drugs will make a significant difference considering the patient's past anticonvulsant history.

Balanced against the time necessary for a search for a new drug regimen for the patient is the matter of prolonging the decisions for surgery. Statistics cited in this volume indicate that the surgical outcome is in part influenced by the length of the seizure history and that further attempts at medical management beyond a point will only prolong the disability of the patient, incurring the risks of side effects and making rehabilitation more difficult.

WHAT IS THE EVIDENCE THAT THE SEIZURE DISORDER IS FOCAL?

The evidence for focality is a standard part of classical clinical neurology and as such will not be evaluated extensively here. However, in the context of the evaluation of a seizure disorder, it should be kept in mind that there may well be a discrepancy between the demonstrable structural lesion and the epileptogenic focus. For example, the demonstration of an enlarged and dilated temporal horn of the lateral ventricle by pneumoencephalography does not, in itself, provide incontrovertible evidence that this region is responsible for the patient's temporal lobe seizures. In reality, then, the clinical investigation of surgical candidates ideally involves the use of all available strategies—clinical, radiographic, and electrophysiological.

In some instances, conflicting localization may be developed through the use of these various approaches and judgments must be made weighing all of the available data. The following subsections will review aspects of each of these approaches.

Clinical Seizure Pattern

The notorious and traditional problem in regard to the clinical seizure pattern is that of reliability, sampling, and documentation. It is platitudinous to state that the patient is generally unable to supply sufficient details of his seizure sequence which is necessary to make valid inference regarding localization. On the other hand, the patient alone can supply information regarding his aura—information which can be so substantial that other procedures only become confirmatory. The subjective nature of the experience makes its reporting particularly vulnerable to the vicissitudes of the art of securing a reliable history. Another facet of the problem of seizure description provided by the patient is the second-order contamination resulting from the reports to him by observers. Embarrassment frequently precludes the patient being told of the details, and it is a common consultation room vignette to have mother and father argue over whether the patient turns to the right or left during the ictus. In spite of these difficulties, an attempt should be made to secure as accurate a description of the seizure as possible from observers. Notoriously, hospital records, both in the progress and nurses' notes, often supply only cryptic comments such as "grand mal" or "brief seizure" without the descriptive elements necessary for localization.

There are two methods of securing more reliable information regarding the seizure pattern. Both depend on the occurrence of a seizure, and this in itself may represent a formidable practical problem. Whether the reduction in seizure frequency frequently observed on admission to the hospital is a function of greater reliability in taking anticonvulsant medication or because of the nonspecific effect of a change in the environment, it is still highly desirable to have something to observe. It is among our practices at UCLA to gradually reduce the anticonvulsant medication or to utilize sleep deprivation in an effort to increase the probability of observing a seizure. We have not had the problem of inducing serious status epilepticus and feel that the information obtained warrants any risk.

The first method of securing reliable data on seizure patterns is that of the "trained observer." The hospital personnel who have the greatest exposure to the patient have the highest probability of witnessing a seizure. Considering the modern hierarchy in a medical center this individual is usually a nurse's aide or a vocational nurse. The training of this observer requires more than casual effort and should be the responsibility of the neurologist rather than the floor supervisor. A disadvantage of this trained observer method is that the seizure sequence may be quite complex and compressed into a short time interval so that observational errors are possible. In addition, a pictorial documentation for multiple-observer study or future analysis is not available.

The other methods of recording the clinical aspects of the seizure basically require some type of pictorial preservation. Motion picture or sequential-frame photography has proved to be impractical simply because of the sporadic and unpredictable nature of the event. There are exceptions in that some patients have a high seizure density or the episodes can be activated by fairly predictable circumstances—various sensory inputs or at predictable times in the wake-sleep cycle. Film does have the advantage over video tape of higher fidelity and resolution. Most centers working with these methods, however, have found that video tape is the more practical method of recording seizures because of the ease of editing and its economy. A further increase in the yield of useful information can be obtained by the split-screen technique of recording the surface EEG along with the clinical behavior of the patient. This type of recording facility is practical only if the number of patients being considered for surgical treatment is fairly high.

Radiological Localization

It is quite unlikely that any medical center would treat epilepsy surgically unless excellent neuroradiological facilities are available. This section, then, will only outline some of the problems that might relate to the choice of a radiological procedure rather than an extensive treatise on the subject. The traditional clinical neurological routine skull series may provide localizing clues—intracranial calcification, an asymmetry of a fossae or hemisphere, bony erosion, etc.,—but it is an unprecedented circumstance that this would constitute the sole radiological evaluation of such a patient.

Isotopic brain scanning, the other currently ubiquitous routine method of evaluation in neurology, in its present form is not likely to provide a great deal of positive information relating to the seizure focus. Certainly the presence of a mass lesion may be demonstrated by the scan and then provide extremely significant data. Although our own clinical experience has been that the brain scan has not been helpful in adult patients except for the rare unanticipated findings, Prensky, Swisher, and De Viro (1973) have recently reported that 6 of 52 children with focal seizures had an increased uptake of the radioisotope on the appropriate side. This uncommon finding may be a manifestation of either an alteration in permeability at the seizure site or an increase in tissue vascularity. Perhaps there is a clue for further research in this area, but at the present time the yield is small.

The major decision regarding radiological localization is in the area of contrast procedures. This decision may well be influenced by the increasing availability of the EMI scanner or similar device based on the same principle. Based on the currently limited experience with this very promising technique, a projection might be possible to provide a greater resolution for some lesions, but the more conventional contrast procedures will still be necessary.

Pneumoencephalography

From a pragmatic point of view, the greatest yield for structural localization has been pneumoencephalography. This is particularly true in temporal lobe epilepsy, where a dilated or distorted temporal horn may be the only radiographic clue. In other areas, the identification of a porencephalic cyst, a region of localized atrophy, or the finding of an unsuspected mass lesion can provide significant and essential data. Although not of a localizing value, the presence of diffuse atrophy and the degree and character of hydrocephalus may also yield information to be considered in the contemplation of surgery. Generalizations about the *value* of pneumoencephalography are difficult in regard to focal seizure disorders. Although our own experience seems marred by a large number of negative studies, the value of this technique in an individual case may be tremendous. The general experience may be epitomized by the report of Brett and Hoare (1969); they found a relatively poor correlation between the EEG studies and pneumoencephalographic findings in patients with mental retardation and focal epilepsy.

Some individuals dealing with the surgical treatment of epilepsy feel that pneumoencephalography is not being performed as frequently as it is indicated and that this procedure is replaced in part by angiography. Our own feeling is that it is still a nearly essential procedure, that the best neuroradiographic technique should be used, and that there should be sufficient flexibility at the time of the procedure so that subtle findings may be enhanced by special views, tomography and laminography. An anesthetic will be required in some patients— particularly the mildly retarded, young patient with a seizure disorder—and a word of caution might be in order about the use of an agent such as ketamine. Bennett, Madsen, Jordan, and Wiser (1973) have reported on both the EEG and clinical activating features of this anesthetic.

Angiography

A great advance in cerebral angiography has taken place over the past decade, in regard to both a greater capacity to define more subtle lesions and a reduction of the past morbidity associated with the procedure. In temporal lobe epilepsy, however, the yield for positive information continues to be less than that of pneumoencephalography, except for the occasional surprise of an aneurysm, arteriovenous malformation, or tumor. It would seem logical that if further advances are to be made in the angiographic demonstration of small lesions responsible for a focal seizure disorder, a still finer technique for resolution will be required. Waddington (1970) has reported on the angiographic findings in 23 patients with focal motor epilepsy without obvious cause. She demonstrated an occlusion of small branches to the motor or premotor area or both in 16 patients, by using a template designed by Ring (1962) for the middle cerebral artery distribution. Although our own group has not yet utilized this technique to the point of surgical exploration, it would seem potentially useful and might be extended to other major cerebral vessel territories.

There are only a few reports on the general aspects of the angiographic findings in patients with focal seizures. Gudmundsson (1966) indicated a 33% incidence of angiographic abnormalities in such patients; Casati, Fieschi, and Ascheri (1970) reported a finding of 29.5%. More recently, Vermess, Stein, Ajmone-Marsan, and Di Chiro (1972) studied patients with focal seizures in the frontal, central, and parietal areas with angiography. In the 26 patients with satisfactory studies, 8 had vascular abnormalities and 2 of these were bilateral. Again, the point was made in this report that there may be a poor correlation between the angiographic changes and the localization of the epileptic focus. Another technique that may provide helpful localizing information in the future is the amalgamation of modern angiographic catheter techniques with the ability to record electroencephalographically from an intravascular site as recently described by Penn, Hilal, Michelsen, Goldensohn, and Driller (1973).

Clinical Neurophysiology

It has been stressed in the preceding section that regardless of the location of an apparently structural lesion, whether based on clinical, pneumoencephalographic, or angiographic evidence, the lesion may not correspond to the site of the epileptogenic focus. The techniques of clinical neurophysiology are then essential in the evaluation of potential surgical candidates. In chapter 5 in this volume, Gloor provides a detailed description of the value and limitations of these techniques. Another recent but somewhat more limited review has been published by Walter (1973). The following will therefore be a brief resume of some of the important principles to be considered as it applies to surgery for seizure disorders.

(1) *The maximum advantage should be derived from clinical EEG in regard to interictal studies.* Basically this involves obtaining high-quality recordings over an adequate period during any one recording session as well as a sampling over time. Serial recordings are to be emphasized since it is a commonplace for interictal electrical abnormalities in some patients to appear focally or lateralized during one recording period and have a different distribution during another.

A selective and individualized use of both special electrodes and activating techniques will increase the yield of useful information, but this requires the laboratory to have had some experience in the use of these procedures.

(2) *A simultaneous record of both the clinical and EEG events during the seizures may provide very useful information.* Securing the record, however, may be technically difficult and time-consuming. Split-screen video tape has proved to be the most practical method with or without telemetry. The restriction in mobility necessary to obtain the video tape of the clinical aspects of the seizure permits hard-wire recording, frequently of a technical quality matching that of the telemetered signal. Notoriously, however, either the surface recording may be marred by artifact during the clinical seizure or the focal abnormality may not be reflected in the scalp tracing.

(3) *Depth electrode studies have proved invaluable, if not essential, in the evaluation of some patients for surgical treatment.* This is particularly the case in those patients with temporal lobe seizures in whom serial recordings have demonstrated bilateral, independent surface spiking approaching a parity between right and left temporal areas. Chronic depth electrode studies have also been helpful in planning for surgical treatment of partial epilepsies outside the limbic system. The experience of the UCLA group has recently been reported in both situations by Crandall (1973) and Walter (1973).

(4) *Electrocorticography, combined with electrical stimulation studies, continues to be the basic technique for planning the area of resection at the time of surgery.* Although electrocorticography is indispensable in the performance of

resection outside of the temporal lobe, there may be cases in which it is not necessary or helpful. For example, there is the limited situation of the patient with temporal lobe seizures in whom a clear-cut focus responsible for the patient's clinical seizures has been established by the use of chronically implanted depth electrodes. If the surgical procedure elected is a maximal, standardized, *en bloc* temporal lobectomy, then it could be argued that electrocorticography at the time of the resection would be superfluous.

A further generalization, apparent from the above brief outline and the more detailed exposition by Gloor in Chapter 5, is that considerable flexibility, technical capability, and experience are required to conduct these types of clinical neurophysiological investigations. This in itself suggests that more than an intermittent or casual opportunity to study these patients is impractical for good medical practice and argues in favor of the specialized center for these procedures.

ARE THERE CONTRAINDICATIONS TO SURGERY?

Two types of consideration are raised by this question: the first a more global one involving such aspects as the patient's general health, age, mental status, etc., and the second a more specific one relating to a possible loss of some function if surgery is performed. In the first category, the following areas may constitute a problem in the clinical investigation of a patient who is a surgical candidate.

Age

The older patient, who has a long history of a seizure disorder, presents a more difficult problem with regard to socieconomic rehabilitation after successful surgery, whereas the young patient might be considered with reluctance because of the statistical evidence that with further maturation some seizure disorders will disappear. There is also the notion that surgical treatment should be considered earlier in the course of the disorder in order to diminish the handicap of frequent seizures, reduce the exposure time to high levels of anticonvulsant drugs, and benefit from a greater ease of rehabilitation. At the present time, the decision in this area must be individualized and based on clinical judgment since there is no solid body of evidence that provides firm guidelines.

Intelligence

A commonly encountered problem in the area of intelligence is the patient who is mentally retarded and who has a medically intractable seizure disorder. The considerations that influence a surgical decision are whether the control of the seizures will assist in the total management and care of the patient and whether a procedure such as chronic depth electrode implantation which requires cooperation on the part of the patient can be undertaken.

For example, there are many retarded patients in whom seizure control would permit greater mobility and ambulation, require less in the way of supervision or nursing care, and offer a greater chance for rehabilitation. Similarly, there are patients with relatively severe degrees of retardation who are able to cooperate in procedures such as depth electrode studies. Since these capacities on the part of such a patient are not necessarily reflected in an IQ score, an individualized judgment, considering all factors, must be made.

Psychosis

Aside from the ongoing discussion of the possible relationship between temporal lobe epilepsy and schizophrenia, the practical problem of psychological evaluation not infrequently concerns a patient who has had a serious psychiatric illness in the past, or who now demonstrates a "schizoid state" or signs of mental illness (see Chapter 16 by Serafetinides). Psychiatric and psychological consultation is obviously essential in this context: ideally, every patient being considered for surgery should have the benefit of this evaluation. Again in a practical way, the decision regarding surgery is made independently of any anticipated improvement in the patient's mental status. The difficulty, however, is in the identification of that small number of patients in every group's series (see Chapter 13) who are seizure-free after surgery, but institutionalized or floridly psychotic.

The second type of contraindication relates to a potential undesirable and handicapping loss of function if a surgical procedure is performed. In most circumstances, particularly with cortical resection, this is decided at the time of surgery, based on electrocorticographic and stimulation studies. However, in surgery for temporal lobe epilepsy, a preoperative evaluation may unearth a contraindication based on the inability of the nonoperated side to maintain adequate memory function.

In its simplest form, the problem is exemplified by the patient in whom a seizure focus has been localized in one temporal lobe—either by serial surface recordings, clues from the contrast procedures, or depth electrode studies. If a temporal lobectomy is the procedure of choice, is there any method of evaluating the "good" side in regard to its functional state? There are two techniques that may provide information in this regard.

(1) *Modified Wada test.* This technique is described in Chapter 5. Briefly, the carotid on the side of the contemplated surgery is injected with a barbiturate, and visual auditory presentations are given to the patient during the period in which the hemisphere supplied by the carotid is "anesthetized." On recovery, the patient's recall of these stimuli is evaluated. Conceptually, if the nonanesthetized temporal lobe is impaired, there will be a deficit in his recent memory, as measured by this test, a fact which may modify the surgical decision.

(2) *Electrical stimulation studies with depth electrodes.* In some situations using depth electrodes implanted in the temporal lobes, it has been observed that a prolonged afterdischarge induced in the hippocampus of the same side as the seizure focus results in a transient, confusional, amnestic state. If the afterdis-

charge does not propagate to the contralateral hippocampus (as can be measured by bilateral implantation), then it can be proposed that the opposite or non-stimulated side is inadequate for ongoing recent memory function. The analogy is that the temporal lobe that is the site of the seizure focus is temporarily nonfunctional during the afterdischarge, instead of being barbituarized as it is in the Wada Test. In our own experience, however, the usefulness of this observation may be limited in that there are some patients in whom afterdischarges cannot be generated in the suspected side.

Both of these procedures are relatively new, and as yet there are insufficient data to provide a statement about their predictive value in preventing memory deficits after surgery. However, even though the statistical evidence is not available, any suspicions evoked by these tests that the "surviving" hippocampus may be inadequate might well influence the decision regarding an *en bloc* temporal lobe resection.

SUMMARY

The evaluation of patients who are candidates for the surgical treatment of epilepsy requires the participation of individuals from a number of disciplines, all with more than a casual interest in seizure disorders. In addition, the facilities and equipment necessary to undertake these investigations are beyond those provided by the average neurological-neurosurgical service. It is to be hoped that further experience and research will provide simpler strategies for making this type of treatment available to a greater number of patients. At the present time, however, these efforts are more appropriately the province of fairly specialized centers.

REFERENCES

Bennett, D. R., Madsen, J. A., Jordan, W. S., and Wiser, W. C. (1973): Ketamine anesthesia in brain-damaged epileptics: Electroencephalographic and clinical observations. *Neurology,* 23:449–460.

Brett, E. M., and Hoare, R. D. (1969): An assessment of the value and limitations of air encephalography in children with mental retardation and with epilepsy. *Brain,* 92:731–742.

Casati, C., Fieschi, C., and Ascheri, C. (1970): Correlazione neuroradiologiche in corso di epilessie ad insorgenza tardiva. *Sist. Nerv.,* 22:21–26.

Crandall, P. H. (1973): Developments in direct recordings from epileptogenic regions in the surgical treatment of partial epilepsies. In: *Epilepsy, Its Phenomena in Man,* edited by M. A. B. Brazier. Academic Press, New York.

Gudmundsson, G. (1966): Epilepsy in Iceland. *Acta Neurol. Scandinav.,* Suppl. 75.

Penn, R. D., Hilal, S. K., Michelsen, W. J., Goldensohn, E. S., and Driller, J. (1973): Intravascular intracranial EEG recording. Technical note. *J. Neurosurg.,* 38:239–243.

Prensky, A. L., Swisher, C. N., and De Viro, D. C. (1973): Positive brain scans in children with idiopathic focal epileptic seizures. *Neurology,* 23:798–807.

Ring, B. A. (1962): Middle cerebral artery, anatomical and radiographic study. *Acta Radiol.,* 57:289–300.

Vermess, M., Stein, S. C., Ajmone-Marsan, C., and Di Chiro, G. (1972): Angiography in "idiopathic" focal epilepsy. *Am. J. Roentgeniol. Rad. Ther. Nucl. Med.,* 115:120–125.
Waddington, M. M. (1970): Angiographic changes in focal motor epilepsy. *Neurology,* 20:879–888.
Walter, R. D. (1973): Tactical considerations leading to surgical treatment of partial epilepsies. In: *Epilepsy, Its Phenomena in Man,* edited by M. A. B. Brazier. Academic Press, New York.
Woodbury, D. M., Penry, J. K., and Schmidt, R. P., editors (1973): *Antiepileptic Drugs.* Raven Press, New York.

Advances in Neurology, Vol. 8, edited by D. P
Purpura, J. K. Penry, and R. D. Walter. Raven
Press, New York © 1975.

5
Contributions of Electroencephalography and Electrocorticography to the Neurosurgical Treatment of the Epilepsies

P. Gloor

INTRODUCTION

At the present state of our knowledge, neurosurgical treatment of focal (partial) epilepsy is dependent on the demonstration that a patient's epileptic seizures originate in a circumscribed area of the brain which can be removed without exposing the patient to the risk of an intolerable neurological deficit. Epileptogenic areas amenable to surgical treatment are almost always localized in the cerebral neocortex and/or limbic structures of the temporal lobe (amygdala and hippocampus).

It is evident that ideal proof of the site of origin of an epileptic seizure can be provided only by direct observation of signs of excessive neuronal discharge at the onset of a spontaneous attack in an electrical recording which permits unequivocal identification of the site of origin of the discharge. Although rigorous fulfillment of this optimal criterion is not possible in clinical practice, electroencephalography is the only method available at present which permits direct demonstration of the presence of neuronal dysfunction responsible for the clinical paroxysmal event.

Demonstration in the EEG of a focal onset of ictal discharge in the record of a spontaneous seizure most closely approximates the ideal requirement of unequivocal identification of the site of origin of an attack. Frequently, however, EEGs show only interictal epileptiform discharges, or ictal records remain uninterpretable for a variety of reasons. Although interictal discharges give less reliable localizing information, they still provide direct and otherwise unobtainable evidence of neuronal dysfunction of an epileptiform type and therefore provide valuable diagnostic information if evaluated critically. The second best diagnostic and localizing evidence is thus represented by unequivocal and localized interictal epileptiform discharge in the EEG, provided its localization agrees with that indicated by well-documented, initial clinical ictal phenomena of definite localizing significance.

Other clinical and paraclinical data—including neurological signs, radiological changes, and the psychological test pattern—often support the localizing evi-

---

Montreal Neurological Institute Reprint No. 1166.

dence obtained from EEG recordings, but their reliability as indicators of the area of seizure onset is not as great. It is important to realize that the localization of maximum structural brain damage need not necessarily correspond with the site of origin of the patient's seizures, although it very frequently does. The nature of the diagnostic data in any given case therefore often forces one to make a localizing diagnosis based on circumstantial evidence. It must then remain a matter of clinical judgment whether the evidence provided by the clinical history and examination, EEG findings, and radiological and psychological data are sufficiently clear-cut to justify surgical therapy.

This chapter presents the strategy of a pragmatic approach to the localization of epileptogenic foci by electroencephalography, stereotactic depth electrode exploration, and electrocorticography, in the light of our experience accumulated over many years at the Montreal Neurological Institute.

INTERICTAL ABNORMALITIES AND THEIR DIAGNOSTIC VALUE

Morphology of Interictal Epileptiform Abnormalities and Limitations of Their Diagnostic Usefulness

Interictal abnormalities in the EEG are the most readily available and verifiable electrographic evidence obtained in epileptic patients. Patients with focal seizures frequently present in their EEGs paroxysmal disturbances localized to the area of the presumed onset of attacks (Jasper and Hawke, 1938; Jasper and Kershman, 1941, 1949; Gibbs, Gibbs, and Fuster, 1948b; Jasper, 1949a,c; Jasper, Pertuiset, and Flanigin, 1951; Penfield and Jasper, 1954). The assumption is usually made that if repeated EEG examinations demonstrate an area from which interictal epileptogenic potentials consistently originate, this corresponds to the most likely site of onset of the patient's spontaneously occurring seizures. On what kind of evidence is this contention based?

First, clinical evidence: it is indeed very common to find that the presumptive localization of a patient's epileptogenic area based on the clinical history and observation coincides with that shown by the interictal EEG abnormalities (Penfield and Jasper, 1954). For instance, a patient with a history of right-sided focal motor Jacksonian attacks may in his EEG show interictal, epileptiform sharp waves localized to the left central region. In patients in whom surgical exploration and treatment is undertaken on the basis of such correlations, the electrocorticogram commonly confirms the previously obtained EEG localization (Jasper et al., 1951; Penfield and Jasper, 1954). This correlation may be further strengthened if electrical stimulation of the cortex within the area giving rise to interictal abnormalities in the EEG and electrocorticogram reproduces the initial event of the patient's habitual attacks (Penfield and Jasper, 1954).

The second type of evidence derives from experimental observations: results of animal studies support a close correlation between the localization of interictal epileptiform abnormality and that of the actual area of onset of spontaneous seizures. When an epileptogenic agent is applied to a circumscribed cortical region, the EEG shows focal sharp waves and spikes localized to the area of the insult and closely resembling those seen in human focal epilepsies (Walker, Johnson, and Kollros, 1945; Pope, Morris, Jasper, Elliott, and Penfield, 1947; Pacella, Kopeloff, and Kopeloff, 1947; Kopeloff, Chusid, and Kopeloff, 1954; Smith and Purpura, 1960). When seizures occur in these animals, they originate from the same region. Furthermore, animal studies show that cortical spikes and sharp waves as they appear in the EEG are the expression of the fundamental neuronal dysfunction in focal epilepsy which appears as a recurrent paroxysmal depolarization shift in intracellular recording (Matsumoto and Ajmone-Marsan, 1964*a;* Prince and Futamachi, 1968; Dichter and Spencer, 1969*a*). This type of dysfunction easily leads to the development of self-sustained seizure activity, presumably when inhibitory braking mechanisms fail (Matsumoto and Ajmone-Marsan, 1964*b;* Prince and Wilder, 1967; Dichter and Spencer, 1969*b;* Ayala, Dichter, Gumnit, Matsumoto, and Spencer, 1973).

Although it is thus reasonable to assume that the location of interictal epileptiform abnormalities is closely related to the area giving rise to the patient's spontaneous attacks, one should remember that the information provided by the interictal EEG is nevertheless partial and may at times even be misleading. Unfortunately, it seems that no well-documented and rigorous statistical study exists which correlates in a group of patients the EEG localization obtained by the analysis of interictal abnormalities with that derived from the recorded onset of the patients' spontaneous attacks. However, demonstration of an epileptogenic focus on the basis of interictal abnormalities alone does not necessarily indicate the region of origin of the patient's habitual seizures. Every experienced electroencephalographer has encountered such exceptions.

We have thus to accept the fact that scalp recordings, especially when these yield only the interictal type of epileptogenic disturbances, provide limited information on the true dimensions of the patient's epileptogenic condition. This is so for a number of reasons.

Only a portion—the smaller part—of the cerebral cortex is accessible to conventional scalp EEG recording. The mesial and inferior surfaces of the cerebral hemispheres, as well as the depths of the fissures and sulci, are not directly accessible. Primary epileptic discharges originating in these areas may therefore be missed altogether, or only projected interictal (or ictal) EEG signs driven from a distant inaccessible site may be recorded. There are no foolproof signs by which to recognize that a scalp-derived potential is projected from such a distant source.

Less frequently appreciated are the difficulties deriving from the biophysical requirements for the appearance of cerebral potentials at the scalp, but these are sufficiently stringent that some types of epileptiform discharges may fail to appear in scalp recordings (Abraham and Ajmone-Marsan, 1958).

One important biophysical factor is the size of the generator surface involved in producing a spike or a sharp wave. Cooper, Winter, Crow, and Walter (1965) have shown that a cortical potential becomes recordable at the scalp not so much by virtue of its amplitude, but because of its synchronization over a minimal area of cortical surface which they have approximately established as being about 6 cm². Thus an epileptogenic discharge synchronously involving an area of lesser extent will be missed in the EEG.

Since the EEG is generated by the activity of synchronized neuronal generators behaving like virtual dipoles oriented at right angles to the cortical surface (Li, Cullen, and Jasper, 1956*a,b;* Spencer and Brookhart, 1961*a,b;* Calvet, Calvet, and Scherrer, 1964), the potential recorded by an electrode in the monopolar mode is proportional to the solid angle subtended by the generator surface[1] at that electrode (Gloor, Vera, and Sperti, 1963; Fourment, Jami, Calvet, and Scherrer, 1965) (Fig. 1). In the bipolar recording mode, the potential measured between two electrodes is proportional to the algebraic difference between the solid angles subtended by the generator surface at the two electrodes of the bipolar pair; therefore, the geometric orientation of the generator surface in relation to the surface on the scalp is of great importance. If the generators of a potential involve a cortical area covering the crowns of gyri which are oriented essentially in parallel to the scalp, the chances of picking up such potentials from the scalp are good (Fig. 1A and B). However, generator surfaces which involve the walls of a sulcus may well escape detection at the scalp because the scalp electrodes subtend the generator surface with a very small, solid angle. This is particularly true if the generator surface involves both walls of a sulcus. In this case, even a potential generated by a large surface may be completely missed at the scalp, for any electrode positioned in front of or behind the sulcus will in fact subtend with an almost equal solid angle both the "positive" and the "negative" side of the generator surface, because the latter is folded upon itself (Fig. 1C).

The requirement of synchronization of potentials within the generator surface is a further limitation. The shorter the potential, the more precise such synchronization must be to produce a potential recordable at the scalp. Since the most diagnostically useful epileptogenic potentials are spikes of short duration, these must be tightly synchronized over a relatively large surface of the cortex or they will escape detection. For slow waves the requirements are much less stringent. A simple example will illustrate this. Assume that a group of neurons in a cortical area is involved in producing delta waves of 400-msec duration. If individual neurons generating this slow wave differ in their synchronization by as much as 50 msec, they still share in the generation of a potential of the same electrical sign for a duration of 300 msec. This shared potential change of 300 msec, if it involves a surface area exceeding 6 cm², is recordable at the scalp as a delta wave of this duration. If, however, the same cortical area produces short spike discharges of a duration of 50 msec, the limits of tolerable asynchrony between various neuronal groups involved in this activity are much narrower; a 50-msec difference in the timing of various neuronal groups within the area would make it impossible to produce a potential recordable at the scalp, since no potential

---

[1] It is important to realize that the term "generator surface" as used here is not identical with "epileptogenic area." The latter may contain a large number of "generator surfaces" of the type discussed here.

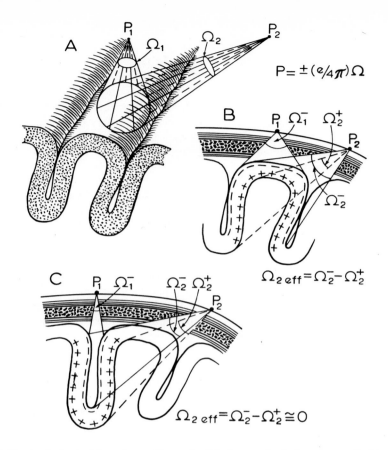

$$P = \pm \left(\frac{e}{4\pi}\right)\Omega$$

$$\Omega_{2\,\text{eff}} = \Omega_2^- - \Omega_2^+$$

$$\Omega_{2\,\text{eff}} = \Omega_2^- - \Omega_2^+ \cong 0$$

FIG. 1. Biophysical principles of recording potentials from a dipole layer as applied to clinical electroencephalography: A potential P when recorded in monopolar fashion to a distant reference point is proportional to the solid angle Ω subtended by a dipole layer at the position of the recording electrode. (Ideally the conducting medium must be homogeneous and the reference point unaffected by the potential created by the dipole layer.) The magnitude of the potential P at any point around the dipole layer is determined by the function expressed by the formula shown in the upper right-hand corner of the figure, where e is the potential across the dipole layer and Ω the solid angle subtended at the recording electrode position.

 A: Illustration of the dependence of the potentials P_1 and P_2 upon the solid angles Ω_1 and Ω_2 subtended at the two electrode positions P_1 and P_2 by a hypothetical dipole layer with a circular circumference occupying the crown of a gyrus.

 B: Dipole layer occupying the crown of a gyrus and its two sides each forming one of the walls of two adjacent sulci. At P_1 the potential depends only on the solid angle Ω_{-1}, since at this point the recording electrode only "sees" a portion of the negative side of the dipole layer. At P_2, two solid angles have to be taken into account, Ω_{-2} and Ω_{+2}, since the electrode at position P_2 "sees" portions of both the negative and the positive sides of the folded dipole layer. The potential P_2 is therefore proportional to the effective solid angle $\Omega_{2\,\text{eff}}$ which equals the difference between Ω_{-2} and Ω_{+2}, the sign of the larger solid angle dictating the electrical sign at P_2.

 C: Illustrates the difficulty of obtaining a surface recording from a dipole layer occupying both walls of a sulcus, since at P_1 the solid angle subtended is extremely small and at P_2 the effective solid angle $\Omega_{2\,\text{eff}}$ is nearly zero, because the solid angles subtended by the positive and negative portions of the dipole layer seen by the electrode at P_2 are nearly equal and their difference thus is nearly zero.

deflection of the same electrical sign would be time-shared under these circumstances. It is important to realize that the actual amplitude of discharges in the cortex will alter this requirement for synchronization very little or not at all. Thus, it is reasonable to conclude that any short epileptogenic spike potential visible in a scalp recording must in fact involve the nearly synchronous firing of a large number of neurons distributed over a relatively large area of cortex. Equally active but relatively asynchronous spike discharges in the same area completely escape detection by scalp recording.

General Recording Principles

EEG examinations of patients considered for surgical therapy must emphasize effective and reliable localization methods. Such methods and their application require of the electroencephalographer and the technologist a good grasp of volume conductor principles as they apply to electroencephalography, as well as a keen understanding of the respective advantages and disadvantages of monopolar and bipolar recording methods. Since these are complementary, both should be used judiciously in every patient and applied so as to maximize reliable localizing information. The localization of scalp-derived potentials must be viewed as a problem of analyzing the distribution and configuration of electrical fields on the scalp from which information on the localization of the neuronal generator involved in the genesis of these potentials can be inferred. The interpreter must make the mental effort to translate the set of potential-versus-time plots provided by a number of EEG channels into meaningful potential maps. He must therefore be able to visualize the three-dimensional configuration of potential fields of significant electrographic events on the scalp if he is to avoid drawing misleading localizing conclusions.

In the analysis of bipolar recordings it is thus important to realize that the amplitude of a wave is only a function of the steepness of the gradient of a particular potential field in the area covered by two adjacent electrodes, and does not by itself carry any reliable localizing information; localization of the peak in such recordings depends on identifying the electrode position at which phase reversals occur. To be meaningful, such phase reversals must be established in montages using long, straight rows of electrodes. In addition, it is important to realize that the phase reversal along such a row of electrodes only indicates where the potential reaches its maximum *in that particular electrode row.* Unless the same potential can be shown to reverse phase at the same electrode in a montage taken at right angles to the initial one, such a phase reversal does not *necessarily* indicate the true localization of the potential peak. In view of this, both longitudinal and transverse bipolar montages should be utilized and angulated runs should be avoided. Also to be avoided are so-called "bipolar" montages made up of a number of disconnected electrode pairs distributed over the scalp, often arranged in various orientations. These may yield results which defy any rational localizing analysis.

In monopolar recordings the choice of the reference point is of great importance. The interpreter must have a proper appreciation of the difficulties that can arise from an active reference. Unfortunately, all commonly used reference electrode sites suffer from a number of disadvantages. Ipsilateral or contralateral ear reference electrode recordings, because two reference points are used (one for the right and the other for the left hemisphere), negate one of the most fundamental principles of monopolar recording, namely that all potentials be referred to a *single* reference point. Interconnecting the ears solves this problem only at the cost of introducing a new one: in this situation it is not possible to lateralize temporal lobe discharge arising near one or the other auricular electrode. Another disadvantage of the ear reference electrode is that the distances between it and the other electrodes on the scalp are very unequal. In the case of a temporal lobe focus, because of relative equipotentiality between temporal scalp electrodes and the ear reference, the paradoxical result may be that the discharge appears in all except the temporal channel near the focus (Gibbs et al., 1948*a*). We therefore prefer to use positions other than the ear as reference points. An electrode placed on the neck over the spinous process of the C_7 vertebra or slightly higher is often very satisfactory. Such a cervical reference electrode, however, sometimes picks up an excessive amount of electrocardiographic artifact. Other points that can be used in such a case are the chin or nose.

Another possibility is the use of average reference recording, an excellent method for recording potentials which are sharply localized and not too high in voltage. However, if some of the signals are of large amplitude and especially if they are synchronized over wide areas of the head, they contribute to the average reference potential. Thus the average reference now injects the signal which one wishes to localize into all channels, with the result that it appears 180° out of phase in those channels connected to inactive or to the least active electrodes. Furthermore, the amplitude of the signal from the active area is reduced by the amount of voltage which it contributes to the average reference. The 180° out-of-phase signal in the inactive areas may at times reach almost the same voltage as that prevailing in the active focus. An experienced electroencephalographer usually does not have too much difficulty in unraveling this situation, especially if he has the benefit of comparing the findings obtained with monopolar and bipolar techniques, but such records are ready traps for the inexperienced or unwary.

Diagnostic Evaluation of Interictal Epileptiform Discharges

Accurate evaluation of the significance of interictal epileptiform abnormality requires adherence to stringent criteria for the description of an epileptiform discharge; otherwise the incidence of misleading false positive findings will become very great indeed. Only definite spikes, sharp waves, and spike-and-wave complexes should be regarded as unequivocal epileptiform abnormalities in the interictal EEG. Paroxysmal slow waves or paroxysmal, rhythmic slow-wave discharges are of less certain diagnostic significance. It is, however, necessary to define spikes and sharp waves more clearly in terms of their "epileptogenicity" than is usually the case. The interpretation of an EEG should involve not only the immediate visual impression of "sharpness" of a potential, since not every potential that appears "sharp" should unquestionably be considered epileptogenic. Additional criteria should underpin the notion of its presumed epileptogenicity.

The proposed International EEG Terminology (Storm van Leeuwen et al., 1966) defines *spikes* as isolated waves (arbitrarily) lasting less than 80 msec, and *sharp waves* as isolated waves with triangular form (arbitrarily) lasting more than 80 and less than 200 msec. These definitions are, however, a lowest common denominator and insufficient for our purposes. Additional criteria, as described by Penfield and Jasper (1954), are that "spikes" and "sharp waves" must be "paroxysmal" and "of high voltage." These authors also describe an asymmetry of wave form, and the frequent slow wave "afterpotential" as further characteristics of epileptogenic spikes and sharp waves. The terms "spike" and "sharp waves" imply a "pointedness" of the wave, but this has nowhere been defined in strict terms. Kooi (1966) insisted on the importance of the rate of voltage change and found that segmental velocities of spikes were of the order of 2 μV/msec or more.

There are thus "sharp"-appearing potentials which experienced clinical electroencephalographers do not regard as epileptiform. The problem is one of rigorously defining those features which distinguish epileptiform "spikes" from other "sharp" potentials. No stringent criteria have as yet been defined; those proposed here largely reflect the personal experience of the author. True epileptic spikes or sharp waves show an abruptly and rapidly rising phase, followed by a less rapidly declining phase after the potential has reached its peak (Fig. 2); therefore, a vertical line drawn through the tip of the spike or sharp wave shows

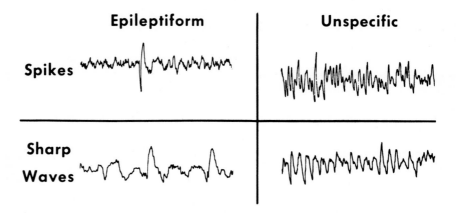

FIG. 2. Examples of "epileptiform" and "unspecific" (i.e., nonepileptiform) spikes and sharp waves taken from EEGs of four patients.

that the wave form, with respect to this line, is "asymmetrical." Frequently the potential is also polyphasic, the main phase being usually surface-negative, followed, and sometimes preceded, by a positive phase. The late positive phase is often a slow wave, which may be followed by a still slower negativity. The duration of the epileptogenic spike or sharp wave compared with that of the constituents of the background activity is distinctly different, usually shorter. It rarely emerges from a perfectly normal background activity. The latter is frequently intermingled with slow waves or at least irregular. In contrast to these typical epileptic spikes and sharp waves, there are those which look sharp to the eye, most often because a single wave which is a constituent of background activity stands out from it by its high amplitude (Fig. 2). Its duration is usually the same or almost the same as that of the waves constituting the ongoing background activity; the wave appears symmetrical with regard to a vertical line drawn through its peak. There are, of course, all kinds of transitional forms between these idealized wave forms which merely represent the two ends of a spectrum.

Another important feature in the evaluation of an interictal epileptiform abnormality is its abundance and consistency in localization. It is particularly essential to ascertain that such potentials can be demonstrated in the same area in repeated examinations. A clear delineation of the areas in which these potentials occur is another helpful criterion.

Correlations Between Interictal EEG Findings and Clinical Data, and Therapeutic Decisions Deriving Therefrom

Since repeated EEG recordings may yield only interictal EEG abnormalities, decisions on further management of the patient's problem must often be based upon such relatively incomplete data. If the clinical localization derived from the observation of spontaneous seizures by trained personnel (physicians, nurses, EEG technologists) is clear and congruent with the EEG localization, surgical therapy can be recommended, especially if ancillary data such as the results of radiological studies and of the psychological testing concur with this localization. The analysis of prognostic factors in temporal lobe epilepsies carried out by Bengzon, Rasmussen, Gloor, Dussault, and Stephens (1968) bears this out. This study has underlined another important factor in prognosis: sometimes the clinical, radiological, psychological, and interictal EEG data concur in their main localizing significance; yet if one of the sets of data indicates involvement of an additional part of the brain, the therapeutic results of removing the presumed main epileptogenic area are, statistically speaking, less than optimal.

In many instances, especially in temporal lobe epilepsy, the clinical localization of the brain region involved may be clear, but lateralization on clinical grounds remains uncertain. Even though the interictal EEG localization may be quite clear in such a case, one should attempt to record a seizure in order to confirm the lateralizing and localizing evidence provided by the interictal EEG abnormality. If such evidence cannot be obtained, decision with regard to surgical therapy must be carefully weighed in the light of the patient's history, neurological, radiological, and psychological findings, the severity of his seizures, and their degree of refractoriness to medical treatment.

Finally, if the clinical localization is clear and the EEG localization in conflict with it, one should attempt to record a seizure. If the conflicting evidence cannot be satisfactorily resolved, surgery should not be contemplated.

ICTAL EEG RECORDS

Methodological Problems

The record of a spontaneous seizure theoretically provides the best diagnostic evidence on the localization of the patient's epileptogenic area. This highly desirable goal often remains elusive, however, because spontaneous seizures by definition are intermittent and unpredictable events and only rarely can focal epileptic seizures be provoked at will.

Even if a seizure *is* recorded, the ictal record often cannot be interpreted because it is obscured by muscle potentials and by movement artifact, which often completely mask the ictal cerebral record.

Furthermore, since only a fraction of the cerebral cortex is directly accessible to conventional scalp EEG recording, some uncertainty often remains about the actual site of origin of a seizure, especially when the first ictal event in the EEG is poorly localized or even generalized, or when it appears in the record only after clinical signs have been in progress for some time. Rapid or almost instantaneous spread over a large area or equally rapid generalization of the seizure discharge may also prevent identification of a focal onset, even when clinical signs point to a focal origin.

Finally, there is always some residual uncertainty about whether all the patient's seizures consistently originate from the same cerebral region.

The number of disappointing negative investigations aimed at obtaining an ictal recording can be reduced to some extent by the following procedures.

(1) *Prolonged recordings* are the simplest of these. The patient's EEG is recorded uninterruptedly for many hours, perhaps an entire day and/or an entire night. A montage must be chosen on a 16-channel instrument which covers all head regions accessible to standard EEG recording. In temporal lobe epileptics, it is useful to insert a pair of sphenoidal electrodes. The procedure, although simple, often taxes the patient's patience beyond his endurance, although boredom can be somewhat relieved by having the patient read or listen to the radio. When planning a prolonged recording, the investigator should be guided by the patient's seizure incidence. This strategy is not very successful if the patient's attacks are infrequent. If the seizures occur in clusters, the patient should be examined at a time when he is seizure-prone.

(2) *Precipitation of seizures* is another useful procedure. In some patients, definite seizure-precipitating stimuli are known. They should be applied while

the patient's EEG is being recorded. However, there are only a few patients with focal seizures for whom precipitating factors are known.

Seizures can be elicited by the intravenous injection of a convulsant drug such as pentylenetetrazol or bemegride. This topic will be dealt with in the section on activation procedures.

(3) *Telemetric recordings* overcome many of the difficulties inherent in prolonged recordings. The procedure is much less stressful on the patient, for he has a wide range of freedom of movement. His behavior on the ward does not need to be in any way restricted by the fact that his EEG is being continuously monitored (Stevens, 1969; Storm van Leeuwen and Kamp, 1969; Porter, Wolf, and Penry, 1971; Ives, Thompson, and Woods, 1973). The main drawbacks of most of the EEG telemetry systems now in existence are the lack of a sufficient number of channels. Costs and the increasing bulk of the transmitter package with increasing number of channels are the main limiting factors in multichannel telemetry. With recent miniaturizing techniques, some of the technological difficulties are now being overcome. Also, multiplexing of a large number of channels onto one carrier track on a tape recorder is now a feasible solution. High quality EEGs can be obtained by demultiplexing the recorded data.

(4) *Patient-monitoring systems with or without computer assistance* can be developed in order to observe ictal events. Such systems are particularly useful in combination with cable or radiotelemetry in order to reduce the tremendous amount of paper that results from an uninterrupted, prolonged recording in which one waits for the elusive and unpredictable ictal event. They are most useful in conjunction with depth electrode recordings and are discussed in a later section.

(5) *Depth electrode recording through stereotactically implanted electrodes* is another effective method which improves the chance of obtaining a useful, interpretable ictal record. This technique is covered in another section of this chapter.

Interpretation of Ictal Records

Interpreting an ictal EEG record requires identification of the earliest detectable ictal event, which is often very discrete. It frequently consists of low-voltage, fast rhythmic activity, often in the 20 to 40 cps band. This activity should be clearly distinguishable from the preceding, ongoing background activity by its different frequency and amplitude (Fig. 3). Most ictal records start with such low-voltage fast activity, if one records in the area of seizure onset. The activity then gradually increases in amplitude as its frequency decreases. During this augmentation of voltage, the spread of the discharge to adjacent regions often becomes evident. If only areas reached by this secondary spread of the discharge are accessible to scalp recording, rhythmic, relatively slow activity may be the first sign of ictal discharge appearing in the scalp EEG. The slower the frequency of the ictal discharge, the greater the likelihood that the actual area of its origin is remote from the scalp electrodes.

Some seizures, especially those of temporal lobe or frontal parasagittal origin,

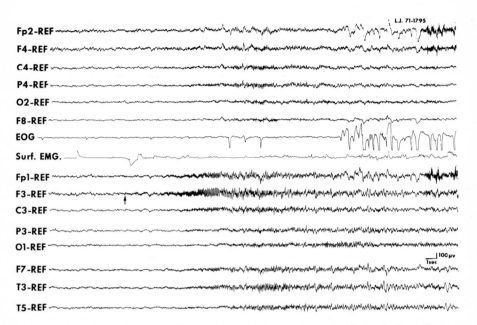

Fp2-REF

F4-REF

C4-REF

P4-REF

O2-REF

F8-REF

EOG

Surf. EMG.

Fp1-REF

F3-REF

C3-REF

P3-REF

O1-REF

F7-REF

T3-REF

T5-REF

LJ. 71-1795

100 μv
1sec

FIG. 3. Example of an ictal record in a patient with focal seizures beginning in the right face. Note the low-voltage fast activity in the left midfrontal (F3) region at the start of the seizure (arrow). The seizure discharge gradually spreads to involve other areas. EOG, vertical electro-oculogram; Surf.EMG, surface electromyogram from the left face; electrode positions labelled according to 10–20 International System.

start with a sudden flattening of the EEG, often associated with a complete suppression of interictal epileptiform abnormality (Jasper et al., 1951; Penfield and Jasper, 1954). Such so-called suppressor onsets may provide localizing evidence if the voltage suppression is localized to a particular area, and especially if flattening is followed by gradually increasing low-voltage, fast rhythmic activity in the same region. Sometimes voltage suppression at seizure onset is quite generalized and thus of little localizing significance.

Postictal slow-wave activity may also provide localizing evidence. It is usually most pronounced in the area which had been most intensely involved in the seizure activity. This very often but not consistently coincides with the area of onset of the seizure discharge. The possibility that postictal slow-wave activity may be greater in an area to which the discharge had spread later during the course of an attack must be kept in mind, and, therefore, postictal localized slow-wave activity is a much less reliable localizing sign than the actual observation of a localized seizure onset in an EEG.

The value of an ictal record is greatly enhanced if an accurate written description of the attending clinical events is available. The patient should therefore be observed by trained personnel familiar with the symptomatology of epileptic seizures. Some clinical manifestations and their correlation with the development of the seizure discharge in the EEG can be clarified and defined with greater precision if a polygraphic recording is taken (Gastaut and Broughton, 1972). This usually, however, implies the sacrifice of some EEG channels for the recording of other biological variables and may therefore make it more difficult to localize adequately the seizure onset in the EEG.

ACTIVATION PROCEDURES AND SPECIAL RECORDING TECHNIQUES DESIGNED TO CLARIFY OR ELICIT INTERICTAL AND/OR ICTAL EEG ABNORMALITIES

Frequently the evidence obtained in the interictal EEG is insufficient either for establishing the presence of unequivocal epileptiform abnormality or for obtaining sufficiently clear-cut localizing evidence. Under such circumstances, simple activation or special recording procedures may bring out latent interictal abnormality or provoke a seizure.

Withdrawal of Anticonvulsant Medication

The simplest activation procedure is the gradual withdrawal of anticonvulsant medication. There are instances when this is clinically contraindicated, especially in patients known to be prone toward status epilepticus. In the protected hospital environment, however, medication can be gradually reduced and finally withdrawn in most patients. One should not expect, however, that the EEG will become more active within 24 or 48 hr after withdrawal. Anticonvulsant drug levels do not fall as quickly as was once surmised, and 5 to 7 days is often required to eliminate the anticonvulsant completely from the patient's system (Buchthal, Svensmark, and Simonsen, 1968; Arnold and Gerber, 1970; Buchthal and Lennox-Buchthal, 1972). After such prolonged drug withdrawal, it is common to see epileptiform abnormality appear in an EEG record of a patient whose previous EEGs were quite uninformative, especially when diphenylhydantoin (Dilantin®) was the anticonvulsant employed. Phenobarbital seems to suppress interictal epileptiform abnormality to a lesser degree. Plasma drug level determinations are useful, since they permit more precise evaluations of the degree of withdrawal. In the case of phenobarbital, there is a significant correlation between drug concentration in brain and in plasma (Sherwin, Eisen, and Sokolowski, 1973).

Hyperventilation and Intermittent Photic Stimulation

These are simple activation procedures which should be carried out in every patient. Although in focal epilepsies, hyperventilation does not precipitate epileptiform discharges as frequently as in generalized seizure disorders, it can be quite effective at times, especially with frontal lobe foci.

Intermittent photic stimulation, however, usually has no effect upon focal epileptiform abnormality, even when the focus is in the occipital region.

Natural or Drug-Induced Sleep

Sleep is useful for activating interictal or ictal epileptiform abnormalities, especially in patients with temporal lobe epilepsy (Gibbs and Gibbs, 1947; Gibbs et al., 1948*a,b;* Gibbs, 1958; Merlis, Grossman, and Henriksen, 1951; Passouant, 1950; Silverman, 1956; Gloor, Tsai, and Haddad, 1958; Niedermeyer and Rocca, 1972). Natural sleep, if it can be obtained under laboratory conditions, is preferable over drug-induced sleep, but if drugs must be used the amounts given should be relatively modest to prevent the appearance of drug-induced EEG changes which may mask the epileptiform abnormality. A modest dose (100 mg) of secobarbital sodium (Seconal®) by mouth given alone or in combination with 25 mg of intramuscular chlorpromazine (Largactil®) (Stewart, 1957) is often quite effective. Most of the abnormalities tend to appear in stages I and II of slow-wave sleep. Activation may persist in deeper stages, but epileptiform activity may become masked in stage IV by high-voltage slow waves. REM sleep is said to activate epileptiform discharges originating in limbic structures of the temporal lobe (Delange, Castan, Cadilhac, and Passouant, 1962; Passouant, Cadilhac, and Delange, 1965; Gastaut and Broughton, 1972), but this can be demonstrated only if all night recordings are carried out (it is not usually necessary to resort to this method).

Intravenous Methohexital Activation

In temporal lobe epilepsy, intravenous injection of subanesthetic or anesthetic doses of methohexital (Brevital®, Brietal®) may bring out epileptiform abnormalities in otherwise uninformative EEG records (Wilder, 1969, 1971; Musella, Wilder, and Schmidt, 1971). Small subanesthetic doses are said to be particularly useful for precipitating generalized spike-and-wave discharges in patients suffering from absence attacks (Gumpert and Paul, 1971; Wilder, Musella, Van Horn, and Schmidt, 1971), but larger amounts inducing a light stage of anesthesia often bring out previously nonexistent focal sharp waves and spikes in temporal lobe epilepsies. The most effective doses range between 0.25 and 1.5 mg/kg, but repeated injections may be needed for optimal effects (Musella et al., 1971). Whether methohexital offers any real advantage over conventional sleep activation is still a matter of controversy (Celesia and Paulsen, 1972; Sherwin and Hooge, 1973).

Intravenous Pentylenetetrazol or Bemegride Activation

Since a focal onset of ictal discharge in the EEG often provides more reliable evidence for the site of origin of a focal seizure than interictal epileptiform abnormalities, one might expect that the artificial precipitation of a seizure by the intravenous injection of a convulsant drug, such as pentylenetetrazol (Metrazol®) (Kaufman, Marshall, and Walker, 1947; Cure, Rasmussen, and Jasper,

1948; Merlis, Henriksen, and Grossman, 1950; Gastaut, 1955; Penfield and Jasper, 1954; Ajmone-Marsan and Ralston, 1957) or bemegride (Megimide®) (Delay, Verdeaux, Drossopoulo, Schuller, and Chanoit, 1956; Rodin, Rutledge, and Calhoun, 1958), should be one of the most diagnostically useful activation procedures in clinical EEG. This expectation is justified, however, only if it can be shown that the intravenous injection of a convulsant drug always activates the epileptogenic mechanism responsible for the patient's spontaneous seizures. Unfortunately this is often not the case. Convulsant drugs produce seizures in normal brains, the thresholds varying greatly from individual to individual. Such purely drug-induced "unspecific" seizures are nearly always generalized, but they may be elicited with drug dosages which are insufficient to precipitate the patient's habitual attacks.

Thus the frequently induced occurrence of a generalized seizure with simultaneous bilateral onset both clinically and in the EEG is a result without diagnostic value. Even if a pentylenetetrazol-induced seizure reproduces the patient's habitual attack, the EEG record is often still uninterpretable because it is totally obscured by muscle artifact from the start; thus a possible focal onset remains undetectable. In other instances the pentylenetetrazol-induced seizure may show a focal onset in the EEG, but the clinical pattern may be sufficiently different from that characterizing the patient's habitual seizures that the diagnostic validity of the drug-induced attack could be questioned. In some instances the difference may merely be one of speed of development of the generalized convulsion out of an initially focal event, but in others the difference between pentylenetetrazol- or bemegride-induced partial seizures and those occurring spontaneously is so great that one has to conclude that the focal attack induced by the drug bears no relationship to the patient's habitual attacks (Bancaud, Talairach, Waltregny, Bresson, and Morel, 1968). The area with the lowest intravenous pentylenetetrazol threshold in such a patient may thus not be the one responsible for his habitual seizures. The conclusion in such a case is almost inescapable that the patient has potentially multifocal epileptogenic disease. Such observations indicate that the interpretation of an ictal record obtained with this activation procedure requires a great deal of critical circumspection.

We have almost totally abandoned this activation procedure because of these many shortcomings, especially since the procedure of intravenous injection of pentylenetetrazol almost always elicits an anxiety reaction from the patient.

Some of these unpleasant side effects of intravenous pentylenetetrazol injection can be counteracted by giving the patient small amounts (1 to 2 mg up to a total cumulative dose of 10 mg) of diazepam (Valium®) through another vein during the procedure. Small amounts are injected repeatedly, if necessary, whenever anxiety becomes a problem or when generalized unspecific pentylenetetrazol-induced epileptiform discharges are elicited. It has been claimed that intravenous diazepam given in this manner counteracts these unspecific generalized convulsive effects of pentylenetetrazol, while leaving the focal epileptogenic abnormality relatively untouched (Torres and Ellington, 1970). In a series of 32 epileptic patients with known or suspected focal seizures in whom we carried out this test, this expectation was not often fulfilled. The diagnostic usefulness of this test is thus limited, but we are convinced that combining diazepam and pentylenetetrazol injection is useful in making the test less stressful for the patient. However, most of the patients receiving diazepam with pentylenetetrazol exhibited unusually high seizure thresholds.

In carrying out an intravenous pentylenetetrazol activation either alone or in combination with diazepam injection, it is advantageous to inject the drug in fractionized amounts by giving 1 mg/kg body weight every 30 sec until the onset of a seizure (Jasper and Courtois, 1953).

Recordings with Basal (Pharyngeal or Sphenoidal) Electrodes

In many temporal lobe epileptics, the epileptogenic area is localized in or extends to the uncinate region on the mesio-basal aspect of the temporal lobe. This area is inaccessible to conventional scalp recording. The need was thus felt many years ago to make at least part of this region accessible to EEG recording by devising special electrodes (basal electrodes). Two types can be used: (1) nasopharyngeal electrodes (Grinker, 1938; Gastaut, 1948; Roubicek and Hill, 1948; MacLean, 1949; Penfield and Jasper, 1954; Rovit, Gloor, and Henderson, 1960), which are inserted through the nose and rest on the mucosa of the pharyngeal roof; and (2) sphenoidal electrodes (Pertuiset and Capdevielle-Arfel, 1951; Penfield and Jasper, 1954; Pampiglione and Kerridge, 1956; Rovit et al., 1960), which have to be inserted transcutaneously and rest with their tips on the ala magna of the sphenoid bone near the foramen ovale. Both the nasopharyngeal and sphenoidal electrodes are located in the immediate vicinity of the uncinate area of the temporal lobe, the former about 2 to 2.5 cm more mesially and anteriorly than the latter (Rovit et al., 1960).

Nasopharyngeal electrodes can be easily and quickly applied by a skillful technician without undue discomfort or risk to the patient. Two electrodes should always be inserted, one through each nostril, since with a single pharyngeal electrode it is impossible to lateralize an abnormality. The chief disadvantage of nasopharyngeal electrodes is their proneness to pick up disturbing artifacts caused by respiratory movements, the carotid pulse, swallowing, or vibration induced by snoring in a sleeping patient. Also, the moist pharyngeal mucosa offers a low-resistance shunt between the two nasopharyngeal electrodes with consequent flatness and a variable loss of resolution of the record derived from this area.

Sphenoidal electrodes, if properly inserted, provide high-quality, high-resolution records (Fig. 4) with very little artifact from a region which represents in most patients suffering from temporal lobe epilepsy their major epileptogenic area (Rovit et al., 1960; Rovit and Gloor, 1960; Rovit, Gloor, and Rasmussen, 1961b). Sphenoidal electrode recordings should be carried out in every patient in whom temporal lobectomy for seizure control is contemplated.

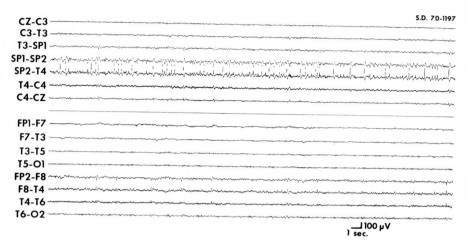

FIG. 4. Sphenoidal electrode and scalp electrode recording of epileptiform activity arising from a right temporal focus. Note the large number of epileptiform spikes and sharp waves at the right sphenoidal electrode, of which only very few appear with low voltage in the right anterior sylvian region at F8. SP1 and SP2 indicate left and right sphenoidal electrodes, respectively.

The insertion of these electrodes should be carried out by a physician, not by technical personnel. For the correct and safe placement of these electrodes, an accurate knowledge of the anatomy of the pterygo-palatine fossa and of the base of the skull in the region of the foramen ovale is mandatory. A proper understanding of the potential risks of inserting needles into the soft tissues of these areas is necessary, as well as a thorough familiarity with the technique of aseptic procedures.

The technique of insertion of a pair of anterior and a pair of posterior sphenoidal electrodes is described in detail by Rovit et al. (1960). Presently, however, we routinely use only one pair of sphenoidal electrodes (the posterior one aimed at the region just posterior to the foramen ovale, according to the description of Rovit et al., 1960). The necessity of using two pairs has been an exceptional situation in our more recent experience.

Sphenoidal electrode recordings offer three main advantages in the EEG evaluation of patients with temporal seizures.

(1) It may reveal definite epileptiform abnormality in patients in whom such abnormality could not be found by use of standard scalp or nasopharyngeal electrode recordings.

(2) It may clarify problems encountered with bitemporal epileptiform disturbances, either by disclosing bitemporal epileptiform firing in a patient in whom previously in scalp EEGs only unilateral epileptiform abnormality had been found, or by demonstrating that the bilateral temporal epileptiform discharges on the scalp are probably secondary to a lateralized mesial temporal epileptogenic focus.

(3) Rarely, a sphenoidal electrode recording may disclose an unsuspected focal discharge apparently responsible for triggering generalized, bilaterally synchronous spike-and-wave discharges (secondary bilateral synchrony).

SPECIAL PROBLEMS AND PROCEDURES

Secondary Bilateral Synchrony

The Concept and EEG Diagnosis of "Secondary Bilateral Synchrony"

It has been known for many years that patients with focal epileptogenic lesions may exhibit EEGs with generalized, bilaterally synchronous discharges, which usually assume a spike and wave form (Penfield and Jasper, 1947; Jasper, 1949*c;* Tükel and Jasper, 1952; Penfield and Jasper, 1954; Rovit, Gloor, and Rasmussen, 1961*a;* Madsen and Bray, 1966; Stewart and Dreifuss, 1967; Gastaut, Mouren, and Paillas, 1968; Niedermeyer, 1968; Gloor, 1969; Niedermeyer, Laws, and Walker, 1969; Lombroso and Erba, 1970; Niedermeyer, Walker, and Burton, 1970). The important role of the focal epileptogenic lesion in these cases is demonstrated by the fact that the surgical removal of the lesion often results in freedom from further attacks. It is assumed that in such instances the generalization of the epileptiform discharges is secondary to focal epileptiform activity in a circumscribed cortical area, hence the term "secondary bilateral synchrony" (Tükel and Jasper, 1952; Penfield and Jasper, 1954). Even though true instances of secondary bilateral synchrony are rare, this possibility must be considered in the differential diagnosis of medically intractable seizure problems in which the EEG shows generalized, paroxysmal, bilaterally synchronous discharges. Unfortunately, however, neither the clinical signs and symptoms nor the standard EEG recordings can give unequivocal evidence that the patient presenting with generalized epileptiform abnormality in his EEG may belong to this category. It is true that in most instances of secondary bilateral synchrony, the EEG deviates to a variable degree from the classical pattern of primary generalized corticoreticular ("centrencephalic") epilepsy with regular symmetrical 3/sec spike-and-wave discharges emerging from a normal background EEG activity (Tükel and Jasper, 1952; Niedermeyer et al., 1970). However, some patients mimic this pattern very closely, and conversely "atypical" spike-and-wave discharges may be found in cases of primary bilateral synchrony. Consistent asymmetries of the spike-and-wave pattern, focal epileptiform discharges in the EEG in addition to the generalized ones, especially if they show a stable localization from one examination to the next, and a demonstration that such a focal discharge may be followed within a fraction of a second by a generalized bilaterally synchronous spike-and-wave discharge are useful hints which suggest a mechanism of secondary bilateral synchrony—but they furnish no proof. Sometimes clinical evidence suggests such a mechanism, e.g., when the seizure pattern in a patient with generalized bilaterally synchronous spike and wave discharge exhibits definite focal features—but again this provides no proof. Conversely, some patients without any clear focal features in their clinical seizure pattern may exhibit generalized epileptiform discharges which depend on a mechanism of secondary bilateral synchrony and are thus amenable to surgical therapy.

In view of these difficulties in diagnosing the condition of secondary bilateral synchrony, it seemed desirable to devise methods whereby it could be differentiated from primary bilateral synchrony. Apart from the method of stereotactic depth electrode exploration used in some centers (Bancaud, Talairach, Bonis, Schaub, Szikla, Morel, and Bordas-Ferer, 1965; Bancaud, 1969; 1971; Niedermeyer et al., 1969), two pharmacological techniques have been used for this purpose. The first is the intracarotid amobarbital and pentylenetetrazol test developed at the Montreal Neurological Institute (Rovit et al., 1961*a*; Gloor, Rasmussen, Garretson, and Maroun, 1964; Garretson, Gloor, and Rasmussen, 1966; Gloor, 1969); the second is the intravenous thiopental test introduced by Lombroso and Erba (1970).

Intracarotid Amobarbital and Pentylenetetrazol Test

In a case of secondary bilateral synchrony, it is assumed that a circumscribed area of the cerebral cortex acts as the pacemaker for the generalized discharges. If this area lies within the territory of one of the carotid arteries, it should be possible to inactivate it temporarily by injection of amobarbital through that carotid artery. Such inactivation of the pacemaker by *unilateral* intracarotid amobarbital should temporarily eliminate the generalized discharges *on both sides,* whereas a similar injection on the side opposite to the pacemaker should affect the discharges only on the side of the injection (Rovit et al., 1961*a*; Gloor, 1969). Conversely, the pacemaker should be the area most sensitive to the perfusion of a convulsant drug such as pentylenetetrazol. Thus unilateral intracarotid injection of fractionized doses of pentylenetetrazol should reveal a lower threshold for the elicitation of EEG and clinical convulsive phenomena when injected on the side of the pacemaker than when injected contralaterally (Gloor et al., 1964; Gloor, 1969). In cases of primary bilateral synchrony, unilateral intracarotid injection of amobarbital should produce mirror effects when injected on the right and the left sides. Also, with unilateral intracarotid injection of fractionized doses of pentylenetetrazol, the clinical and electrographic thresholds should be the same on the left and right sides in cases of primary bilateral synchrony.

The results of these tests can, however, be interpreted reliably only if strict methodological criteria are observed. [For a detailed description of the technique, see Garretson et al. (1966).] An important prerequisite is that the amount of drug delivered to the ipsilateral hemisphere is the same with the left- and right-sided injections. This can be achieved only when the drugs are injected directly into the internal carotid artery by means of a catheter placed into that vessel. Injections into the common carotid artery are not satisfactory, because the injectate may divide differently between the internal and external carotid circulation on the two sides. Also, it is necessary to visualize the carotid circulation of the patient in order to be aware of possible asymmetries of vascular supply which are to be expected particularly in the territory of the anterior cerebral circulation. These may by themselves produce asymmetries of the test results. A 2-cc angiogram is preferable for these investigations rather than the usual 10-cc injection of contrast medium given rapidly under high injection pressure, which tends to produce considerable imbalance in normal cerebral hemodynamics resulting in a filling of vascular territories which under normal conditions may not be irrigated by the injected vessel. This is particularly important because amobarbital and pentylenetetrazol are injected in small amounts and at speeds which are unlikely to produce any significant imbalance of hemodynamics. This ensures, as much as possible, a unilateral distribution of the drug, unless, for instance, a single carotid artery feeds both anterior cerebral circulations.

The amounts of amobarbital given are 50 mg in 2 cc saline, injected over a period of 6 sec. Pentylenetetrazol is injected in fractionized amounts of 1 cc containing 1 mg (or rarely 0.25 mg) of drug delivered every 5 sec. The patients should be adequately sedated before the test by drugs which do not produce any great alterations of the EEG, e.g., an intramuscular injection of 10 mg of morphine plus 25 mg of chlorpromazine. Sedation ensures a stable background firing in the EEG; this is important because the generalized discharges in these patients are very sensitive to arousal stimuli. For this reason it is impossible to obtain reliable results if the intracarotid injection is used to determine concurrently the lateralization of speech or of memory function.

Since intracarotid amobarbital and pentylenetetrazol tests necessitate the simultaneous incannulation of the two main arterial supply vessels of the brain, the potential risks of the procedure must be weighed against the potential benefits for the patient. We feel that this test is indicated only in patients in whom surgical therapy for seizures is contemplated and in whom the decision to operate is largely dependent on the outcome of these tests.

In the case of primary bilateral synchrony, one of three response types is observed with unilateral intracarotid injection of amobarbital: (1) no reduction in the rate at which the spike-and-wave discharges occur, with or without a slight to moderate reduction of the amplitude of the paroxysmal discharges on the side of the injection (Fig. 5); (2) diminution or arrest of spike-and-wave discharges on both sides, the decrease in discharge rate being either sudden or gradual; or (3) ipsilateral or bilateral activation of paroxysmal epileptiform discharge which, on rare occasions, may be associated with minor clinical manifestations resembling an absence attack. The EEG in this instance consists of a sudden appearance of 2 to 3/sec, rhythmic, paroxysmal slow waves or slow sharp waves, sometimes associated with a few spike-and-wave forms with maximum amplitude in the frontal region. Even when these discharges are bilateral, they always predominate on the injection side. This response lasts only for a few seconds and is followed by response (1) or (2), described above.

In primary bilateral synchrony, the intracarotid pentylenetetrazol test shows

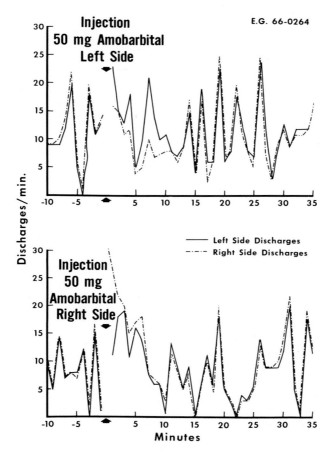

FIG. 5. Response of generalized, bilaterally synchronous discharges to unilateral intracarotid injection of 50 mg of amobarbital in a case of primary bilateral synchrony. Note the lack of a decrease in number of discharges after injection and the short-lived ipsilateral activation immediately after injection (clearly documented in this graph only for the right side).

equality or near equality of electrographic and/or clinical seizure thresholds on the two sides (Fig. 6). Sometimes such unilateral pentylenetetrazol injection induces continuous spike-and-wave activity throughout the remainder of the pentylenetetrazol injection without the precipitation of a generalized tonic-clonic convulsion. This is associated with a clinical state resembling a prolonged absence attack. In other instances, a generalized convulsion ensues.

In secondary bilateral synchrony, the response to unilateral injection of amobarbital is characterized by *bilateral* disappearance of epileptiform abnormality if the injection is carried out on the side of the pacemaker (Fig. 7). Paroxysmal discharges often reappear first on the injected side or bilaterally after approximately 4 to 20 min. Injection of amobarbital on the side contralateral to that

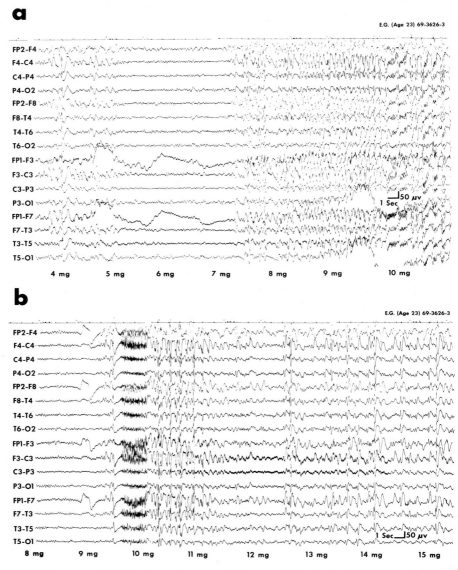

FIG. 6. Response of bilaterally synchronous discharges to fractionized unilateral intracarotid injection of pentylenetetrazol in a case of primary bilateral synchrony (same patient as in Fig. 5). The thresholds for the initiation of continuous seizure activity with left-sided *(a)* and right-sided *(b)* injections are virtually identical (injected cumulative amounts of pentylenetetrazol indicated at bottom of figure).

containing the pacemaker does not arrest the paroxysmal discharges; only the amplitude of the discharges is reduced on the injected side (Fig. 7).

Intracarotid pentylenetetrazol injection in cases of secondary bilateral synchrony discloses a marked difference in thresholds between the two sides, the

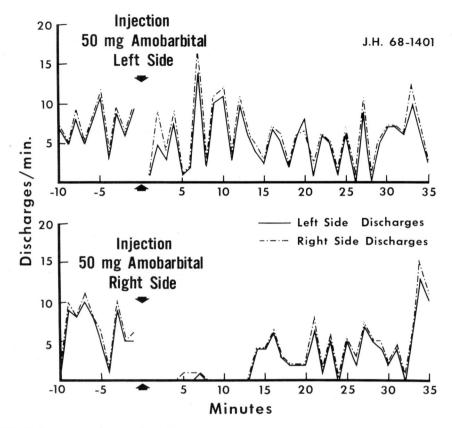

FIG. 7. Response of generalized bilaterally synchronous discharges to unilateral intracarotid injection of 50 mg of amobarbital in a case of secondary bilateral synchrony. Note the lack of diminution of paroxysmal discharges on both sides following left-sided injection, and suppression of discharges on both sides after right-sided injection. After the latter, the discharges on the right side return slightly earlier than those on the left.

threshold being lower with injection on the side on which amobarbital injection had produced a bilateral arrest of paroxysmal activity (Fig. 8). The degree of threshold asymmetry varies from patient to patient, but usually in cases of secondary bilateral synchrony these are of the order of at least 3 to 2, 2 to 1, or frequently even more. Injection on the side of the pacemaker should ideally reproduce the patient's habitual seizure pattern, but this is not always the case.

In addition to these two well-defined response patterns which are characteristic of primary and of secondary bilateral synchrony, the test results often show responses which cannot easily be pigeonholed into one of these two categories. The number of patients with this kind of results is in fact rather large. Thus one may find instances in which the test provides evidence that areas in both hemispheres exert some control upon the bilateral discharges yet this effect may be more pronounced on one side than the other. In other instances the test results

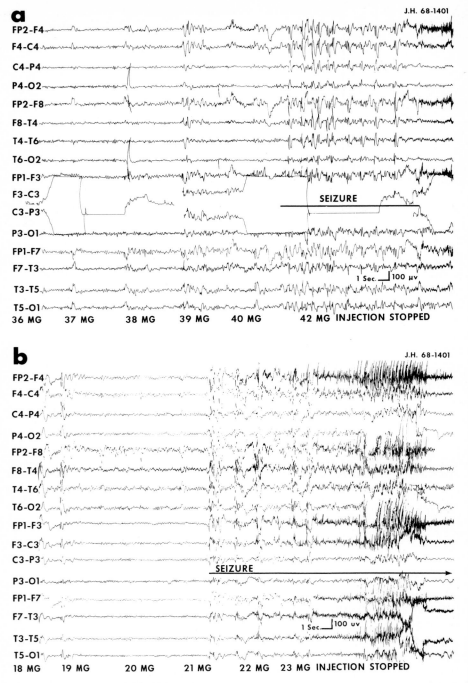

FIG. 8. Response of generalized bilaterally synchronous discharges to fractionized unilateral intracarotid injection of pentylenetetrazol in a case of secondary bilateral synchrony (same patient as in Fig. 7). On the left side *(a)* the convulsive threshold is reached only after 42 mg of pentylenetetrazol; on the right side *(b)*, 21 mg is sufficient to precipitate a clinical seizure.

with intracarotid amobarbital may be asymmetrical but there may be no, or a conflicting type of, asymmetry with the pentylenetetrazol test or vice versa. Focal features appearing as local accentuations of the diffuse epileptogenic process or a focal mechanism which appears to be independent of the generalized discharges may be revealed by the tests. It is probable that in all these instances there is diffuse or multifocal brain disease, most likely due to widespread structural brain lesions, which have not affected the brain in a homogeneous manner. This would account for asymmetries and/or the focal accentuations of the epileptogenic process revealed by the intracarotid tests. There is probably no sharp limit between these cases and those of "true secondary bilateral synchrony."

A number of patients in whom these tests have been carried out have been operated on in an attempt to arrest their seizures, some in spite of the fact that the intracarotid amobarbital and pentylenetetrazol test did not support the hypothesis of secondary bilateral synchrony. The decision to operate on these patients was reached on the basis of clinical evidence. A recent analysis of the surgical followup results in these operated patients (Rasmussen et al., *in preparation*) indicates that whenever the test pattern indicated that one hemisphere was more epileptogenic than the other, the postoperative results were better than when no lateralizing features were revealed by these tests. In some of the operated patients, the test results did not fulfill the critieria for secondary bilateral synchrony, but nevertheless indicated that one hemisphere was more epileptogenic than the other. The therapeutic results in this group were comparable to those obtained in patients with a test pattern indicative of secondary bilateral synchrony.

This follow-up analysis also demonstrated the importance of the carotid angiogram for the predictive value of the test results, in those cases in which the tests indicated a lateralizing predominance of the epileptogenic mechanism or suggested classical secondary bilateral synchrony. If the cerebral circulation is symmetrical, the predictive value of an asymmetry of the test results is good. If the circulation is asymmetrical, the test results are reliable only if they lateralize the epileptogenic process to the hemisphere opposite that of the carotid artery which supplies more of the two anterior quadrants of the brain than the other carotid artery; if the circulatory asymmetry is of the reverse type, however, the success rate of surgical therapy was low.

The Intravenous Thiopental Test

In 1970, Lombroso and Erba proposed a test based on the intravenous injection of a small amount of thiopental (Pentothal®) as a procedure whereby secondary bilateral synchrony can be differentiated from primary bilateral synchrony. Small amounts (0.5 or 1 mg/kg body weight) of thiopental are injected intravenously and the responses of the background activity and of the paroxysmal discharges are observed. For the interpretation of the test, it is important that the patient not be allowed to fall asleep.

Lombroso and Erba have distinguished four response types.

Type 1 is characterized by bilateral, symmetrical, abundant beta activity elicited by intravenous thiopental and an arrest or marked depression of the bilateral synchronous spike-and-wave discharges on both sides. This response is typical for primary bilateral synchrony in patients with primary generalized epilepsy.

Type 2 is characterized by an asymmetrical beta response after thiopental injection, with decreased or absent beta activity over one hemisphere or in a circumscribed area. This is associated with depression of generalized spike-and-wave discharges, but persistence of unilateral or focal epileptiform discharges in the area of depressed beta activity. This response type is typical for cases of secondary bilateral synchrony. The lateralization and sometimes localization of the presumed pacemaker is indicated by the area showing depressed beta activity and persistent epileptiform discharge.

Type 3 is characterized by delayed, fleeting, or absent thiopental-induced beta activity on both sides and the persistence or even enhancement of the bilateral synchronous spike-and-wave discharges. This response type is typical for primary bilateral synchrony encountered in patients with diffuse brain lesions.

Type 4 is an equivocal response which cannot be classified according to the above criteria.

According to Lombroso and Erba (1970), who have used this test mainly in a population of epileptic children, the predictive value of the criteria has been vindicated by favorable results of surgical therapy in patients with Type 2 responses and by failure of surgical therapy in cases with Type 3 responses.

Exploration with Stereotactically Implanted Depth Electrodes

Indications for Depth Electrode Implantation

The results obtained using traditional methods of clinical and EEG investigations are not always sufficient to localize the area of onset of the patient's seizures with certainty. In such a situation, one is forced either to renounce surgical therapy, even in the face of a complete failure of medical treatment, or to consider the implantation of multilead electrodes into selected areas of the brain (Bickford, 1956; Walker and Ribstein, 1957; Ajmone-Marsan and Van Buren, 1958; Ribstein, 1960; Bates, 1963; Crandall, Walter, and Rand, 1963; Fischer-Williams and Cooper, 1963; Rand, Crandall, and Walter, 1964; Bancaud et al., 1965; Niedermeyer et al., 1969; Bancaud, Geier, Talairach, and Scarabin, 1973). Since it is impossible to implant electrodes at all possible sites from which seizures could originate, one must, before resorting to this technique, have relatively good indications as to the *probable* area of onset. Thus the clinical and scalp EEG results must be sufficiently informative to allow one to make at least broad distinctions between frontal, temporal, or other localized cortical mechanisms. Patients with bilateral temporal foci in whom the side of seizure onset cannot be established on the basis of repeated scalp and sphenoidal electrode recordings are the most obvious candidates for depth electrode studies. Other foci which lend themselves to stereotactic exploration are those which, because of their location on the mesial surface of the hemisphere or the orbital surface of the frontal lobe, are inaccessible to direct scalp recordings.

Depth electrode investigations should not be undertaken lightly. The implantation of multiple electrodes in a patient's brain, including areas which will not be removed in a subsequent surgical procedure, carries some risks which, even though statistically small, must be considered. The most obvious ones are infection along the electrode track which finally may reach the meninges or the brain, and hemorrhage caused by the rupture of a vessel by the penetrating electrode. Correct surgical and aseptic techniques and adequate arteriographic demonstration of the patient's individual cerebral vascular anatomy before implantation minimize these risks very greatly (Talairach, Szikla, Tournoux, Prossalentis, Bordas-Ferer, Covello, Iacob, and Mempel, 1967). It is not yet completely clear to what extent the minimal damage inflicted by the depth electrodes to brain areas which are not subsequently removed may be of clinical significance, but as of now there is no evidence of untoward effects caused by electrode implantation alone. Since the surgical and radiological procedures involved in stereotactic depth electrode implantation cannot be covered in this chapter, the reader is referred to the publications of Crandall et al. (1963), Rand et al. (1964), Talairach et al. (1967), and Bancaud et al. (1973).

Methodology

The electrodes, which should be as thin as possible, are made of sheaves of thin wires cut at various predetermined lengths and covered with a nontoxic and nonirritating insulating material. Each thin wire leads to a separate contact. There should be multiple contacts in each electrode strand. The distances between contacts should be no more than 0.5 mm for areas situated in gray matter; in areas presumably located in white matter the distances can be larger. The electrodes must be inserted as atraumatically as possible in a manner which ensures that, once implanted, they do not produce additional damage, since it is often necessary to leave these electrodes in place for several weeks. They must be firmly fixed to the skull to prevent their displacement after implantation. To avoid infection it is advantageous to have the lead wires run subcutaneously for some distance from their point of emergence through the skull before bringing them out through the skin. The contact surfaces of the electrodes must be made of a nontoxic metal (Fischer, Sayre, and Bickford, 1961; Cooper, Osselton, and Shaw, 1969): stainless steel, for example, is relatively inexpensive and quite satisfactory; gold may also be used. Under no circumstances should the resistance of the electrodes be measured with an ordinary DC-operated ohmmeter once they are implanted, since this would produce electrolytic lesions in the brain.

Target sites should be chosen carefully in the light of the clinical and EEG information which is available. It is advantageous to implant the electrodes in symmetrical positions with as much accuracy as possible. Temporal lobe depth electrodes should provide for contacts in neocortical as well as limbic areas. The latter should include the amygdala, hippocampus, and parahippocampal gyrus.

In the hippocampal area, both anterior and posterior positions should be sampled.

The best montages for recording are bipolar chains linking successive electrode contacts. Monopolar recordings usually are less satisfactory. It is advantageous, at least in a few instances, to record simultaneously from both the scalp and depth electrodes. This is most easily achieved by using two 16-channel EEG machines, one recording from the depth of the brain and the other from the scalp. If the two machines can be synchronized with a digital clock, this greatly facilitates the identification of corresponding segments of the records in the two paper charts.

The main purpose of depth electrode recordings is to localize as accurately as possible the area of onset of the patient's habitual seizures. Although interictal abnormalities such as random spikes and sharp waves provide useful background information, no therapeutic decisions should be made based only on this information. It is therefore very important to record *several* of the patient's spontaneous seizures and to determine the lateralization and localization of the onset of the attack and the consistency of this localization from one seizure to the next. The recording technique must be tailored to meet these requirements. Prolonged "conventional" type recordings are the most obvious choice. They suffer, however, from the disadvantage that one generates a tremendous amount of paper, much of it containing redundant, relatively unimportant information showing only interictal epileptiform abnormality. Radiotelemetry makes these prolonged recordings more acceptable to the patient, but most of the existing systems do not provide enough channels. Thus exclusive use of telemetry recording is not a desirable option with such limited systems. Telemetry recordings of the conventional type do not reduce the amount of paper or redundant data; on the contrary, they usually aggravate these problems. One can, of course, elect to inspect only the ictal records of seizures observed by hospital personnel or of which the patient himself was aware. Even under the best conditions, however, small and often very revealing minor seizures are missed under these circumstances. These may have no or only very discrete clinical accompaniments, but are still diagnostically very useful.

This problem can be solved by a patient-monitoring system, using logic circuitry or computer programs, which scrutinizes the record and identifies segments of the EEG which most probably contain a seizure (Ives, Thompson, Gloor, and Olivier, *in preparation*). Those parts of the record containing a probable seizure are saved and are available for later playback. The system must be biased in favor of recording "false positives" in order not to miss any of the true seizures, and it must be organized so that a delay mechanism is included which

→

FIG. 9. Seizure activity recorded with 8-channel radiotelemetry and detected by computer in a patient with stereotactically implanted depth electrodes. This record was photographed directly from the playback of the recording on the computer terminal. The lower half of the figure is a direct continuation of the record shown in the upper half. The first 4 channels record the activity from the depth of the left temporal lobe, channels 5 to 8 the activity from the depth of the right temporal lobe (channel 1, left amygdala; channel 2, left anterior hippocampus; channels 3 and

4, left parahippocampal gyrus and posterior hippocampus; channel 5, right amygdala; channel 6, right anterior hippocampus; channels 7 and 8, right parahippocampal gyrus and posterior hippocampus). The seizure discharge starts in the right parahippocampal gyrus (channel 7) and then spreads to involve mainly the hippocampal and parahippocampal region on the right and left side, as well as the left amygdaloid region.

permits incorporation of several seconds or, preferably, even minutes of the preictal record into the playback of the ictal episode. We have had some preliminary experience with this type of approach and, although our system is still under development, it has proved to be very useful, even though we cannot as yet be absolutely sure that it may not miss some of the seizures exhibiting an unexpected electrographic pattern (Fig. 9). The system can also be turned on for recording either by a nurse or the patient himself whenever a seizure occurs or has taken place. By using a suitably long delay of several minutes, the record of the entire seizure, including its onset, can thus be retrieved.

The implantation of stereotactic depth electrodes also affords the opportunity to stimulate electrically the various contact points within the brain in an attempt to reproduce the patient's habitual seizure or elements of it. If this is successful, the electrical concomitants of the seizure can be observed and compared with those seen during spontaneous seizures. If the localization of the point of stimulation reproducing the patient's habitual seizure coincides with the area of onset observed in spontaneous attacks, the likelihood is good of having thus identified the patient's principal epileptogenic region.

The technique for these stimulations is simple. A constant current stimulator should be used, because accurate threshold measurements of afterdischarges and of clinical responses are essential for the correct interpretation of the stimulation results. Voltage thresholds are meaningless as long as one cannot be sure that the impedance of every electrode pair stimulated is identical. Pulse duration should be kept at 0.5 msec or less to minimize or avoid local damage due to electrolytic lesions (Lilly, Hughes, Alvord, and Galkin, 1955; Lilly, 1961). For the same reason, biphasic pulses should be used. The frequency can be set at 60 cps. Effective stimulation intensities for these parameters range from about 500 μA to 4 mA. By systematically stimulating all electrode pairs sequentially for 3 to 6 sec at a time, a threshold map showing the hierarchy of responsiveness of various areas can be established, taking into account both electrographic responses (as evidenced by afterdischarges) and clinical stimulation effects.

A word of caution, however, should be added with regard to these stimulations. Since not all areas stimulated will finally be included in the surgical removal, care must be taken not to produce any permanent changes in the brain through electrical stimulation. Short biphasic pulses minimize the danger of local damage in the electrode-brain contact area. In addition, the kindling effect, which has now been amply documented in animal experiments (Goddard, 1967; Goddard, McIntyre, and Leech, 1969; Racine 1972a,b), must be kept in mind. These experiments showed that repeated stimulation of the same contact in daily sessions in all animal species tested results in the development of a profound and permanent lowering of afterdischarge thresholds, both at the point of stimulation and in distant areas. This type of stimulation also leads to the occurrence of generalized convulsions with stimulation intensities which were originally so low that they did not produce any electrographic or behavioral response. A relatively small number of repeated stimulations may already produce this permanent change if repeated afterdischarges are elicited (Racine, Burnham, Gartner, and Levitan, 1973). However, so-called massed trials in which repeated stimulations are carried out at short intervals in one single session produce a negligible kindling effect (Goddard et al., 1969). Prudence therefore dictates that depth electrode stimulations in patients should be carried out in one single session, if possible, and that the number of repeated stimulations of the same contacts, especially if they evoke afterdischarges, should be kept to the minimum required for obtaining adequate diagnostic information. Repeated stimulation sessions spread over a series of days should be avoided.

Diagnostic Evaluation of Depth Electrode Recordings

Indwelling depth electrodes afford the opportunity to record, with a minimum of artifactual contamination, the entire sequence of the patient's habitual seizures.

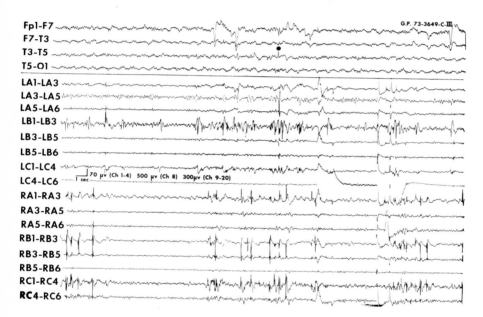

FIG. 10. Combined scalp (first 4 channels) and depth electrode recordings (next 16 channels) in a patient with temporal lobe epilepsy. The record from the depth and from the scalp electrodes was taken with two 16-channel EEG instruments which were synchronized by a digital clock. Only 4 channels of the 16-channel scalp recording are shown in this figure. Note the widespread spike-and-sharp-wave discharges in the depth of the temporal lobe on both sides, of which only one discharge is clearly reflected in the scalp recording in the left temporal region, as indicated by the black circle between channels 2 and 3. This was one of the few discharges which involved the left temporal neocortex at the lateral surface in the 2nd temporal convolution (LA5). LA and RA, anterior depth electrode array with the deepest contacts LA_1 and RA_1 in the left and right amygdala, respectively; LB and RB, intermediate depth electrode array with the deepest contacts LB_1 and RB_1 in the left and right hippocampus, respectively; LC and RC, posterior depth electrode array with contacts LC_1 and RC_1 in the left and right subicular regions of the parahippocampal gyrus, respectively. Contacts 1, 2, and 3 are 0.5 cm apart; all other contacts are 1 cm apart. The three depth electrode strands have been inserted through a horizontal approach penetrating the temporal lobe through the second temporal convolution. Electrode numbers 5 and 6 are in or near the cortex of the second temporal convolution. Electrode designations for the first 4 channels refer to positions of the standard 10–20 International System.

The main emphasis of these studies should be to record several of these. If anticonvulsant medication is withdrawn and the patient monitored constantly for 24 hr, it is usually possible to record at least 10 or more seizures in every patient. The interictal abnormalities, although usually very abundant in these records, have less diagnostic importance. It is a common observation that only few of them appear in simultaneous scalp records (Fig. 10). Such interictal discharges are helpful in that they allow evaluation of the extent and degree of bilaterality of the epileptogenic condition, but therapeutic decisions with regard to surgical treatment should be based primarily on the evidence provided by the recording of spontaneous seizures. In most patients, the clinical seizures have a very stereotyped electroencephalographic onset, from the point of view of both localization and electrographic pattern (Fig. 11). If one includes minor seizures which are associated with only very minimal clinical manifestations, it is quite possible to record in one patient as many as 100 ictal episodes; if all of them show the same area of onset, surgical therapy can obviously be recommended on the basis of strong objective criteria. One interesting aspect of these depth electrode recordings has been to show how many minimal clinical seizure manifestations completely escape the detection of even the most astute clinical observer. Unmistakable ictal discharges involving deep structures are sometimes associated with only very minute clinical changes, as for instance a very slight but stereotyped visceral sensation, some very simple behavioral automatism such as head-scratching or behavioral patterns not normally recognized as seizures. For example, one of our patients drank or asked for water each time a localized seizure discharge in limbic structures of the left temporal lobe occurred.

The final diagnostic evaluation of the results obtained with depth electrode exploration is based on the localization of the onset of spontaneous clinical seizures, including minimal ones which are recognized as seizure activity only because of the availability of concomitant depth electrode recordings. The localization of onset of electrographic seizures without any clinical accompaniments adds useful additional information. This localizing evidence derived from the recording of spontaneous seizures is further strengthened when electrical stimulation through deep contacts elicits the patient's aura or a full-blown habitual seizure with afterdischarge occurring or beginning in the same location as the initial electrographic events of the patient's spontaneous seizures (Figs. 11 and 12).

Conversely, if a patient shows multiple areas of seizure onset, surgical treatment may not be advisable. This is particularly true if some of the patient's seizures start on the right and some on the left side. In the face of a medically completely intractable seizure problem, however, a very occasional contralateral onset of a minor seizure may not be an absolute contra-indication to surgery, if it could be demonstrated that all or nearly all of the spontaneous seizures of the kind which are socially disabling to the patient always originated from the same side and from the same area.

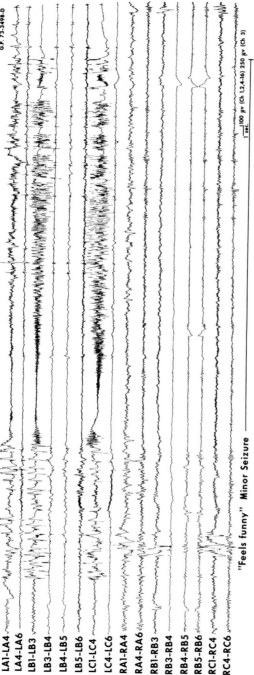

FIG. 11. Record of a spontaneous minor clinical seizure occurring in a patient with bilateral stereotactically implanted depth electrodes in the temporal lobes (same patient as in Fig. 10; for identification of electrode positions, see legend to Fig. 10). Note the onset of the seizure discharge from the left hippocampus (LB_1) and subiculum (LC_1) with virtually simultaneous lower voltage involvement of the left amygdala (LA_1). There was no spread of seizure activity to the contralateral side or toward the surface of the temporal lobe.

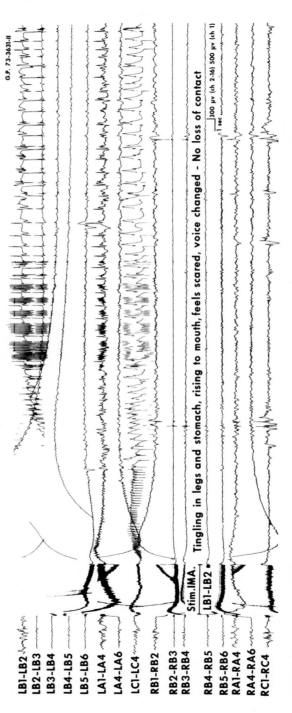

FIG. 12. Minor clinical seizure evoked by left anterior hippocampal stimulation (LB$_1$–LB$_2$) with a 1-mA current in a patient with bilateral, stereotactically implanted depth electrodes in the temporal lobes (same patient as in Figs. 10 and 11; for identification of electrode positions, see legend to Fig. 10). The electrically evoked seizure discharge had the same distribution as that shown in Fig. 11, which had arisen spontaneously. The clinical manifestations were similar to those observed in many of the recorded spontaneous minor seizures which had arisen from the same area.

ELECTROCORTICOGRAPHY

Purpose and Technique

The main purpose of electrocorticographic recording is to outline as accurately as possible the precise localization and extent of the epileptogenic area during the neurosurgical procedure.

The technical requirements for this method are relatively simple and straight-forward and have been described by a number of authors (Walker et al., 1947; Jasper, 1949*b;* Marshall and Walker, 1949; Penfield and Jasper, 1954; Ajmone-Marsan and Baldwin, 1958; Magnus, de Vet, van der Marel, and Meyer, 1962; Bates, 1963; Ajmone-Marsan, 1973). A sufficiently large number of electrodes (16) are required to cover the entire exposed cortical area with an adequate recording grid. The electrodes must be movable to make it possible to place them wherever this appears necessary. The simplest method to achieve this is to mount them on the tip of a thin silver rod covered with an insulating material and mounted on a ball joint which allows freedom of movement in all directions. An array of 16 electrodes can thus be mounted in four parallel rows on a rack (see Fig. 2 of Chapter 7) which can be attached to the patient's skull by means of a vertical metal bar screwed into or clamped to the bone edge at the craniotomy site. The electrodes at each end of a row can be replaced by flexible wire electrodes plugged into special outlets at the side of the electrode rack. These wire electrodes can be slipped into otherwise inaccessible regions such as the undersurface of the temporal or frontal lobe or the mesial surface of the hemisphere. The electrode rack also provides for plug-ins for reference electrodes which consist of small metal clamps attached to the bone edge of the craniotomy. The contact area of the electrode is made of a smooth ball of carbon or of silver–silver chloride surrounded by a cotton ball soaked in Elliott's solution. In addition to these surface electrodes, acute depth electrodes for recordings from deeper portions of the brain, usually the deep temporal structures (amygdala and hippocampus) are used. These are made of blunt needles and contain silver–silver chloride ring-shaped contact areas 1 cm apart over a distance of 3 cm (see Fig. 3 of Chapter 7).

It is advantageous to arrange the surface electrodes in a simple geometric pattern with nearly equal interelectrode distances in the horizontal and vertical direction. This permits recording along a row of electrodes in a straight line. If four parallel rows of four equidistant electrodes are used, bipolar electrode re-cordings in "horizontal" and "vertical" montages at right angles to each other can be carried out. This makes it possible to localize phase reversals of relevant abnormal potentials accurately to a particular electrode site. This is not possible when the bipolar recordings are run in only one direction. Erroneous localization could also result from montages that would use electrodes placed at quite unequal distances from each other, or in placements which may result in angulated bipolar chains of electrodes. Montages must be kept simple and straightforward in order to avoid errors in interpretation, especially since the latter must be carried out quickly while the record is running off the machine. Monopolar recordings should be used to clarify ambiguous or unclear localizations seen in bipolar recordings.

Any standard EEG recording apparatus with at least 12 channels is adequate for electrocorticography. It is advantageous to use a few simple preset runs which can be selected by a master switch. This helps to avoid errors that may occur when montages have to be selected by manual dialing of each individual electrode position. This is particularly important in electrocorticography, because the record must be interpreted immediately as the record is running off the machine. The electroencephalographer must be very experienced in interpreting records of epileptic patients in order to give quick and reliable diagnostic interpretations. It is equally important that the neurosurgeon have an adequate understanding of electrophysiological recording principles. This should include a working knowledge of the common sources of artifacts and of the methods used to avoid or correct them. The neurosurgeon must also be prepared to devote at least half an hour, and frequently longer, to the recording of the electrocorticogram.

The electrocorticogram should be recorded in the awake, locally anesthetized patient. Stress and anxiety can be reduced by giving the patient 10 μg of fentanyl and 2.5 mg of droperidol every 2 hr. These drugs exert no visible effect on the electrocorticogram. All general anesthetics have great drawbacks. If, however, the patient must be anesthetized because of lack of cooperation, preference should be given to short-acting barbiturate anesthetics, at least for the duration of the electrocorticogram, and the anesthesia should be kept as light as possible. Gaseous anesthetics such as halothane and nitrous oxide often eliminate the epileptiform abnormality completely. Even under barbiturate anesthesia, the epileptiform abnormality may well disappear or be more restricted than under normal conditions.

Electrocorticographic Patterns

Normal activities in the electrocorticogram of an awake patient are easily identified. As in the scalp EEG, the alpha rhythm predominates in the parieto-occipital regions and beta activity is frequently seen in the central areas. The former reacts to opening and closing of the eyes, the latter to voluntary movements or to the intention to carry out such movements. The alpha rhythm is more irregular and less abundant in the temporal region, a quite sharp demarcation line being seen often between suprasylvian and infrasylvian cortical regions, even in patients in whom there is little or no known temporal lobe pathology. It is rare to see the μ-rhythm in the central regions assume the same form as it does in the scalp EEG; it is usually much more irregular and its sharp components may simulate epileptic discharges. It is useful to test, under these conditions, whether this sharp activity in the central region responds well to individual finger movements of the contralateral hand, since this serves to distinguish these pseudo-spikes or sharp waves related to the μ-rhythm from true epileptiform discharges.

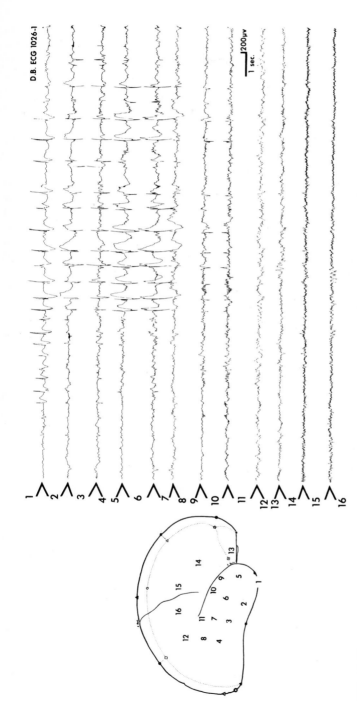

FIG. 13. Electrocorticogram taken from a patient with temporal lobe epilepsy. The positions of the electrodes are shown on the insert on the left side. Note the sequence of spike-and-wave discharges starting at electrode 1 on the undersurface of the right temporal lobe, spreading to the lateral surface, especially in the region of the second temporal convolution (electrodes 3 and 6), and to a lesser extent in the first temporal convolution (electrode 10). There was no spread to the cortex above the fissure of Sylvius (electrodes 13 to 16). (From P. Gloor, discussion in: *Aggression and Defense*, edited by C. D. Clemente and D. B. Lindsley, University of California Press, 1967.)

Abnormal activities in the electrocorticogram (Fig. 13) are essentially the same as those seen in the scalp EEG. Most of the epileptiform abnormalities recorded in electrocorticography are of the interictal type. The same criteria as in the scalp EEG serve to identify epileptiform abnormalities in the electrocorticogram. Brief spikes are seen much more often in the electrocorticogram than in the scalp EEG. For the biophysical reasons described earlier, such very brief epileptic spikes often cannot be recorded on the scalp. Otherwise the wave forms and features of the epileptiform activity on the exposed cortex are very similar to those seen in scalp recording (Fig. 13). Some of the spikes and especially some of the sharp waves may be conducted into relatively normal cortex from the primary epileptogenic area. Such conducted discharges are not always easy to identify; they usually, however, are somewhat blunter and longer in duration (because of time dispersion of afferent impulses), and appear in the midst of normal or relatively normal background activity. Primary epileptogenic discharge in the electrocorticogram almost never emerges from normal background activity. There is usually also some objective evidence that the brain is structurally abnormal in the region of the primary focus. Sometimes conducted epileptiform discharge can be recognized on the strength of the observation that it disappears when the intensity of the primary epileptogenic activity lessens only to reappear again upon recrudescence of the latter (Fig. 13).

Nonepileptiform abnormalities in the form of theta and delta waves and depression of the background activity are frequently seen in areas of cortical pathology. Although these features do not indicate the presence of an epileptic focus, they are nevertheless useful in outlining areas of brain damage.

Spontaneous electrographic or clinical seizures may also be recorded during electrocorticography, and often furnish the most reliable localizing signs which can be obtained during this procedure; their fortuitous occurrence, however, is infrequent.

Activation methods can also be helpful in electrocorticography. As in scalp electroencephalography, hyperventilation may sometimes bring out an otherwise nonexistent or unclear abnormality. In temporal lobe epileptics, the spike discharges are often activated by an intravenous injection of approximately 30 to 40 mg of methohexital of sufficient strength to anesthetize the patient lightly (Wilder, 1971). Such activation does not, however, occur invariably and barbiturate anesthesia may well mask the epileptiform abnormality instead of activating it. It should therefore be given only at the end of the pre-excision electrocorticogram.

Intravenous pentylenetetrazol activation is not recommended during an open craniotomy because it may easily lead to a generalized convulsion.

Electrical Stimulation

During the neurosurgical exploration of the epileptic brain in the awake patient, it is important to map out clinical and electrographic responses obtained with local electrical stimulation of the cortex, or of deep structures (usually the amygdala and hippocampus) into which depth electrodes have been inserted. One of the purposes of electrical stimulation is to localize areas concerned with motor and sensory functions and with speech, since encroachment upon these by surgical removal must be avoided.

Another purpose of electrical stimulation is to try to elicit the initial ictal event characterizing the patient's habitual seizures. This may be a sensory or psychic aura or a focal motor phenomenon (Penfield and Jasper, 1954). If the area from which such responses are elicited coincides with the region exhibiting the most active epileptic discharge, one can be more certain of having localized the patient's epileptogenic focus. Such a clinical response may be associated with a local or spreading afterdischarge (Fig. 14). The diagnostic value of the elicitation of the patient's initial ictal event is less if an afterdischarge occurs, especially if it spreads to distant areas, for the elicitation of the clinical symptomatology may in this case not be related to activation of local convulsive activity at the site stimulated, but may reflect the involvement of distant areas to which the discharge spread (Fig. 14).

It is important to record the electrocorticogram during electrical stimulation of the brain, because the stimulation may elicit afterdischarges; this, as already mentioned, is useful for the interpretation of clinical stimulation responses, and it also serves to warn the surgeon that one approaches the patient's convulsive threshold. The strength of stimulation must then be increased only if further information is necessary, and it must be carried out only with small increments in intensity.

Afterdischarges (Fig. 14) consist of rhythmic, usually stereotyped activity which may assume a variety of forms: high-frequency spikes, rhythmic sharp waves, spike-and-wave sequences, and others. The wave pattern is always distinctly different from the prestimulation activity at the same electrode sites. Afterdischarges usually end abruptly. They may remain localized or may spread slowly or occasionally with great rapidity to other regions. They represent electrically induced seizure activity which may or may not be associated with clinical signs or symptoms. The localization of the areas from which afterdischarges can be elicited are of doubtful validity in outlining the patient's epileptogenic region (Penfield and Jasper, 1954; Ajmone-Marsan, 1973). It is not uncommon that afterdischarges may be elicited from areas where quite normal electrocorticographic activity is recorded and where no spontaneous epileptiform activity is seen. If such afterdischarges are associated with clinical manifestations, these are usually quite different from those which the patient experiences in his habitual attacks. Very gross differences in afterdischarge thresholds between various areas may provide some suggestive evidence as to the localization of the patient's epileptogenic area, particularly if the low threshold area coincides with the region exhibiting active interictal epileptogenic discharges, but such differences are difficult to interpret, partly because each afterdischarge is followed by a very prolonged change in afterdischarge threshold. It would thus be hazardous to base any surgical decision on afterdischarge thresholds. More valid probably is the observation of a long-lasting afterdischarge associated with the patient's initial ictal symptoms and signs when it is elicited from and/or involves the region of the brain giving rise to active interictal epileptiform discharges (Walker, 1949).

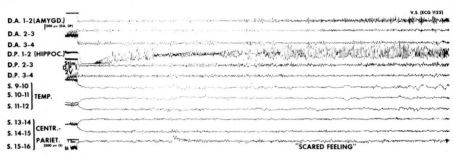

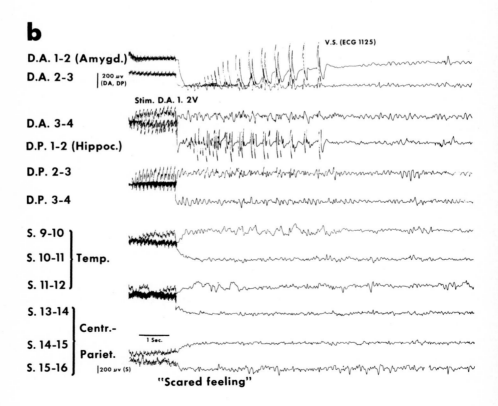

Postexcision Electrocorticogram

The electrocorticogram should be repeated after the excision of the epileptogenic area to determine if all epileptiform abnormality has been eliminated from the cortical electrogram. The effects of surgical trauma on the postexcision cortical electrogram are usually mild. Minimal to moderate slow-wave abnormality may be seen at the border of the excision. Very high voltage delta activity may occasionally appear in the postexcision record. This always raises the question of some ischemic complication in the area bordering the excision or of a white matter lesion underlying the cortex.

Two types of residual epileptogenic abnormalities must be distinguished: (1) the persistence of preexisting epileptogenic abnormality in areas not included in the excision because the area involved could not have been removed without causing an unacceptable neurological deficit; and (2) the appearance after cortical excision of epileptiform abnormality in regions where, prior to removal, this abnormality had been absent. It is difficult to account for this "activation by partial excision" (Penfield and Jasper, 1954), which is most frequently seen in rather widespread, diffuse cortical lesions.

The recording of postexcision electrocorticograms is of importance because of the relatively unfavorable long-range prognostic significance of persistent epileptiform abnormality in the postexcision electrocorticogram. We maintain this point of view in spite of the fact that some authors have doubted or denied that the postexcision electrocorticogram contains any useful prognostic information (Ajmone-Marsan and Baldwin, 1958; Gibbs, Amador, and Rich, 1958; Walker, Lichtenstein, and Marshall, 1960). Statistical follow-up studies in our series have shown that successful surgical therapy of focal epilepsy is more likely when the postexcision electrocorticogram contains no, or very minimal, residual epileptiform abnormality. Conversely, a large amount of residual epileptiform abnormality impairs the prognostic outlook (Jasper et al., 1951; Penfield and Jasper, 1954; Jasper, Arfel-Capdevielle, and Rasmussen, 1961; Bengzon et al., 1968).

←

FIG. 14. Electrical stimulation in the depth of the temporal lobe during electrocorticography which elicited the patient's habitual aura of fear.

a: Stimulation in the hippocampus produced an afterdischarge in the hippocampus which was not associated with any subjective or objective clinical manifestations; 17 sec later, the discharge spread to involve the amygdala. At that moment the patient spontaneously said that she had her "scared feeling." There was no spread of the afterdischarge to the surface of the temporal lobe.

b: Direct stimulation of the amygdala produced a brief afterdischarge and immediately evoked the feeling of fear. Again there was no spread of the afterdischarge to the temporal surface.

It seems clear that the evocation of the feeling of fear was dependent upon invasion of the amygdaloid grey matter by epileptic afterdischarge.

DA, anterior depth electrode with 4 contacts 1 cm apart, the deepest contact being located in the amygdala; DP, posterior depth electrode with 4 contacts 1 cm apart, the deepest contact being located in the hippocampus. The depth electrodes, illustrated in Fig. 3 of Chapter 7, were inserted through the second temporal convolution. S 9 to 16, surface cortical recording; S 9 to 12, on the surface of the temporal lobe; S 13 to 16, in the centro-parietal region. (From P. Gloor. In: *The Neurobiology of the Amygdala,* edited by B. Eleftheriou, Plenum Press, New York, 1972.)

These relationships are, however, of a statistical nature and the predictive value of the postexcision electrocorticogram for a given individual patient is relative.

The occurrence of spikes and sharp waves in the insula uncovered after temporal lobectomy represents a special case. Such insular spike and sharp wave activity has negligible prognostic significance: no statistically significant difference was found in the incidence of favorable outcomes of temporal lobectomy between patients with and without such abnormality (Silfvenius, Gloor, and Rasmussen, 1964). This is important, for the surgical removal of insular cortex is a hazardous procedure which may result in manipulation hemiplegia, presumably brought about by tugging on the middle cerebral vessels which may produce thrombosis or ischemia in the lenticulostriate arteries (Penfield, Lende, and Rasmussen, 1961).

POSTOPERATIVE ELECTROENCEPHALOGRAMS

The importance of the postoperative EEG is similar to that of the postexcision electrocorticogram. It serves to verify whether significant epileptiform abnormality remains after the removal, for its persistence is a factor which impairs the long-range prognostic outlook (Jasper et al., 1951; Penfield and Jasper, 1954; Jasper et al., 1961; Bengzon et al., 1968). Theoretically it would appear desirable to repeat the EEG under the same circumstances in which the preoperative EEGs were recorded. For instance, the absence of residual epileptiform abnormality in a waking postoperative record is relatively meaningless in a patient in whom the epileptiform abnormality had preoperatively been seen only during sleep. Also, if the abnormality had been present only when the patient was completely withdrawn from anticonvulsant medication, it would theoretically be desirable to repeat the postoperative EEG under identical conditions. It is obviously often impossible to satisfy these ideal conditions, and the postoperative EEG examination therefore suffers from a number of shortcomings. Nevertheless, it is useful to establish a baseline postoperative record about 10 days to 2 weeks following operation and then, if feasible, to carry out yearly follow-up EEG recordings. Early postoperative epileptiform abnormality often disappears over the years, often associated with a progressive lessening of seizure incidence. Of course the reverse may be seen, especially in patients with recurrent seizures. Thus postoperative EEGs taken a year or two after operation have more prognostic validity than those obtained earlier.

Postoperative EEGs sometimes show unspecific sharp background activity in the neighborhood of the excision. This is most often the case in the central region after temporal lobe removals that may or may not have encroached upon the suprasylvian cortex. Such activity is sometimes merely an exaggerated μ-rhythm which appears more like that in an electrocorticogram because of the presence of a skull defect in this area. In other instances, however, the sharp activity appears to be a genuine disturbance of the local background activity. For lack of a better term, one usually calls this a sign of "neighborhood irritation," a term partially vindicated by its occasional association with the occurrence of so-called "neighborhood" seizures in the early postoperative period. Like the latter, this abnormality is usually not indicative of an enduring epileptogenic condition, especially if such abnormality had not been seen in the preoperative recordings.

REFERENCES

Abraham, K., and Ajmone-Marsan, C. (1958): Patterns of cortical discharges and their relation to routine scalp electroencephalography. *Electroencephalogr. Clin. Neurophysiol.,* 10:447–461.

Ajmone-Marsan, C. (1973): Electrocorticography. In: *Handbook of Electroencephalography and Clinical Neurophysiology,* edited by A. Rémond, Volume 10, Part C. Elsevier, Amsterdam.

Ajmone-Marsan, C., and Baldwin, M. (1958): Electroencephalography. In: *Temporal Lobe Epilepsy,* edited by M. Baldwin and P. Bailey. Charles C Thomas, Springfield, Ill.

Ajmone-Marsan, C., and Ralston, B. L. (1957): *The Epileptic Seizure: Its Functional Morphology and Diagnostic Significance: A Clinical Electroencephalographic Analysis of Metrazol-Induced Attacks.* Charles C Thomas, Springfield, Ill.

Ajmone-Marsan, C., and Van Buren, J. M. (1958): Epileptiform activity in cortical and subcortical structures in the temporal lobe of man. In: *Temporal Lobe Epilepsy,* edited by M. Baldwin and P. Bailey. Charles C Thomas, Springfield, Ill.

Arnold, K., and Gerber, N. (1970): The rate of decline of diphenylhydantoin in human plasma. *Clin. Pharmacol. Ther.,* 11:121–134.

Ayala, G. F., Dichter, M., Gumnit, R. J., Matsumoto, H., and Spencer, W. A. (1973): Genesis of epileptic interictal spikes. New knowledge of cortical feedback systems suggests a neurophysiological explanation of brief paroxysms. *Brain Res.,* 52:1–17.

Bancaud, J. (1969): Physiopathogenesis of generalized epilepsies of organic nature (stereo-electroencephalographic study). In: *Physiopathogenesis of the Epilepsies,* edited by H. Gastaut, H. Jasper, J. Bancaud, and A. Waltregny. Charles C Thomas, Springfield, Ill.

Bancaud, J. (1971): Rôle du cortex cérébral dans les épilepsies 'généralisées' d'origine organique. Apport des investigations stéréotaxiques (SEEG) à la discussion de la conception 'centrencéphalique'. *Presse Méd.,* 79:669–673.

Bancaud, J. Geier, S., Talairach, J., and Scarabin, J. M. (1973): *E.E.G. et S.E.E.G. dans les Tumeurs Cérébrales et l'Epilepsie.* Edifor, Paris.

Bancaud, J., Talairach, J., Bonis, A., Schaub, G., Szikla, G., Morel, P., and Bordas-Ferer, M. (1965): *La Stéréo-électroencéphalographie dans l'Epilepsie.* Masson, Paris.

Bancaud, J., Talairach, J., Waltregny, A., Bresson, M., and Morel, P. (1968): L'activation par le Mégimide dans le diagnostic topographique des épilepsies corticales focales (étude clinique et EEG et SEEG). *Rev. Neurol. (Paris),* 119:320–325.

Bates, J. A. V. (1963): Special investigation techniques. Indwelling electrodes and electrocorticography. In: *Electroencephalography,* edited by D. Hill and G. Parr. Macmillan, New York.

Bengzon, A. R. A., Rasmussen, T., Gloor, P., Dussault, J., and Stephens, M. (1968): Prognostic factors in the surgical treatment of temporal lobe epileptics. *Neurology,* 18:717–731.

Bickford, R. G. (1956): The application of depth electrography in some varieties of epilepsy. *Electroencephalogr. Clin. Neurophysiol.,* 8:526–527.

Buchthal, F., and Lennox-Buchthal, M. A. (1972): Phenobarbital: Relation of serum concentration to control of seizures. In: *Antiepileptic Drugs,* edited by D. M. Woodbury, J. K. Penry, and R. P. Schmidt. Raven Press, New York.

Buchthal, F., Svensmark, O., and Simonsen, H. (1968): Relation of EEG and seizures to phenobarbital in serum. *Arch. Neurol.,* 19:567–572.

Calvet, C., Calvet, M. C., and Scherrer, J. (1964): Etude stratigraphique corticale de l'activité EEG spontanée. *Electroencephalogr. Clin. Neurophysiol.,* 17:109–125.

Celesia, G. G., and Paulsen, R. E. (1972): Electroencephalographic activation with sleep and methohexital. *Arch. Neurol.,* 27:361–363.

Cooper, R., Osselton, J. W., and Shaw, J. C. (1969): *EEG Technology.* Butterworths, London.

Cooper, R., Winter, A. L., Crow, H. J., and Walter, W. G. (1965): Comparison of subcortical, cortical and scalp activity using chronically indwelling electrodes in man. *Electroencephalogr. Clin. Neurophysiol.,* 18:217–228.

Crandall, P. H., Walter, R. D., and Rand, R. W. (1963): Clinical applications of studies on stereotactically implanted electrodes in temporal-lobe epilepsy. *J. Neurosurg.,* 20:827–840.

Cure, C., Rasmussen, T., and Jasper, H. (1948): Activation of seizures and electroencephalographic disturbances in epileptic and in control subjects with "Metrazol." *Arch. Neurol. Psychiatry,* 59:-691–717.

Delange, M., Castan, P., Cadilhac, J., and Passouant, P. (1962): Etude du sommeil de nuit au cours d'épilepsies centrencéphaliques et temporales. *Rev. Neurol.,* 106:106–113.

Delay, J., Verdeaux, G. and J., Drossopoulo, G., Schuller, E., and Chanoit, P. (1956): Un neurostimulant épileptogène, la mégimide. *Presse Méd.,* 64:1525–1527.

Dichter, M., and Spencer, W. A. (1969a): Penicillin-induced interictal discharges from the cat hippocampus. I. Characteristics and topographical features. *J. Neurophysiol.,* 32:649–662.

Dichter, M., and Spencer, W. A. (1969b): Penicillin-induced interictal discharges from the cat hippocampus. II. Mechanisms underlying origin and restriction. *J. Neurophysiol.,* 32:663–687.

Fischer, G., Sayre, G. P., and Bickford, R. G. (1961): Histological changes in the cat's brain after introduction of metallic and plastic-coated wire. In: *Electrical Stimulation of the Brain,* edited by D. E. Sheer. University of Texas Press, Austin.

Fischer-Williams, M., and Cooper, R. A. (1963): Depth recording from the human brain in epilepsy. *Electroencephalogr. Clin. Neurophysiol.,* 15:568–587.

Fourment, A., Jami, L., Calvet, J. and Scherrer, J. (1965): Comparaison de l'EEG recueilli sur le scalp avec l'activité élémentaire des dipoles corticaux radiaires. *Electroencephalogr. Clin. Neurophysiol.,* 19:217–229.

Garretson, H., Gloor, P., and Rasmussen, T. (1966): Intracarotid amobarbital and Metrazol test for the study of epileptiform discharges in man: A note on its technique. *Electroencephalogr. Clin. Neurophysiol.,* 21:607–610.

Gastaut, H. (1948): Présentation d'une électrode pharyngée bipolaire. *Rev. Neurol. (Paris),* 80:623–624.

Gastaut, H. (1955): Technique, indications and result of Metrazol activation. *Electroencephalogr. Clin. Neurophysiol.,* Suppl. 4:120–136.

Gastaut, H., and Broughton, R. (1972): *Epileptic Seizures: Clinical and Electrographic Features, Diagnosis and Treatment.* Charles C Thomas, Springfield, Ill.

Gastaut, H., Mouren, P., and Paillas, J. E. (1968): A propos de la "bisynchronie secondaire" en électroencéphalographie: paroxysmes bilatéraux synchrones et symétriques révélateurs d'un abscès temporal. *Rev. Neurol. (Paris),* 119:295–298.

Gibbs, E. L., and Gibbs, F. A. (1947): Diagnostic and localizing value of electroencephalographic studies in sleep. *Res. Publ. Assoc. Nerv. Ment. Dis.,* 26:366–376.

Gibbs, E. L., Fuster, B., and Gibbs, F. A. (1948a): Peculiar low temporal localization of sleep-induced seizure discharges of psychomotor type. *Arch. Neurol. Psychiatry,* 60:95–97.

Gibbs, E. L., Gibbs, F. A., and Fuster, B. (1948b): Psychomotor epilepsy. *Arch. Neurol. Psychiatry,* 60:331–339.

Gibbs, F. A. (1958): Abnormal electrical activity in the temporal region and its relationship to abnormalities of behavior. *Res. Publ. Assoc. Nerv. Ment. Dis.,* 36:278–292.

Gibbs, F. A., Amador, L., and Rich, C. (1958): Electroencephalographic findings and therapeutic results in surgical treatment of psychomotor epilepsy. In: *Temporal Lobe Epilepsy,* edited by M. Baldwin and P. Bailey. Charles C Thomas, Springfield, Ill.

Gloor, P. (1969): Neurophysiological bases of generalized seizures termed centrencephalic. In: *The Physiopathogenesis of the Epilepsies,* edited by H. Gastaut, H. Jasper, J. Bancaud, and A. Waltregny. Charles C Thomas, Springfield, Ill.

Gloor, P., Rasmussen, T., Garretson, H., and Maroun, F. (1964): Fractionized intracarotid Metrazol injection. A new diagnostic method in electroencephalography. *Electroencephalogr. Clin. Neurophysiol.,* 17:322–327.

Gloor, P., Tsai, C., and Haddad, F. (1958): An assessment of the value of sleep-electroencephalography for the diagnosis of temporal lobe epilepsy. *Electroencephalogr. Clin. Neurophysiol.,* 10:633–648.

Gloor, P., Vera, C. L., and Sperti, L. (1963): Electrophysiological studies of hippocampal neurons. I. Configuration and laminar analysis of the "resting" potential gradient, of the main-transient response to perforant path, fimbrial and mossy fiber volleys and of "spontaneous" activity. *Electroencephalogr. Clin. Neurophysiol.,* 15:353–378.

Goddard, G. V. (1967): Development of epileptic seizures through brain stimulation at low intensity. *Nature,* 214:1020–1021.

Goddard, G. V., McIntyre, D. C., and Leech, G. K. (1969): A permanent change in brain function resulting from daily electrical stimulation. *Exper. Neurol.,* 25:295–330.

Grinker, R. R. (1938): Method for studying and influencing cortico-hypothalamic relations. *Science,* 87:73–74.

Gumpert, J., and Paul, R. (1971): Activation of the electroencephalogram with intravenous Brietal (methohexitone): The findings in 100 cases. *J. Neurol. Neurosurg. Psychiatry,* 34:646–648.

Ives, J. R., Thompson, C. J., and Woods, J. F. (1973): Acquisition by telemetry and computer analysis of 4-channel long term EEG recordings from patients subject to "petit mal" absence attacks. *Electroencephalogr. Clin. Neurophysiol.,* 34:665–668.

Jasper, H. H. (1949*a*): Electrical signs of epileptic discharge. *Electroencephalogr. Clin. Neurophysiol.,* 1:11–18.

Jasper, H. H. (1949*b*): Electrocorticograms in man. *Electroencephalogr. Clin. Neurophysiol.,* Suppl. 2:16–29.

Jasper, H. H. (1949*c*): Etude anatomo-physiologique des épilepsies. *Electroencephalogr. Clin. Neurophysiol.,* Suppl. 2:99–111.

Jasper, H. H., Arfel-Capdevielle, G., and Rasmussen, T. (1961): Evaluation of EEG and cortical electrographic studies for prognosis of seizures following surgical excision of epileptogenic lesions. *Epilepsia,* 2:130–137.

Jasper, H., and Courtois, G. (1953): A practical method for uniform activation with intravenous Metrazol. *Electroencephalogr. Clin. Neurophysiol.,* 5:443–444.

Jasper, H. H., and Hawke, W. A. (1938): Electro-encephalography. IV. Localization of seizure waves in epilepsy. *Arch. Neurol. Psychiatry,* 39:885–901.

Jasper, H. H., and Kershman, J. (1941): Electroencephalographic classification of the epilepsies. *Arch. Neurol. Psychiatry,* 45:903–943.

Jasper, H. H., and Kershman, J. (1949): Classification of the EEG in epilepsy. *Electroencephalogr. Clin. Neurophysiol.,* Suppl. 2:123–131.

Jasper, H. H., Pertuiset, B., and Flanigin, H. (1951): EEG and cortical electrograms in patients with temporal lobe seizures. *Arch. Neurol. Psychiatry,* 65:272–290.

Kaufman, I. C., Marshall, C., and Walker, A. E. (1947): Activated electroencephalography. *Arch. Neurol. Psychiatry,* 58:533–549.

Kooi, K. A. (1966): Voltage-time characteristics of spikes and other rapid electroencephalographic transients: Semantic and morphological considerations. *Neurology,* 16:59–66.

Kopeloff, N., Chusid, J. G., and Kopeloff, L. M. (1954): Epilepsy produced in macaca mulatta with commercial aluminum hydroxide. *Electroencephalogr. Clin. Neurophysiol.,* 6:303–306.

Li, C. L., Cullen, C., and Jasper, H. (1956*a*): Laminar microelectrode analysis of cortical unspecific recruiting responses and spontaneous rhythms. *J. Neurophysiol.,* 19:131–143.

Li, C. L., Cullen, C., and Jasper, H. (1956*b*): Laminar microelectrode studies of specific somatosensory cortical potentials. *J. Neurophysiol.,* 19:111–130.

Lilly, J. C. (1961): The balanced pulse-pair form. In: *Electrical Stimulation of the Brain,* edited by D. E. Sheer. University of Texas Press, Austin.

Lilly, J. C., Hughes, J. R., Alvord, E. C., Jr., and Galkin, T. W. (1955): Brief non-injurious electric waveform for stimulation of the brain. *Science,* 121:468–469.

Lombroso, C. T. and Erba, G. (1970): Primary and secondary bilateral synchrony in epilepsy. A clinical and electroencephalographic study. *Arch. Neurol.,* 22:321–334.

MacLean, P. (1949): A new nasopharyngeal lead. *Electroencephalogr. Clin. Neurophysiol.,* 1:110–112.

Madsen, J. A., and Bray, P. F. (1966): The coincidence of diffuse electroencephalographic spike-wave paroxysms and brain tumours. *Neurology,* 16:546–555.

Magnus, O., de Vet, A. C., van der Marel, A., and Meyer, E. (1962): Electrocorticography during operations for partial epilepsy. *Develop. Med. Child. Neurol.,* 4:35–48.

Marshall, C., and Walker, A. E. (1949): Electrocorticography. *Johns Hopkins Hosp. Bull.,* 85:344–359.

Matsumoto, H., and Ajmone-Marsan, C. (1964*a*): Cortical cellular phenomena in experimental epilepsy: Interictal manifestations. *Exper. Neurol.,* 9:286–304.

Matsumoto, H., and Ajmone-Marsan, C. (1964*b*): Cortical cellular phenomena in experimental epilepsy: Ictal manifestations. *Exper. Neurol.,* 9:305–326.

Merlis, J. K., Grossman, C. H., and Henriksen, G. F. (1951): Comparative effectiveness of sleep and Metrazol-activated electroencephalography. *Electroencephalogr. Clin. Neurophysiol.,* 3:71–78.

Merlis, J. K., Henriksen, G. F., and Grossman, C. (1950): Metrazol activation of seizure discharges in epileptics with normal routine electroencephalograms. *Electroencephalogr. Clin. Neurophysiol.,* 2:17–22.

Musella, L., Wilder, B. J., and Schmidt, R. P. (1971): Electroencephalographic activation with intravenous methohexital in psychomotor epilepsy. *Neurology,* 21:594–602.

Niedermeyer, E. (1968): Considérations diagnostiques à propos de l'épilepsie généralisée dite "centrencéphalique." *Rev. Neurol. (Paris),* 118:514–522.

Niedermeyer, E., Laws, E. R., Jr., and Walker, A. E. (1969): Depth EEG findings in epileptics with generalized spike-wave complexes. *Arch. Neurol.,* 21:51–58.

Niedermeyer, E., and Rocca, U. (1972): The diagnostic significance of sleep electroencephalograms in temporal lobe epilepsy. *Europ. Neurol.,* 7:119–129.

Niedermeyer, E., Walker, A. E., and Burton, C. (1970): The slow spike-wave complex as a correlate of frontal and frontotemporal post-traumatic epilepsy. *Europ. Neurol.,* 3:330–346.

Pacella, B. L., Kopeloff, L. M., and Kopeloff, N. (1947): Electroencephalographic studies on induced and excised epileptogenic foci in monkeys. *Arch. Neurol. Psychiatry,* 58:693–703.

Pampiglione, G., and Kerridge, J. C. (1956): EEG abnormalities from the temporal lobe studied with sphenoidal electrodes. *J. Neurol. Neurosurg. Psychiatry,* 19:117–129.

Passouant, P. (1950): Séméiologie électroencéphalographique du sommeil normal et pathologique. *Rev. Neurol. (Paris),* 83:545–559.

Passouant, P., Cadilhac, J., and Delange, M. (1965): Indications apportées par l'étude du sommeil de nuit sur la physiopathologie des épilepsies. *Int. J. Neurol.,* 5:207–216.

Penfield, W., and Jasper, H. H. (1947): Highest level seizures. *Res. Publ. Assoc. Res. Nerv. Ment. Dis.,* 26:252–271.

Penfield, W., and Jasper, H. H. (1954): *Epilepsy and the Functional Anatomy of the Human Brain.* Little, Brown, Boston.

Penfield, W., Lende, R. A., and Rasmussen, T. (1961): Manipulation hemiplegia: An untoward complication in the surgery of focal epilepsy. *J. Neurosurg.,* 18:760–776.

Pertuiset, B., and Capdevielle-Arfel, G. (1951): Deux techniques particulières d'exploration basale. Les électrodes sphéno-ptérygoidiennes et orbitaires. *Rev. Neurol. (Paris),* 84:606–612.

Pope, A., Morris, A. A., Jasper, H., Elliott, K. A. C., and Penfield, W. (1947): Histochemical and action potential studies on epileptogenic areas of cerebral cortex in man and the monkey. *Res. Publ. Assoc. Res. Nerv. Ment. Dis.,* 26:218–233.

Porter, R. J., Wolf, A. A., and Penry, J. K. (1971): Human electroencephalographic telemetry. *Am. J. EEG Technol.,* 11:145–159.

Prince, D. A., and Futamachi, K. J. (1968): Intracellular recordings in chronic focal epilepsy. *Brain Res.,* 11:681–684.

Prince, D. A., and Wilder, B. J. (1967): Control mechanisms in cortical epileptogenic foci. "Surround" inhibition. *Arch. Neurol.,* 16:194–202.

Racine, R. J. (1972a): Modification of seizure activity by electrical stimulation: I. Afterdischarge threshold. *Electroencephalogr. Clin. Neurophysiol.,* 32:269–279.

Racine, R. J. (1972b): Modification of seizure activity by electrical stimulation: II. Motor seizure. *Electroencephalogr. Clin. Neurophysiol.,* 32:281–294.

Racine, R. J., Burnham, W. M., Gartner, J. G., and Levitan, D. (1973): Rates of motor seizure development in rats subjected to electrical brain stimulation: Strain and interstimulation interval effects. *Electroencephalogr. Clin. Neurophysiol.,* 35:553–556.

Rand, R. W., Crandall, P. H., and Walter, R. (1964): Chronic stereotactic implantation of depth electrodes for psychomotor epilepsy. *Acta Neurochir.,* 11:609–630.

Ribstein, M. (1960): *Exploration du cerveau humain par électrodes profondes. Electroencephalogr. Clin. Neurophysiol.,* Suppl. 16.

Rodin, E. A., Rutledge, L. T., and Calhoun, H. D. (1958): Megimide and Metrazol. A comparison of their convulsant properties in man and cat. *Electroencephalogr. Clin. Neurophysiol.,* 10:719–723.

Roubicek, J., and Hill, D. (1948): Electroencephalography with pharyngeal electrodes. *Brain,* 71:77–87.

Rovit, R. L., and Gloor, P. (1960): Temporal lobe epilepsy—A study using multiple basal electrodes. II. Clinical EEG findings. *Neurochirurgia,* 3:19–34.

Rovit, R. L., Gloor, P., and Henderson, L. R. (1960): Temporal lobe epilepsy—A study using multiple basal electrodes. I. Description of method. *Neurochirurgia,* 3:5–18.

Rovit, R. L., Gloor, P., and Rasmussen, T. (1961a): Intracarotid amobarbital in epilepsy. *Arch. Neurol.,* 5:606–626.

Rovit, R. L., Gloor, P., and Rasmussen, T. (1961b): Sphenoidal electrodes in the electroencephalographic study of patients with temporal lobe epilepsy: An evaluation. *J. Neurosurg.,* 2:151–158.

Sherwin, A. L., Eisen, A. A., and Sokolowski, C. D. (1973): Anticonvulsant drugs in human epileptogenic brain: Correlation of phenobarbital and diphenylhydantoin levels with plasma. *Arch. Neurol.,* 29:73–77.

Sherwin, I., and Hooge, J. P. (1973): Comparative effectiveness of natural sleep and methohexital. Provocative tests in electroencephalography. *Neurology,* 23:973–976.

Silfvenius, H., Gloor, P., and Rasmussen, T. (1964): Evaluation of insular ablation in surgical treatment of temporal lobe epilepsy. *Epilepsia,* 5:307–320.

Silverman, D. (1956): Sleep as a general activation procedure in electroencephalography. *Electroencephalogr. Clin. Neurophysiol.,* 8:317–324.

Smith, T. G., and Purpura, D. P. (1960): Electrophysiological studies on epileptogenic lesions of cat cortex. *Electroencephalogr. Clin. Neurophysiol.,* 12:59–82.

Spencer, W. A., and Brookhart, J. M. (1961*a*): Electrical patterns of augmenting and recruiting waves in depths of sensorimotor cortex of cat. *J. Neurophysiol.,* 24:26–49.

Spencer, W. A., and Brookhart, J. M. (1961*b*): A study of spontaneous spindle waves in sensorimotor cortex of cat. *J. Neurophysiol.,* 24:50–65.

Stevens, J. R. (1969): Localization of epileptic focus by protracted monitoring of EEG by radio telemetry. *Epilepsia,* 10:420.

Stewart, L. F. (1957): Chlorpromazine: Use to activate electroencephalographic seizure patterns. *Electroencephalogr. Clin. Neurophysiol.,* 9:427–440.

Stewart, L. F., and Dreifuss, F. E. (1967): "Centrencephalic" seizure discharges in focal hemispheral lesions. *Arch. Neurol.,* 17:60–68.

Storm van Leeuwen, W., Bickford, R., Brazier, M., Cobb, W. A., Dondey, M., Gastaut, H., Gloor, P., Henry, C. E., Hess, R., Knott, J. R., Kugler, J., Lairy, G. C., Loeb, C., Magnus, O., Oller Daurella, L., Petsche, H., Schwab, R., Walter, W. G., and Widén, L. (1966): Proposal for an EEG terminology by the terminology committee of the International Federation for Electroenceph-alography and Clinical Neurophysiology. *Electroencephalogr. Clin. Neurophysiol.,* 20:293–320.

Storm van Leeuwen, W., and Kamp, A. (1969): Radio telemetry of EEG and other biological variables in man and dog. *Proc. Royal Soc. Med.,* 62:451–453.

Talairach, J., Szikla, G., Tournoux, P., Prossalentis, A., Bordas-Ferer, M., Covello, L., Iacob, M., and Mempel, E. (1967): *Atlas d'Anatomie Stéréotaxique du Télencéphale.* Masson, Paris.

Torres, F., and Ellington, A. (1970): Metrazol Valium combination for EEG activation. *Electroencephalogr. Clin. Neurophysiol.,* 28:93–94.

Tükel, K., and Jasper, H. (1952): The electroencephalogram in parasagittal lesions. *Electroencephalogr. Clin. Neurophysiol.,* 4:481–494.

Walker, A. E. (1949): Electrocorticography in epilepsy. A surgeon's appraisal. *Electroencephalogr. Clin. Neurophysiol.,* Suppl. 2:30–37.

Walker, A. E., Johnson, H. C., and Kollros, J. J. (1945): Penicillin convulsions. The convulsive effects of penicillin applied to the cerebral cortex in monkey and man. *Surg. Gyn. Obst.,* 81:692–701.

Walker, A. E., Lichtenstein, R. S., and Marshall, C. (1960): A critical analysis of electroencephalogra-phy in temporal lobe epilepsy. *Arch. Neurol.,* 2:172–182.

Walker, A. E., Marshall, C., and Beresford, E. N. (1947): Electrocorticographic characteristics of the cerebrum in posttraumatic epilepsy. *Res. Publ. Assoc. Res. Nerv. Ment. Dis.,* 26:502–515.

Walker, A. E., and Ribstein, M. (1957): Chronic depth recording in focal and generalized epilepsy, an evaluation of the technique. *Arch. Neurol. Psychiatry,* 78:44–45.

Wilder, B. J. (1969): Activation of epileptic foci in psychomotor epilepsy. *Epilepsia,* 10:418.

Wilder, B. (1971): Electroencephalogram activation in medically intractable epileptic patients. Acti-vation technique including surgical follow-up. *Arch. Neurol.,* 25:415–426.

Wilder, B. J., Musella, L., Van Horn, G., and Schmidt, R. P. (1971): Activation of spike and wave discharge in patients with generalized seizures. *Neurology,* 21:517–527.

Advances in Neurology, Vol. 8, edited by D. P
Purpura, J. K. Penry, and R. D. Walter. Raven
Press, New York © 1975.

6
Pathologic Aspects of Epilepsy with Special Reference to the Surgical Pathology of Focal Cerebral Seizures

Gordon Mathieson

INTRODUCTION

This chapter is concerned with the pathology of epilepsy. The term pathology is, for our present purposes, interpreted in a restrictive sense and is considered to include the morphology of lesions, discussion of their probable etiology and pathogenesis, and some reference to their prognosis. This account is not intended as a critical review of factors such as genetic background and environmental influence which belong more appropriately in the earlier discussion of epidemiology in this volume (Chapter 1). Experimental animal models of epilepsy have been the subject of a previous volume (Purpura, Penry, Tower, Woodbury, and Walter, 1972) and will not be considered here.

Cerebral seizures are one manifestation, often a prominent or indeed predominant feature of a whole host of metabolic derangements, either temporary and correctable, or terminal, occurring in patients who are not habitual epileptics and in whom no question of neurosurgical therapy arises. Conditions such as hypoglycemia, overhydration during intravenous therapy, and advanced uremia belong in these categories. They lie outside the scope of this account. Intrinsic disorders of brain metabolism, such as Lafora's disease, have a distinctive cerebral pathology which may be demonstrated by cerebral biopsy but are not amenable to surgical therapy and by their diffuse nature are not likely ever to become so. They are not considered in this chapter.

A wide range of lesions, diverse with respect to their etiology, morphology, and likely outcome, is found in patients with habitual focal cerebral seizures who may be considered for surgical treatment. Added to this diversity is the observation that, in some cases, no convincing morphologic lesion is found. The disorder of brain function which results in the clinical syndrome of habitual seizures cannot, therefore, be neatly equated with a well-delineated morphologic substratum. In the case of focal cerebral seizures, the principal subject of this chapter, the discharge arises in one or more collections of viable neurons which may constitute a morphologically inconspicuous part of a much more extensive and readily recognizable lesion complex, for example, an arteriovenous malformation or glioma. A distinction must therefore be made between the histopathology of the non-neuronal element and the neuronal focus. The point has been put succinctly by Hughlings Jackson (1874): "No one can suppose that a tumour discharges. When we say that a tumour 'causes' convulsions, the only meaning the expression can have is that the tumour *leads* to instability of grey matter, which forms part of sensorimotor processes representing movements. The discharge causing the convulsion is of this unstable grey matter."

In many instances, this non-neuronal element gives a fairly clear-cut indication, at least to a first approximation, of the etiology, pathogenesis, and likely behavior of the lesion complex—for example in cases of tumor, vascular malformation, or hamartoma. In other instances, such as chronic focal encephalitis, assessing etiology and likely prognosis is more difficult. In yet other cases, changes in neuronal population with accompanying gliosis are the sole histopathologic features, and the other (causal) element in the lesion complex must be inferred—as being, for example, an episode of anoxia, with or without local ischemia, occurring in the perinatal period.

This chapter comprises a detailed pathologic study and analysis of material derived from just over 500 consecutive patients operated on for focal seizures together with a review of the relevant literature.

SURVEY OF PATHOLOGIC FINDINGS IN 503 CONSECUTIVE PATIENTS OPERATED ON FOR FOCAL CEREBRAL SEIZURES, 1961–70

Method

All patients in Montreal Neurological Hospital operated on for focal epilepsy during the decade 1961–70 were listed, their clinical records reviewed briefly, and the pathologic observations made at the time by both surgeon and pathologist reviewed in detail, the slides being restudied in an attempt to obtain consistency in interpretation and nomenclature. Operations were carried out on 506 patients. Tissue from three cases was not available for study and the cases have been excluded from this survey; the clinical and operative diagnoses on these three patients were arteriovenous malformation, arachnoid cyst, and postabscess scarring. Cases in which no histopathologic abnormality could be demonstrated or in which changes were trivial and probably of no causal significance have been retained, since they are considered to be important in overall evaluation of surgical rationale. This part of the chapter is therefore based on a study of 503 cases.

It should be emphasized that the patients in this series had cortical excisions or lobectomies carried out with the primary aim of reducing or abolishing the seizure tendency. Patients known to have had seizures as part of their neurologic syndrome but in whom the major aim of surgery was other than the relief of seizures, for example, clinically diagnosed intracranial tumor, were excluded. Of course, this distinction is to some extent arbitrary, since, clearly, the fresh onset of focal seizures in adult life gives rise to a strong diagnostic suspicion of tumor. To exclude all patients in whom a diagnosis of neoplasm was established by histopathologic examination would be even more arbitrary and would not reflect the wide spectrum of pathologic diagnoses found in patients selected for surgical treatment of their epileptic seizures. The patients in this study may be succinctly described as habitual epileptics thought likely to benefit from surgical therapy according to the criteria set forth elsewhere in this volume.

All material was studied by ordinary light microscopy after staining with a standard survey stain (either hematoxylin phloxin-safranin or hematoxylin and eosin) and a battery of stains including Holzer's method, phosphotungstic acid hematoxylin, Luxol fast blue-cresyl violet, Heidenhain's method for myelin, Bodian's silver method, and Cajal's gold chloride sublimate. Blocks were taken from each separate piece of tissue submitted by the surgeon; multiple blocks were taken from larger specimens. Serial sections were not used.

Tabular Summary and Analysis of Findings

The sites of surgical excision have been tabulated according to conventional neuroanatomic lobes, except that removals of Rolandic motor and sensory cortex, as delineated by cortical stimulation under local anesthesia, have been designated as "central" rather than apportioning them between frontal and parietal lobes. In each lobar site except central, some cases had formal lobectomies, while others had quite limited cortical excisions. The frequency of epileptic involvement on both sides of the Sylvian fissure, with removals involving both frontal and temporal lobes, seemed to merit a separate listing for such cases. Other cases with multiple lobe involvement, including patients coming to hemispherectomy, are listed separately; most such patients had massively destructive lesions as described by Rasmussen and Gossman (1963).

Inspection of Table 1, which correlates age at onset of seizures with lobe(s) involved, shows the preponderance of temporal lobe cases, forming three fifths of all cases. They are distantly followed by multilobe cases, combined frontal and temporal cases, frontal cases, and central cases. Parietal and especially occipital lobe cases are infrequent, the latter forming just under 1% of the whole series.

Table 2 presents the proportion of patients developing seizures below a specified age by lobe of involvement. Multilobed cases characterized for the most part by very destructive lesions, and further analyzed in Table 5, had a notably early age of onset: all 51 cases had begun having seizures by their 21st birthday.

Patients with central lesions, by contrast, tended to have seizures of relatively late onset: in less than 30% seizures had commenced by their 21st birthday and in less than 65%, by the age of 41. Reference to Table 5 shows that 19 of these 34 cases with central removals had gliomas which account for their late onset.

Table 3 shows that some three fifths of cases were operated on between the ages of 11 and 30. Again, multilobe and occipital cases were the subjects of early operation, while 41.2% and 31.3% of central and parietal cases, respectively, were over the age of 40 at the time of operation.

Table 4 lists all diagnoses made by histopathologic examination of tissue

TABLE 1. *Distribution of cases in 10-year sample, 1961–70, by age at onset of seizures and site (number of cases)*

Site	Age at onset								
	0–5	6–10	0–10	11–20	21–30	31–40	41–50	51+	All ages
Frontal	11	8	19	17	5	4	2	0	47
Temporal	71	61	132	103	38	18	9	1	301
Frontal and temporal	10	13	23	16	5	2	2	1	49
Central	4	2	6	4	3	9	10	2	34
Parietal	0	5	5	4	1	2	1	3	16
Occipital	2	2	4	1	0	0	0	0	5
Multilobe (mostly destructive lesions)	25	16	41	10	0	0	0	0	51
All sites	123	107	230	155	52	35	24	7	503

TABLE 2. *Proportion of cases in 10-year sample, 1961–70, with onset of seizures under certain ages, by site of lesion*

Site	Percentage of cases with onset			
	under 11 yr	under 21 yr	under 31 yr	under 41 yr
Frontal	40.4	76.6	87.2	95.7
Temporal	43.9	78.1	91.0	97.0
Frontal and temporal	46.9	79.6	89.8	93.9
Central	17.6	29.4	38.2	64.7
Parietal	31.3	56.3	62.5	75.0
Occipital	80.0	100		
Multilobe	80.4	100		
All sites	45.7	76.5	86.8	93.8

removed at operation on the 503 cases in the series. The range is wide. Some diagnoses may be regarded as precise and indicative of their etiology, e.g., tuberculoma, while others are more in the nature of descriptive labels which leave the etiology open to further interpretation, e.g., cortical neuronal loss and gliosis. Cases listed as showing minor abnormality (78 out of 503, 15.5%) had either subpial gliosis or perivascular rarefaction and gliosis in the white matter or both. Of the 503 consecutive cases studied, no abnormality could be found in 99 (19.7%). This observation is the subject of further analysis in Table 9 and subsequent discussion.

In Table 5, the lobar distribution of lesions has been correlated with the histopathologic diagnosis. For brevity and simplicity, some lesions appearing infrequently in Table 4 have been grouped together in subsequent tables as "all other lesions." The expression "pathologic category" has been used advisedly, since some of the terms are descriptive and inevitably lacking in etiologic precision, and may indeed represent the end stage of disparate pathologic processes.

Cerebral contusions are well known to occur most frequently in the frontal and temporal lobes, irrespective of their potential epileptogenicity, and this distribution is reflected in Table 5, only one patient having had a central contusion and none occurring in the parietal or occipital lobes. Most subacute or chronic focal encephalitic lesions involved multiple lobes, but in two cases there was only histologic evidence to implicate one frontal lobe and the adjacent central region. Of the three cases of Sturge-Weber disease (encephalo-facial angiomatosis), one was frontal and one temporal, contrary to the more usual occipital situation of the cerebral component of this disease. Cases characterized by ulegyria and those considered to be the end stage of infarction occurring in early life were almost exclusively multilobed in distribution. Of the 79 cases with only minor histopathologic abnormality, 64 were in the temporal lobe. Similarly, 78 out of the 99 cases in which no abnormality was detected histologically had temporal lobe removals. These puzzling cases are further analyzed in Table 9.

Tables 6 and 7 relate the age at onset of seizures and the age at operation,

TABLE 3. *Distribution of cases in 10-year sample, 1961–70, by age at operation and site of lesion (number of cases)*

Site	Age at operation								All ages
	0–5	6–10	0–10	11–20	21–30	31–40	41–50	51+	
Frontal	0	5	5	17	11	9	4	1	47
Temporal	0	1	1	99	97	56	35	13	301
Frontal and temporal	1	0	1	20	12	9	6	1	49
Central	0	2	2	6	4	8	11	3	34
Parietal	0	0	0	6	3	2	2	3	16
Occipital	0	2	2	2	0	1	0	0	5
Multilobe (mostly gross destructive lesions)	3	8	11	30	7	3	0	0	51
All sites	4	18	22	180	134	88	58	21	503

TABLE 4. *Histopathologic diagnoses established in 10-year sample,*
1961–70

Meningo-cerebral cicatrix and remote cerebral contusion	27
Posttraumatic cerebral atrophy	1
Residuum of cerebral abscess and/or pyogenic meningitis	6
Tuberculoma	1
Parasitic cyst	1
Subacute or chronic encephalitis (by histologic criteria)	8
Gliomas	80
Tumors, other than glioma	11
Remote tumor excision (probably complete)	2
Hamartomas	4
Tuberous sclerosis and formes frustes	10
Vascular malformations	14
Sturge-Weber disease and formes frustes	3
Arteriolosclerosis	2
Remote cerebral infarct, other than in early life	2
Residuum of infarct in early life	
by history probably perinatal	12
by history probably postnatal	1
Cortical neuronal loss and gliosis	55
Cortical neuronal loss and gliosis with glial nodules and	
epilepsia partialis continuans clinically	2
Cortical neuronal loss and gliosis and hippocampal	
sclerosis	21
Hippocampal sclerosis	46
Ulegyria	15
Destruction and gliosis predominantly of white matter	2
Minor abnormality[a]	78
No histopathologic abnormality found	99
All cases	503

[a] See text for definition.

respectively, to the various categories of lesion diagnosed microscopically. Certain features stand out. Patients with subacute or chronic encephalitis all became ill by their 10th year, as did patients presenting with epilepsia partialis continuans in whom glial nodules were a prominent feature of the cortical abnormality. Indeed, the two conditions may be related. The gliomas (which were nearly all astrocytomas or oligodendrogliomas or tumors with a mixture of both astrocytes and oligodendrocytes) gave rise to seizures in nearly equal numbers of patients in each of the first 5 decades, but only two occurred in the 51+ age group. This may well reflect the preponderance of anaplastic gliomas, i.e., glioblastoma multiforme, in the older age group and their exclusion from this series as not giving rise to habitual epilepsy in the sense of this study.

Many factors are involved in determining the time that elapses between the onset of seizures and their operative treatment. In addition to trials of medication, there are social factors and the ease of access to a suitable neurosurgical facility, which have no bearing on the biology of the disease process. Nevertheless, the interval between onset of seizures and operation has been set out in Table 8. In 69 of the 503 patients in the series, seizures had occurred for more than 20 years.

TABLE 5. Distribution of cases from 10-year sample, 1961–70, in certain pathologic categories by site of lesion (number of cases)

Pathologic category	Site of lesion							
	frontal	temporal	frontal and temporal	central	parietal	occipital	multi-lobe	All sites
Meningo-cerebral cicatrix and remote cerebral contusion	7	4	9	1	0	0	6	27
Subacute and chronic encephalitis	1	0	0	1	0	0	6	8
Vascular malformation	2	6	1	2	2	0	1	14
Sturge-Weber disease and formes frustes	1	1	0	0	0	0	1	3
Hamartoma	0	1	1	1	1	0	0	4
Tuberous sclerosis and formes frustes	5	3	1	0	1	0	0	10
Glioma	12	38	5	19	4	2	0	80
Cortical neuronal loss and gliosis	3	37	8	2	1	0	4	55
Cortical neuronal loss and gliosis with glial nodules and epilepsia partialis continuans clinically	0	0	0	1	0	0	1	2
Cortical neuronal loss and gliosis and hippocampal sclerosis	0	20	1	0	0	0	0	21
Ulegyria	0	0	0	0	0	1	14	15
Hippocampal sclerosis	0	42	2	0	0	0	2	46
Residuum of infarct in early life	0	0	0	0	0	0	13	13
Minor abnormality	2	64	11	1	0	0	0	78
All other lesions	7	6	1	5	5	1	3	28
No abnormality found	7	79	9	1	2	1	0	99
All lesions	47	301	49	34	16	5	51	503

TABLE 6. *Distribution of cases in certain pathologic categories by age at onset of seizures (number of cases)*

Pathologic category	Age at onset of seizures								All ages
	0–5	6–10	0–10	11–20	21–30	31–40	41–50	51+	
Meningo-cerebral cicatrix and remote cerebral contusion	2	3	5	15	6	1	0	0	27
Subacute and chronic encephalitis	4	4	8	0	0	0	0	0	8
Vascular malformation	1	0	1	7	4	1	1	0	14
Sturge-Weber disease and formes frustes	2	0	2	1	0	0	0	0	3
Hamartoma	2	0	2	1	0	1	0	0	4
Tuberous sclerosis and formes frustes	6	3	9	1	0	0	0	0	10
Glioma	5	9	14	14	15	20	15	2	80
Cortical neuronal loss and gliosis	15	16	31	19	3	2	0	0	55
Cortical neuronal loss and gliosis with glial nodules and epilepsia partialis continuans clinically	2	0	2	0	0	0	0	0	2
Cortical neuronal loss and gliosis and hippocampal sclerosis	7	6	13	6	2	0	0	0	21
Ulegyria	11	2	13	2	0	0	0	0	15
Hippocampal sclerosis	18	13	31	10	3	2	0	0	46
Residuum of infarct in early life	6	5	11	2	0	0	0	0	13
Minor abnormality	17	24	41	28	6	2	1	0	78
All other lesions	1	4	5	9	1	2	6	5	28
No abnormality found	24	18	42	40	12	4	1	0	99
All lesions	123	107	230	155	52	35	24	7	503

Five patients of the 80 diagnosed as having a glioma had had seizures for 21 years or more; although astrocytomas are known sometimes to behave in a very indolent fashion, the possibility exists that in some of these cases neoplasia supervened on a preexisting focus of gliosis.

Cases Without Convincing Histopathologic Abnormality

Table 5 records that in 99 of the whole series of 503 cases no abnormality was found on microscopic examination of the excised tissue. In a further 78 cases, the only changes that could be found were considered to be minor and unlikely to play any role in the genesis of the patient's epilepsy. The latter group, of course, involves a subjective judgement of what pathologic role such changes might play. Nevertheless, it is disturbing for the pathologist to gaze at field after field of

TABLE 7. *Distribution of cases in certain pathologic categories by age at operation (number of cases)*

Pathologic category	Age at operation								All ages
	0–5	6–10	0–10	11–20	21–30	31–40	41–50	51+	
Meningo-cerebral cicatrix and remote cerebral contusion	0	0	0	10	9	4	4	0	27
Subacute and chronic encephalitis	2	3	5	3	0	0	0	0	8
Vascular malformation	0	0	0	4	4	4	2	0	14
Sturge-Weber disease and formes frustes	0	2	2	1	0	0	0	0	3
Hamartoma	0	0	0	2	1	1	0	0	4
Tuberous sclerosis and formes frustes	0	1	1	6	3	0	0	0	10
Glioma	0	2	2	16	10	26	20	6	80
Cortical neuronal loss and gliosis	0	1	1	25	13	6	7	3	55
Cortical neuronal loss and gliosis with glial nodules and epilepsia partialis continuans clinically	1	0	1	1	0	0	0	0	2
Cortical neuronal loss and gliosis and hippocampal sclerosis	0	0	0	9	7	3	0	2	21
Ulegyria	0	5	5	7	2	1	0	0	15
Hippocampal sclerosis	0	0	0	19	15	9	2	1	46
Residuum of infarct in early life	1	2	3	8	1	1	0	0	13
Minor abnormality	0	0	0	28	31	10	8	1	78
All other lesions	0	1	1	5	5	5	6	6	28
No abnormality found	0	1	1	36	33	18	9	2	99
All lesions	4	18	22	180	134	88	58	21	503

apparently normal brain tissue in about 20% of specimens removed during the surgical therapy of focal seizures. Several factors may operate, either singly or in combination in these cases:

(1) Pathologist observer error. A loss of, say, 10% of cortical neurons would probably not be detectable, especially if there was no confirmatory reactive gliosis, but the pathophysiologic effects of such a loss might be considerable. None of our cases has been subject to quantitative histology, and the methodologic problems and establishment of normals would be formidable.

(2) The techniques customarily used do not show all neural structures. Dendrites and synaptic organization, for example, are not displayed.

(3) Removal of small amounts of brain by suction may deny the pathologist an essential part of the specimen.

(4) The pathologist may miss a small lesion by injudicious selection of blocks.

TABLE 8. *Interval between onset of seizures and operation in patients forming 10-year sample, 1961–70, by certain pathologic categories (number of cases)*

Pathologic category	Interval (yr)						All intervals
	0–5	6–10	11–15	16–20	21–25	26+	
Meningo-cerebral cicatrix and remote cerebral contusion	11	5	6	1	3	1	27
Subacute and chronic encephalitis	7	1					8
Vascular malformation	6	5	1	1	1		14
Sturge-Weber disease and formes frustes		3					3
Hamartoma	1		3				4
Tuberous sclerosis and formes frustes	2	3	3		2		10
Glioma	42	21	11	1	2	3	80
Cortical neuronal loss and gliosis	7	17	8	13	3	7	55
Cortical neuronal loss and gliosis with glial nodules and epilepsia partialis continuans clinically	1		1				2
Cortical neuronal loss and gliosis and hippocampal sclerosis	2	5	2	6	3	3	21
Ulegyria	4	5	1	5			15
Hippocampal sclerosis	5	13	12	9	1	6	46
Residuum of infarct in early life	6	3	1	2	1		13
Minor abnormality	15	19	20	14	2	8	78
All other lesions	17	5	1	3	2		28
No abnormality found	18	29	18	13	7	14	99

This is unlikely and can be avoided by the use of serial sections as practised by Falconer, Serafetinides, and Corsellis (1964).

(5) The essential abnormality may be biochemical rather than structural. The studies of van Gelder, Sherwin, and Rasmussen (1972) are instructive in this respect. They found low levels of glutamic acid and taurine contrasting with high levels of glycine in epileptogenic cortical foci, as identified by electrocorticography, when compared with surrounding peripheral cortex. Tissue from some of these foci showed no histopathologic abnormality.

(6) The essential discharging focus may be elsewhere than the site of surgical removal.

To investigate this problem further, the histopathologic findings in a series of temporal lobe cases were compared with the observations recorded by the surgeon at the time of operation. The results are given in Table 9. Discrete focal lesions such as tumors and hamartomas are not in contention and have been omitted from the table, which covers 117 otherwise consecutive temporal lobe cases operated on over the 5-year period 1961 through 1965. Observations on the temporal neocortex and on the hippocampus have been tabulated. The technique of surgical removal by suction has precluded a systematic study of the amygdaloid nucleus; in some instances, the hippocampus, although clearly identified by the surgeon and partially removed by him, had not been suitably prepared for microscopic examination. In 20 of the 117 cases, the records did not lend themselves to a confident, unequivocal classification in this form.

Table 9 shows that in only two of the 97 cases tabulated was the surgeon in

TABLE 9. *Comparison of surgical observations and histopathologic findings in certain cases of temporal lobe removals, 1961 through 1965 (number of cases)*

Histopathologic findings	Observations at operation					
	objective surgical abnormality in neocortex	objective surgical abnormality in hippocampus	objective surgical abnormality in both neocortex and hippocampus	doubtful or no objective surgical abnormality	insufficient data to tabulate	Totals
Neocortical neuronal loss and gliosis only (hippocampus not examined)	10	1	9	0	4	24
Neocortical neuronal loss and gliosis and hippocampal sclerosis	1	2	10	0	1	14
Hippocampal sclerosis only	1	11	6	0	4	22
Minor abnormality histologically, hippocampus examined histologically	3	2	3	0	0	8
Minor abnormality histologically, hippocampus not examined histologically	9	6	7	0	2	24
No abnormality histologically, hippocampus examined histologically	1	0	1	0	3	5
No abnormality histologically, hippocampus not examined histologically	9	1	2	2	6	20
Totals	34	23	38	2	20	117

any doubt about the presence of abnormality in some temporal region; in neither of these two cases was the hippocampus examined histologically. Twelve cases showing no histologic abnormality but lacking histologic study of the hippocampus were reported by the surgeon as having neocortical abnormality in nine cases, hippocampal abnormality in one, and both neocortical and hippocampal abnormality in two. The lack of agreement between histopathologist and surgeon, therefore, can only to a small extent be attributed to failure to examine the hippocampus histologically. A similar conclusion can be drawn from that part of the table dealing with minor histologic abnormalities.

Clues to Etiology from the Clinical History

The largest etiologic problem is presented by those cases which have diffuse atrophic lesions of varying extent involving the temporal or the frontal and temporal lobes. The clinical records of 132 consecutive patients in these categories

TABLE 10. *Incidence of difficult birth and febrile convulsions in childhood, as recorded in the clinical histories of patients with other than discrete focal lesions in the temporal, and frontal and temporal lobes, 1961 through 1965 (number of cases)*

Site of surgical excision	Birth history			Febrile convulsions		Totals
	difficult birth	history uncertain	history normal	occurred in childhood	did not occur in childhood	
Temporal	22	71	24	24	93	117
Frontal and temporal	2	9	4	3	12	15

were studied in a search for etiologic clues. The views of Earle, Baldwin, and Penfield (1953) regarding transtentorial herniation at birth as a cause of brain damage, especially of medial temporal structures ("incisural sclerosis"), and the opinions of Falconer and his colleagues (Meyer, Falconer, and Beck, 1954; Falconer, Serafetinides, and Corsellis, 1964; Falconer, 1968) on the significance of febrile convulsions in childhood, made a survey of the early medical history of these patients mandatory. The criteria for "difficult birth" are hard to establish when taken as part of a clinical history years later, but neonatal asphyxia, very prolonged labor, and prematurity were considered to be reasonable indicators. Unfortunately, 71 of the 117 temporal lobe cases had to be listed as "birth history uncertain"; 9 of the 15 frontal and temporal cases were similarly listed. The results given in Table 10 indicate an almost equal incidence of difficult birth and febrile convulsions in childhood.

Comparison with Published Series

Early accounts of the pathology of focal epilepsy consisted for the most part of individual case reports with emphasis on their value in establishing localization of cerebral function, e.g., Jackson and Beevor (1889) and Jackson and Colman (1898).

Foerster and Penfield (1930) made a systematic study of cases of posttraumatic seizures, recording seven cases in detail, and emphasizing the proliferation of connective tissue and blood vessels in the excised meningo-cerebral scars. A wider range of pathology, comprising expanding and atrophic lesions, was analyzed by Penfield and Jasper (1954). Of 64 cases with astrocytoma, 70% had seizures, while of 103 cases of glioblastoma only 37% had seizures, a difference that the authors ascribe largely to the difference in the time scale in progression of the tumors. These authors illustrate ulegyria (microgyria) and stress the importance of circulation in the border zone of the lesion as a potential trigger mechanism for seizures.

Falconer and his colleagues have described their pathologic findings in patients with focal epilepsy arising in temporal lobe structures in a series of papers (Meyer, Falconer, and Beck, 1954; Falconer and Cavanagh, 1959; Falconer, Serafetinides, and Corsellis, 1964; Falconer and Taylor, 1968), their studies being facilitated by the surgical technique of block resection, which permits systematic tissue sampling and anatomically oriented serial sectioning. Some 24% of their patients had small, tumor-like lesions, 47% had mesial temporal sclerosis, 13% had focal scarring, and 22% had what the authors termed equivocal lesions; in these, the nerve cells were normal and only subpial and white matter gliosis was present (Falconer et al., 1964). It is interesting that one fifth of cases showing no significant abnormality should occur in a series scrutinized in such detail pathologically; this corresponds well with the incidence of negative findings in this present series. In their 1968 paper, Falconer and Taylor record no lesion or only nonspecific gliosis in 25% of cases.

Green and Scheetz (1964) carried out unilateral temporal lobectomy in 78 patients (out of over 2,500 screened) and found 14 neoplasms, 50 "chronic atrophic lesions," and, in 14 cases (17.9%), no demonstrable pathology. Some 20.5% of their patients had a history of difficult birth (not further defined).

In a valuable postmortem study, Margerison and Corsellis (1966) examined the brains of 55 patients out of a population of 650 institutionalized epileptics who had been investigated clinically and electroencephalographically. Of these autopsied patients, 26 were considered on clinical grounds to have had temporal lobe epilepsy; hippocampal sclerosis was found in 22 of these. In 13 patients considered not to have had temporal lobe epilepsy, no hippocampal sclerosis was found in 8. The correlation between hippocampal sclerosis demonstrated at autopsy and the clinical diagnosis of temporal lobe epilepsy is significant at the 0.01 level. In 21 of the 22 patients with hippocampal sclerosis, hypoxic damage was seen elsewhere in the brain; the cerebellum was affected in 14, the amygdaloid nucleus in 14, and the thalamus in 11. Of the 14 patients in whom hippocampal damage was restricted to the end folia, there was hypoxic damage elsewhere in only 6 cases. The mean age at onset of seizures in patients with classical Ammon's horn sclerosis was 6 years, whereas in end folium sclerosis it was 16 years (difference significant at the 0.01 level). Thus patients with an early onset of seizures tend to have classical Ammon's horn sclerosis and hypoxic damage elsewhere in the brain.

SELECTED LESIONS

Many of the neuropathologic observations recorded in the preceding section differ in no essential way from those which may be made on material from a nonepileptic population. The point has been put forcefully by Crome (1955) in connection with diffuse lesions of the temporal lobes. It is even more cogent when applied to discrete lesions such as vascular malformations and gliomata. We have nothing to add to the detailed descriptions of brain tumors given by Rubinstein (1972) and by Russell and Rubinstein (1971). Other lesions, however, present in novel ways or otherwise merit description, illustration, and discussion.

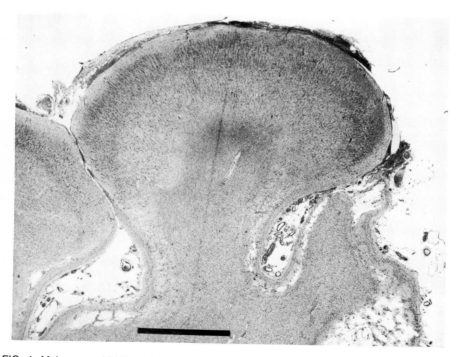

FIG. 1. Male, normal birth and early development, febrile illness at 1 year of age, onset of seizures at 3½ yr. Left homonymous hemianopsia and left cortical-type sensory deficit. Excision of right occipital, temporal, and parietal lobes at 23 yr. Pathologically, extensive ulegyria. Luxol blue-cresyl violet stain. Scale marker 2 mm.

Ulegyria

This term is applied to an individual gyrus or group of gyri (sclerotic microgyria) which, on section, have a mushroom-like shape. This is the end result of destruction of the cortex forming the walls and depths of sulci with sparing of the cortical crown of the gyrus (Fig. 1). The stem of the deformed gyrus is intensely gliosed (Fig. 2) and may, in extreme cases, show linear cavitation.

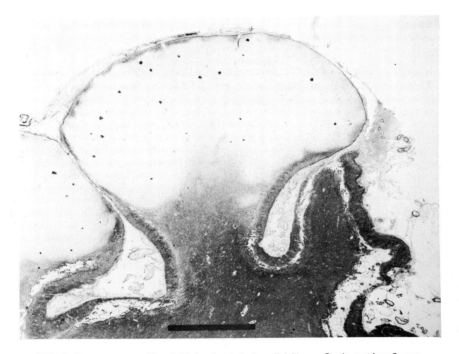

FIG. 2. Same case as Fig. 1. Holzer's stain for glial fibers. Scale marker 2 mm.

Ulegyria may occur in arterial boundary zones or within the territory of distribution of individual arteries as described by Norman, Urich, and McMenemy (1957) and by Norman (1963). Such lesions are attributed by these authors to impaired arterial perfusion consequent on arterial compression, often combined with systemic hypoxia occurring during difficult childbirth (see also Figs. 3 and 4), but may occur in the course of febrile illness in early childhood as illustrated in Figs. 1 and 2.

In the present series, cases with ulegyria as the pathologic substratum tended to have seizures at an early age (11 out of 15 under 6 years and all but two before their 11th birthday, Table 6), but operation was deferred until after 21 years in three cases (Table 7).

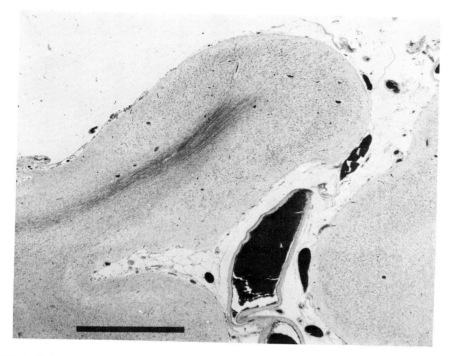

FIG. 3. Male, face presentation and forceps delivery, seizure on second day of life, onset of habitual seizures at 3 yr; left-sided weakness. Right hemispherectomy at 7 yr. Pathologically, multiple foci of ulegyria. Luxol blue-cresyl violet stain. Scale marker 2 mm.

Residuum of Infarction Occurring in Early Life

Fairly well demarcated destructive lesions occurring within the territory of the larger cerebral arteries are most readily and appropriately identified as infarcts. Most of these in the present series were in middle cerebral artery territory, but a few were clearly in the region of posterior cerebral artery supply. Narrow margins with an abrupt change from total devastation to apparently normal brain was the rule (Fig. 5), but occasionally a narrow rim of ulegyria was also present. In most instances the clinical history recorded that hemiparesis was apparent within the first few months of life, while seizures developed several years later.

Extensive cavitation, unilocular or with branching strands giving a multiloculated appearance, is frequent in these infarcts, and gives rise to the term porencephalic cyst. Such lesions are examples of encephaloclastic porencephaly differing in origin from the "prenatal porencephalies" or "schizencephalies" as distinguished by Yakovlev and Wadsworth (1946).

The etiology of these infarcts is not clear. In many instances there is a history of perinatal distress and asphyxia, but this is not invariable. Clark and Linell (1954) have reported a case of neonatal embolus occluding one internal carotid

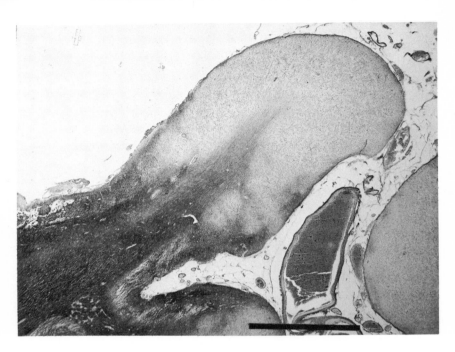

FIG. 4. Same case as Fig. 3. Holzer's stain for glial fibers. Scale marker 2 mm.

and middle cerebral artery and producing cerebral infarction in a neonate; they considered the embolus as probably composed of necrotic placenta. Crome (1958) described multilocular cystic encephalomalacia in an infant dying at the age of 3½ months in whom organized venous thrombi were present and branches of the middle cerebral artery showed rather cribriform subendothelial connective tissue proliferation which the author regarded as likely to be the sequel of old thrombosis. Norman and Urich (1957) have recorded dissecting aneurysm of the stem of the middle cerebral artery occurring in a 6-month-old infant associated with the abrupt onset of hemiparesis and persistent seizures, but such cases must be rare.

Lesions of blood vessels were not commonly found in the material of the present series. An exception was in a child who developed right hemiparesis associated with mastoiditis at 14 months: seizures began at 4 years; operation at 8 years revealed a cavitated lesion in the left cerebrum; histologically pial vessels had thickened walls, some with mineral deposition (Fig. 6).

Hamartomas

These may be neuronal, glial, meningeal, or any combination of these types. Cavanagh (1958) has drawn attention to "certain small tumours encountered in the temporal lobe" of patients operated on for temporal lobe seizures by Falconer

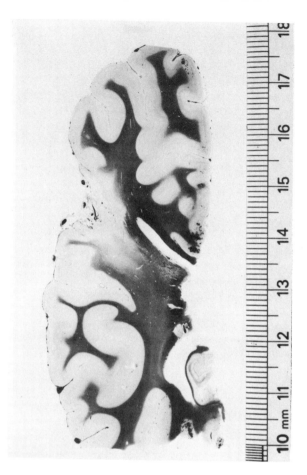

FIG. 5. Female, right-sided weakness noted at 18 months of age, frequent seizures began at 7 yr. Hemispherectomy at 14 yr. Pathologically, old infarct involving left central, parietal, temporal, and lateral occipital lobes. Coronal section of specimen. Luxol blue-cresyl violet stain. Scale in mm.

at the Guy-Maudsley Neurosurgical Unit. At the time of reporting, such lesions were found in 10 to 12% of temporal lobes removed for seizures. In some cases the abnormality took the form of multiple nodular clusters of cells. In two, neurons took part in the lesion and gave a diagnostic impression of tuberous sclerosis although the other features of this disease were not observed. In the present series, similar cases have been classified as formes frustes of tuberous sclerosis and are discussed below. In the other six cases the cellular cluster were glial, both astrocytes and oligodendrocytes being identified. The author regarded all such lesions as hamartomas partly because of their static biologic behavior; whether they might form the starting point for an aggressive glial neoplasm is uncertain.

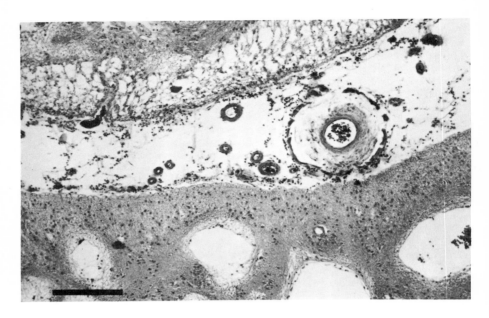

FIG. 6. Male, onset of hemiplegia at 14 months during mastoiditis, seizures began at 4 yr. Operation at 8 yr showed cavitated lesion. Photomicrograph shows thickened pial vessel with mineral deposition and underlying fenestrated cortex. Hematoxylin, phloxin, and safranin stain. Scale marker 200 microns.

Another form of arguably hamartomatous lesion with a prominent neuronal component is the ganglioglioma, fully depicted by Rubinstein (1972). The abundant connective tissue element seen in the indolent forms is shown in Fig. 7.

In meningiomatosis, well-defined segments of cortex are replaced by stretches of tissue resembling meningioma with scattered psammoma bodies and occasional included neurons (Figs. 8 and 9).

Tuberous Sclerosis and Formes Frustes

Patients with the fully developed syndrome of tuberous sclerosis are readily recognizable clinically. The value of surgical excision of one or more of their cortical tubers is problematic, although in carefully selected cases good results with respect to seizures may be obtained as reported by Perot, Weir, and Rasmussen (1966). There are, however, occasional patients in whom operation for focal cerebral seizures yields tissue which, on gross and microscopic examination, shows changes indistinguishable from the cerebral lesions of tuberous sclerosis, although there may be no other clinical or laboratory evidence of the disease complex (Figs. 10–14). The lesions are distinct from those of pachygyria using the criteria laid down by Norman (1963). Most of the patients are within the normal intelligence range. Some, however, are mildly to moderately retarded.

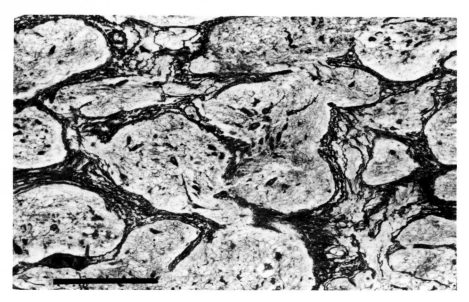

FIG. 7. Male, onset of seizures at 15 yr of age. Mass removed from left frontal lobe at 17 yr. Pathologically, ganglioglioma. Photomicrograph shows sparse stellate neurons embedded in glial tissue traversed by anastomosing strands of connective tissue. Laidlaw's silver method. Scale marker 200 microns.

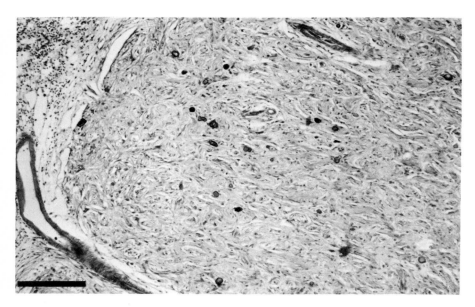

FIG. 8. Female, seizures began at 2 yr of age, equivocal left-sided neurologic signs, right-sided cerebral atrophy in pneumogram. Operation at 17 yr revealed stony hard tissue replacing part of right central cortex. Histopathologically, meningiomatosis. Photomicrograph shows meningioma-like tissue replacing cortex; leptomeninges at left. Hematoxylin, phloxin, and safranin stain. Scale marker 200 microns.

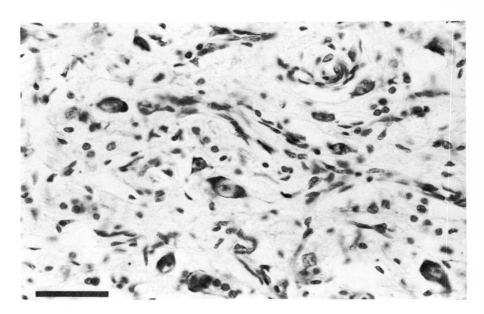

FIG. 9. Same case as Fig. 8. Included neurons in meningiomatosis. Cresyl violet stain. Scale marker 50 microns.

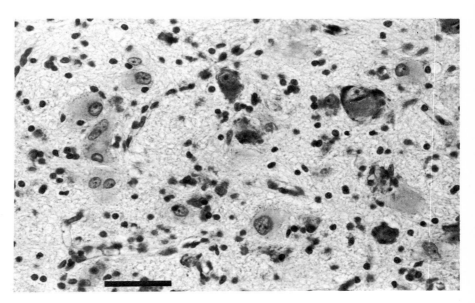

FIG. 10. Male aged 12 yr, uncontrolled seizures and moderate mental retardation, other features of tuberous sclerosis present. Operation: left frontal lobectomy guided by consistent EEG focus. Photomicrograph shows haphazardly arranged abnormal neurons and glia from cortical tuber. Luxol blue-cresyl violet stain. Scale marker 50 microns.

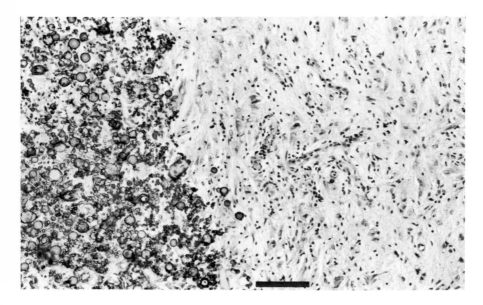

FIG. 11. Tuberous sclerosis, complete complex. Calcareous deposits on left of field, proliferating glia on right. Cresyl violet stain. Scale marker 100 microns.

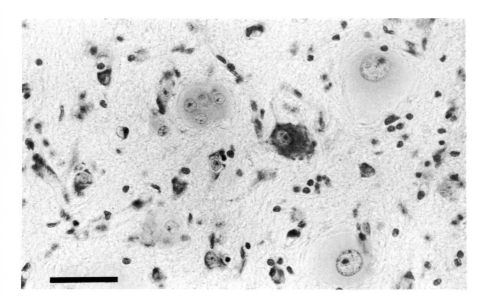

FIG. 12. Male aged 17 yr, seizures began at 4 yr, poorly controlled by medication, patient not mentally retarded—"a good pupil at school." Operation revealed two nodules each about 1 cm in diameter in the left intermediate frontal region. Photomicrograph shows tuberous sclerosis-like features, large astrocytes—one multinucleate—and neurons; compare with Fig. 10. Luxol blue-cresyl violet stain. Scale marker 50 microns.

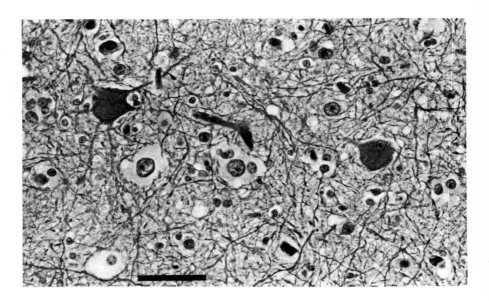

FIG. 13. Same case as Fig. 12. Neurons and neurites (darkly stained) and abnormal astrocytes (pale-staining cytoplasm) in cortical tuber. Bodian's silver method. Scale marker 50 microns.

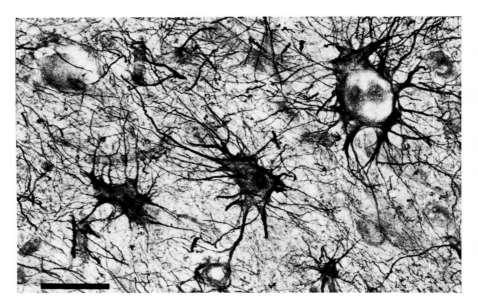

FIG. 14. Same case as Figs. 12 and 13. Monster astrocytes, one of which is binucleate. Cajal's method for astrocytes. Scale marker 50 microns.

Kofman and Hyland (1959) relate the story of a man with the cutaneous and cerebral changes of tuberous sclerosis who retained normal intelligence and was regularly employed at the age of 62, despite frequent seizures and occasional epileptic status.

Encephalitic Lesions

Epileptic seizures of various patterns occur in the course of acute and subacute encephalitides. Such patients would not be considered for surgery (with the possible exception of herpes simplex encephalitis and then only for diagnostic purposes). There are, however, a few patients in whom very slowly ingravescent neurologic deficits develop in association with recurrent focal seizures and in whom tissue obtained at operation shows changes strongly suggestive of encephalitis (Figs. 15–18). Rasmussen, Olszewski, and Lloyd-Smith (1958) reported three such cases and Aguilar and Rasmussen (1960), in a retrospective survey, subsequently identified 32 examples from a consecutive series of 449 patients operated on for seizures.

Inclusion bodies have rarely been found in these cases and none were seen in the present series. The disease differs in both clinical and pathologic features from

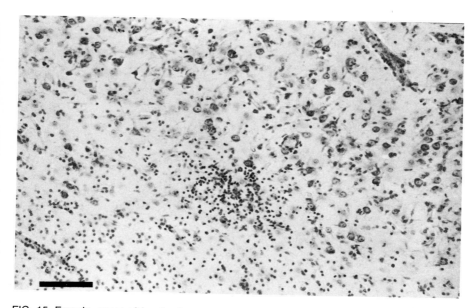

FIG. 15. Female, onset of focal seizures and gradually progressive hemiplegia at 4 yr of age, afebrile and never unconscious. On admission at 7 yr had left flaccid hemiplegia with hyperreflexia and frequent focal seizures involving left face, arm, and leg. Right hemispherectomy. Histopathologically, chronic encephalitis involving gray matter. Photomicrograph shows glial nodule at corticomedullary junction and diffuse microglial hyperplasia. Cresyl violet stain. Scale marker 100 microns.

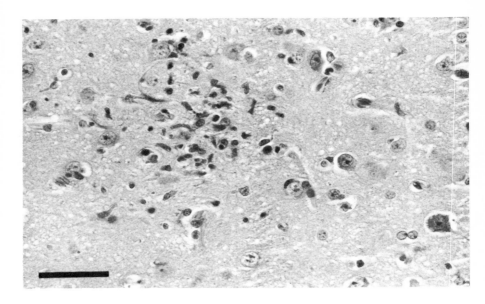

FIG. 16. Chronic encephalitis. Cortical glial nodule. Hematoxylin and eosin stain. Scale marker 50 microns.

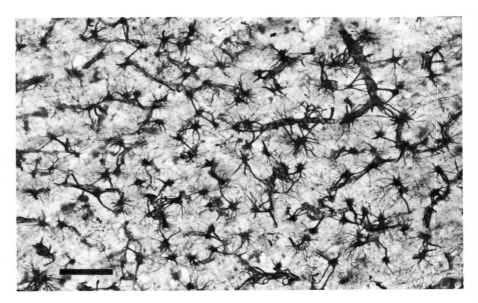

FIG. 17. Chronic encephalitis. Diffuse cortical gliosis. Cajal's method for astrocytes. Scale marker 100 microns.

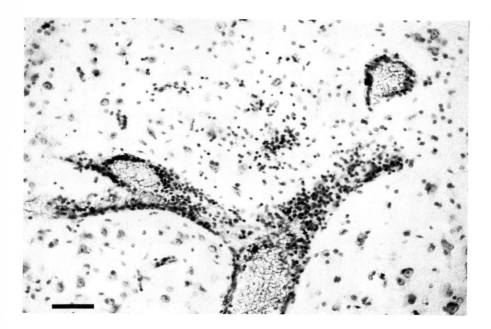

FIG. 18. Chronic encephalitis. Same case as Fig. 15. Perivenular cuffing by lymphocytes and glial nodule. Cresyl violet stain. Scale marker 100 microns.

subacute sclerosing panencephalitis. Standard virologic isolation techniques for a wide range of viruses, and serologic tests, have so far been negative, so that proof of the infectious nature and specific etiology of these cases is unfortunately not available. Animal inoculation in a manner suitable to establish transmissibility, as with the slow virus diseases of the nervous system (Gajdusek, 1967), has not to date (1974) proved successful.

An alternative view of these histopathologic findings is that the inflammatory element is secondary to a noninfectious process producing neuronal breakdown. The features, however, are unlike those seen in authenticated cases of ictal brain damage (see below, discussion of etiologic considerations). Moreover, some cases classified as encephalitic in the present series have never had generalized seizures but presented clinically as epilepsia partialis continuans.

DISCUSSION

Etiologic Considerations

Only a few aspects of this vast field can be considered here. The genesis of low-grade neoplasia, the origin of hamartomata, and the genetics of tuberous sclerosis lie outside the scope of this account. The genetics of seizure susceptibility in general have been discussed elsewhere by McKhann and Shooter (1969) and by Metrakos and Metrakos (1969).

Two problems call for special comment: the question of ictal brain damage and the pathogenesis of nondiscrete temporal lobe lesions, frequently referred to as hippocampal or Ammon's horn sclerosis. The two problems are intertwined inasmuch as medial temporal structures are, by common consent, especially vulnerable to damage, although the mechanism and sequence of events involved is the subject of controversy.

The long, circuitous history of the views held on the significance of Ammon's sclerosis since its first description in 1825 is succinctly described by Falconer (1970). More recently, Earle et al. (1953) hypothesized that the sclerosis of infero-medial temporal structures found in 100 of 157 temporal lobe excisions resulted from compression of vessels, particularly the anterior choroidal artery, by transtentorial uncal herniation during childbirth—hence their term "incisural sclerosis." In the same year, Sano and Malamud (1953) described hippocampal sclerosis in 29 of 50 institutionalized epiletics at autopsy; 11 of these had severe brain malformations and were mentally retarded; 16 of the remaining 18 had psychic ictal phenomena. Falconer et al. (1964) reported a 40% incidence of febrile convulsions occurring within the first 3 years of life in the 47 cases of temporal lobe epilepsy who had mesial temporal sclerosis diagnosed at operation and verified histologically.

Thus both perinatal brain damage (asphyxial and/or mechanical) and febrile convulsions in childhood (perhaps in subjects with a low seizure threshold on a genetic basis) are regarded as major etiologic factors in focal seizures of temporal lobe origin. These views are not mutually exclusive, and the proponents of neither school of thought claim that one mechanism causes all cases. It may be that the proportion due to each varies from population to population.

There is considerable evidence in the literature that repeated major seizures and especially status epilepticus can produce brain damage. The single case reported by Meyer, Beck, and Shepherd (1955) showed widespread lesions, but these were most severe in the hippocampus, hippocampal gyrus, first temporal gyrus, and medial orbital and anterior cingulate regions; the patient was a child. The five cases reported by Fowler (1956) were between 10 months and 2 years of age, previously healthy but neurologically devastated following prolonged convulsions associated with non-neurologic infections. Norman (1964), in describing the cerebral lesions in 11 children dying in status epilepticus, reported that cerebral cortical and hippocampal lesions were as severe in edematous as in nonedematous brains, suggesting that herniation phenomena were not an essential mechanism. Lyon, Dodge, and Adams (1961) discuss in great detail acute encephalopathies of obscure origin in young children, characterized clinically by fever, impaired consciousness, and convulsions; histologic examination of the brains of these patients showed either no abnormality or acute anoxic changes in the pyramidal layer of the hippocampus and in the cerebral cortex.

Norman (1966), in discussing the birth asphyxia verus postepileptic encephalopathy controversy, remarks on the association of neonatal asphyxia with hippocampal-amygdaloid lesions in which there is selective involvement of the h2 sector, a pattern not seen in postepileptic brain damage.

There has been considerable investigation of selective hippocampal vulnerability in animals. Friede (1966), in a histochemical study, demonstrated a sharp chemical border between Rose's fields h1 (Sommer's sector) and h2. That hippocampal pyramidal neurons are selectively vulnerable to agents other than anoxia has been shown by Purpura and Gonzalez-Monteagudo (1960), who used methoxypyridoxine to produce changes in end-blade neurons in paralyzed, artificially ventilated cats. Using a different model, Meldrum and Brierley (1972) produced lesions in h1 as well as h3–5 in adolescent baboons by administration of allylglycine. The problems posed by selective vulnerability (pathoclisis) even in a single brain structure are complex: they remain of great importance for the understanding of the genesis of epilepsy in man.

Prognosis: The Limited Role of the Surgical Pathologist

The pathologist can make only a modest contribution to the assessment of the seizure patient's prognosis following operation. A tissue diagnosis should settle definitively whether or not a progressive disease process is present; this is important in view of the relative frequency of occurrence of otherwise occult gliomas, usually indolent astrocytomas or occasionally oligodendrogliomas. In the case of essentially static lesions, it is not yet clear to what extent the prognosis is affected by the nature of their pathology. Falconer (1973), in presenting the results of temporal lobectomy in two series each of 100 patients, reports that improvement in both seizure tendency and social adaptation was greater in those cases found to have mesial temporal sclerosis than in patients harboring hamartomas or cryptic tumors. In his second series, 16 of 100 cases had a preoperative psychosis. In 12 the psychosis persisted after operation; none of these 12 had mesial temporal sclerosis but 6 had hamartomas. Possibly the presence of a hamartoma in one temporal lobe increases the likelihood of others being present elesewhere in the brain or of some subtle diffuse cortical abnormality, but so far there is no direct evidence that this is so. Nevertheless, the frequency of cerebral lesions indistinguishable from those of tuberous sclerosis in the present series may indicate a more widespread disorder of brain development in such cases.

CONCLUSION

A multiplicity of lesions, widely differing in both etiology and structure, give rise to focal epilepsy. Roughly one third (33.9%) of a series of over 500 consecutive cases treated surgically according to criteria laid down elsewhere in this book had some form of discrete focal lesion; these included posttraumatic meningocerebral cicatrix, gliomas (usually well differentiated and sometimes very small), hamartomas, vascular malformations, tuberous sclerosis-like lesions, and the residua of infarcts occurring in early life. In a further third of cases (35.2%), histopathologic examination either failed to show any abnormality microscopically (19.7%) or revealed minor changes not considered etiologically significant (15.5%). Some of these may be accounted for by injudicious histologic sampling; in others the lesion may not be detectable by light microscopy, e.g., minor degrees of neuronal loss or subtle biochemical abnormalities.

The remaining third (30.9%) had lesions which were less circumscribed and in some cases rather diffuse and widespread. In one category of these, atrophic cortical lesions in which, microscopically, only cortical neuronal loss and gliosis were seen, etiologic diagnosis must be based on the clinical history and, to some extent, on hypothesis. Hippocampal sclerosis was observed in 15.3% of all cases. Ulegyria was a common finding in patients with extensive hemispheral lesions involving several lobes of the brain. In a small number of patients, the excised tissue presented the histopathologic features of a subacute or chronic encephalitis but, to date, virologic studies have proved negative.

Two theoretically preventable etiologic mechanisms occur: birth injury in the form of perinatal asphyxia and/or transtentorial herniation (incisural sclerosis), and cerebral anoxia consequent upon febrile convulsions occurring in childhood.

ACKNOWLEDGMENTS

I am indebted to the surgeons whose operative material I have studied. Part of this work was done while I was on sabbatical leave in the Department of Pathology, University of Aberdeen, Professor A. L. Stalker, Chairman.

REFERENCES

Aguilar, M. J., and Rasmussen, T. (1960): Role of encephalitis in pathogenesis of epilepsy. *Arch. Neurol.*, 2:663–676.
Cavanagh, J. B. (1958): On certain small tumours encountered in the temporal lobe. *Brain*, 81:389–405.
Clark, R. M., and Linell, E. A. (1954): Case report: Prenatal occlusion of the internal carotid artery. *J. Neurol. Neurosurg. Psychiatry*, 17:295–297.
Crome, L. (1955): A morphological critique of temporal lobectomy. *Lancet*, 1:882–884.
Crome, L. (1958): Multilocular cystic encephalopathy of infants. *J. Neurol. Neurosurg. Psychiatry*, 21:146–152.
Earle, K. M., Baldwin, M., and Penfield, W. (1953): Incisural sclerosis and temporal lobe seizures produced by hippocampal herniation at birth. *Arch. Neurol. Psychiatry*, 69:27–42.
Falconer, M. A. (1968): The significance of mesial temporal sclerosis (Ammon's horn sclerosis) in epilepsy. *Guy's Hosp. Rep.*, 117:1–12.
Falconer, M. A. (1970): Historical review: The pathological substrate of temporal lobe epilepsy. *Guy's Hosp. Rep.*, 119:47–60.
Falconer, M. A. (1973): Reversibility by temporal lobe resection of the behavioural abnormalities of temporal-lobe epilepsy. *N. Engl. J. Med.*, 289:451–455.
Falconer, M. A., and Cavanagh, J. B. (1959): Clinicopathological considerations of temporal lobe epilepsy due to small focal lesions. A study of cases submitted to operation. *Brain*, 82:483–504.
Falconer, M. A., Serafetinides, E. A., and Corsellis, J. A. N. (1964): Etiology and pathogenesis of temporal lobe epilepsy. *Arch. Neurol.*, 10:233–248.
Falconer, M. A., and Taylor, D. C. (1968): Surgical treatment of drug-resistant epilepsy due to mesial temporal sclerosis. *Arch. Neurol.*, 19:353–361.

Foerster, O., and Penfield, W. (1930): The structural basis of traumatic epilepsy and results of radical operation. *Brain,* 53:99–120.

Fowler, M. (1957): Brain damage after febrile convulsions. *Arch. Dis. Child.,* 32:67–76.

Friede, R. L. (1966): The histochemical architecture of the Ammon's horn as related to its selective vulnerability. *Acta Neuropath.,* 6:1–13.

Gajdusek, D. C. (1967): Slow virus infections of the nervous system. *N. Engl. J. Med.,* 276:392–400.

Green, J. R., and Scheetz, D. G. (1964): Surgery of epileptogenic lesions of the temporal lobe. *Arch. Neurol.,* 10:135–148.

Jackson, J. H. (1874): On the scientific and empirical investigation of epilepsies. *Medical Press and Circular,* 18:475. Reprinted in: *Selected Writings of John Hughlings Jackson,* Vol. 1, edited by J. Taylor (1931). Hodder and Stoughton, London.

Jackson, J. H., and Beevor, C. E. (1889): Case of tumour of the right temporo-sphenoidal lobe bearing on the localisation of the sense of smell and the interpretation of a particular variety of epilepsy. *Brain,* 12:346–357.

Jackson, J. H., and Colman, W. S. (1898): Case of epilepsy with tasting movements and "dreamy state"—very small patch of softening in the left uncinate gyrus. *Brain,* 21:580–590.

Kofman, O., and Hyland, H. H. (1959): Tuberous sclerosis in adults with normal intelligence. *Arch. Neurol.,* 81:43–48.

Lyon, G., Dodge, P. R., and Adams, R. D. (1961): The acute encephalopathies of obscure origin in infants and children. *Brain,* 84:680–708.

Margerison, J. H., and Corsellis, J. A. N. (1966): Epilepsy and the temporal lobes. A clinical, electroencephalographic and neuropathological study of the brain in epilepsy, with particular reference to the temporal lobes. *Brain,* 89:499–530.

McKhann, G. M., and Shooter, E. M. (1969): Genetics of seizure susceptibility. In: *Basic Mechanisms of the Epilepsies,* edited by H. H. Jasper, A. A. Ward, and A. Pope. Little, Brown, Boston.

Meldrum, B. S., and Brierley, J. B. (1972): Neuronal loss and gliosis in the hippocampus following repetitive epileptic seizures induced in adolescent baboons by allylglycine. *Brain Res.,* 48:361–365.

Metrakos, J. D., and Metrakos, K. (1969): Genetic studies in clinical epilepsy. In: *Basic Mechanisms of the Epilepsies,* edited by H. H. Jasper, A. A. Ward, and A. Pope. Little, Brown, Boston.

Meyer, A., Beck, E., and Shepherd, M. (1955): Unusually severe lesions in the brain following status epilepticus. *J. Neurol. Neurosurg. Psychiatry,* 18:24–33.

Meyer, A., Falconer, M. A., and Beck, E. (1954): Pathological findings in temporal lobe epilepsy. *J. Neurol. Neurosurg. Psychiatry,* 17:276–285.

Norman, R. M. (1963): Malformations of the nervous system, birth injury and diseases of early life. In: *Greenfield's Neuropathology,* 2nd edition, edited by W. Blackwood and others. Edward Arnold, London.

Norman, R. M. (1964): The neuropathology of status epilepticus. *Med. Sci. Law,* 4:46–51.

Norman, R. M. (1966): The pathogenesis of temporal lobe epilepsy. In: *Biological Factors in Temporal Lobe Epilepsy, Clinics in Developmental Medicine No. 22,* edited by C. Ounsted, J. Lindsay, and R. Norman. The Spastics Society and Heinemann Medical Books, London.

Norman, R. M., and Urich, H. (1957): Dissecting aneurysm of the middle cerebral artery as a cause of acute infantile hemiplegia. *J. Path. Bact.,* 73:580–582.

Norman, R. M., Urich, H., and McMenemy, W. H. (1957): Vascular mechanisms of birth injury. *Brain,* 80:49–58.

Penfield, W., and Jasper, H. (1954): *Epilepsy and the Functional Anatomy of the Human Brain.* Little, Brown, Boston.

Perot, P., Weir, B., and Rasmussen, T. (1966): Tuberous sclerosis; Surgical therapy for seizures. *Arch. Neurol.,* 15:498–506.

Purpura, D. P., and Gonzalez-Monteagudo, O. (1960): Acute effects of methoxypyridoxine on hippocampal end-blade neurons; An experimental study of "special pathoclisis" in the cerebral cortex. *J. Neuropathol. Exp. Neurol.,* 19:421–432.

Purpura, D. P., Penry, J. K., Tower, D., Woodbury, D. M., and Walter, R., editors (1972): *Experimental Models of Epilepsy,* Raven Press, New York.

Rasmussen, T., and Gossman, H. (1963): Epilepsy due to gross destructive brain lesions. *Neurology,* 13:659–669.

Rasmussen, T., Olszewski, J., and Lloyd-Smith, D. (1958): Focal seizures due to chronic encephalitis. *Neurology,* 8:435–445.

Rubinstein, L. J. (1972): *Atlas of Tumor Pathology. Second ser., Fasc. 6. Tumors of the Central Nervous System.* Armed Forces Institute of Pathology, Washington, D.C.

Russell, D. S., and Rubinstein, L. J. (1971): *Pathology of Tumours of the Nervous System,* 3rd edition. Edward Arnold, London.

Sano, K., and Malamud, N. (1953): Clinical significance of sclerosis of the cornu Ammonis. *Arch. Neurol. Psychiatry,* 70:40–53.

van Gelder, N. M., Sherwin, A. L., and Rasmussen, T. (1972): Amino acid content of epileptogenic human brain: Focal versus surrounding regions. *Brain Res.* 40:385–393.

Yakovlev, P. I., and Wadsworth, R. C. (1946): Schizencephalies. A study of the congenital clefts in the cerebral mantle. *J. Neuropath. Exp. Neurol.,* 5:116–130.

Advances in Neurology, Vol. 8, edited by D. P
Purpura, J. K. Penry, and R. D. Walter. Raven
Press, New York © 1975.

7
Cortical Resection in the Treatment of Focal Epilepsy

Theodore Rasmussen

INTRODUCTION

The surgical treatment of epilepsy has a lengthy and colorful history (Marshall, 1951). The list of discarded surgical procedures bears eloquent testimony to the many fanciful ideas concerning the nature of epilepsy that were held by both medical and nonmedical people well into this century, as well as to the desperation of the epileptic patient in his search for relief. Cortical resection has stood the test of time and has earned a secure and gradually enlarging role around the world in the treatment of selected patients with medically refractory focal epilepsy.

Although some of the pioneer neurosurgeons during the early decades of the modern neurosurgical era resected lesions and areas of cortex in an attempt to alleviate focal seizures (Starr, 1893; Horsley, 1886, 1892, and 1909; Krause, 1909–1912), the present technique of cortical resection in the treatment of focal epilepsy stems from Otfrid Foerster's operations of the 1920's (Foerster, 1925, 1926). However, it was Wilder Penfield's scholarly, scientific, and persistent efforts, stimulated by his studies with Foerster (Foerster and Penfield, 1930*a,b*) and joined by Herbert Jasper's electroencephalographic genius, that have largely been responsible for the development of cortical resection as a valuable therapeutic technique for a selected group of patients with focal cerebral seizures (Penfield and coauthors, 1930 to 1955).

Neurosurgical Hypothesis

Continuing analysis and study of patients operated on since 1928 by Penfield, his associates, and successors have gradually told us that small, discrete epileptogenic foci are rare in these patients (Penfield and Steelman, 1947; Penfield and Flanigin, 1950; Penfield and Paine, 1955; Rasmussen and coauthors, 1958 to 1974). The great majority were found to have epileptogenic areas of considerable extent with the region of lowest threshold giving the local sign to the attack pattern.

Follow-up studies, however, have indicated that success in stopping the seizures is correlated with the completeness of the removal of epileptogenic cortex, and excisions limited to restricted foci of lowest seizure threshold usually failed to provide a satisfactory reduction in seizure tendency. Reoperation and more

---

Montreal Neurological Institute Reprint No. 1169.

complete excision of the epileptogenic area often reduced the patient's seizure tendency enough further to convert an unsuccessful into a successful result.

By January 1, 1972, 129 patients in the Montreal Neurological Institute surgical seizure series with nontumoral lesions had undergone one and occasionally two or three reoperations (Fig. 1). In most of these patients the initial operation had produced a moderate but inadequate reduction in seizure tendency. Following the additional removal of epileptogenic cortex, 29 patients (25%) became seizure-free, either immediately after discharge from the hospital or after a few attacks in the early postoperative months or years, and have remained so. An additional 13 patients (11%) became seizure-free for periods of 3 to 18 years, then experienced late recurrence of rare or occasional attacks. In 18 more patients (16%) there was a marked but not quite complete reduction of seizure tendency, so that the patients continued to have only up to 1 to 2% as many attacks as preoperatively. Thirty-one patients (27%) thus had a marked but not quite complete reduction of seizure tendency following operation.

Thus, half of these patients experienced a reasonably satisfactory reduction in seizure tendency as a result of additional removal of epileptogenic cortex after an inadequate reduction had been produced by the original, more limited cortical excision.

The surgical aim, therefore, is to identify and map out the total epileptogenic area of the cortex and to remove the involved cortex as completely as possible without running too great a risk of producing a significant neurologic deficit or of increasing one that is already present.

Cortical Excision for Non-tumoral Epileptogenic Lesions

Results of reoperation - 1928 through 1971

Seizure free since discharge	13 pts. (11%)	29 pts. (25%)		
Became seizure free after some early attacks	16 pts. (14%)		60 pts. (52%)	115 pts. with follow-up data of 2-39 yrs. after last operation
Free 3 or more years then rare or occasional attacks	13 pts. (11%)	31 pts. (27%)		
Marked reduction of seizure tendency	18 pts. (16%)			
Moderate to no reduction of seizure tendency	55 pts. (48%)			median 13 yrs.
Inadequate data	11 pts.			
Postoperative deaths	3 pts.			
Total	**129 pts.**			

FIG. 1.

SURGICAL PROCEDURE

Preoperative Preparation

The patient's anticonvulsant medication is managed so as to have the epileptiform activity in the EEG as active as possible and yet under sufficient control that the patient is not having seizures so frequently as to interfere with the operation or result in a postictal state in the cortical EEG. In some patients, all anticonvulsant medications are stopped during the preoperative study and the patient is kept off all anticonvulsants until the final postexcision cortical EEG is completed. More frequently, it has been advisable to keep the patient on a partial dose of his anticonvulsant medication for protection against too frequent seizures or status during the preoperative study and the medication is stopped only on the morning or afternoon of the day before surgery. Occasionally it is advisable to maintain some anticonvulsant medication until oral intake is stopped preoperatively. In rare instances it is necessary to give phenobarbital (sodium Luminal®) by injection after oral intake is stopped in order to keep the attacks controlled enough so that the cortical EEG will show the epileptiform activity and not simply postictal depression.

Cortisone or dexamethasone is given orally for 24 hours preoperatively and intravenously during the operation and postoperatively until oral intake is resumed.

Anesthesia

In order to have the maximum possibility of eradicating the epileptogenic cortex as completely as possible with minimum risk of producing a neurologic deficit, the operation, up to the closure, is carried out under local anesthetic if the patient is over 13 to 14 years old. In younger children and in the rare adult whose cooperation is unpredictable, the patient is lightly anesthetized with intravenous sodium methyl hexital (Brietal®) and fentanyl citrate (Sublimaze®) prior to injection of the local anesthetic into the scalp.

Adults

The patient is visited by the anesthetist on the afternoon before operation to establish good rapport. Pentobarbital (Nembutal®), secobarbital (Seconal®), or diazepam (Valium®) is used the night before operation, if necessary, for sleep. On arrival in the operating suite in the morning, the patient is given 0.4 mg of atropine subcutaneously and an intravenous setup established. The patient is then suitably postured on the operating table in as comfortable a position as possible, placing a Stryker (artificial fat) pillow under the hip.

Droperidol (tranquilizer) and fentanyl (analgesic) are then given intermittently through the intravenous, set as necessary to keep the patient in a drowsy, relaxed state. If there is any significant unavoidable discomfort, Brietal, the shortest-acting barbiturate anesthetic agent, is given for a few minutes as needed.

The patient is normally alert and cooperative during the EEG and stimulation procedures and during the cortical resection and postexcision EEG recording. Some, however, become fatigued and drowsy and must be roused periodically in order to check speech and motor functions during the cortical excision.

Children

Children below the age of 12 to 13 are given secobarbital or pentobarbital the evening before operation and, on the morning of operation, atropine as well. The patient is lightly anesthetized with a general anesthetic and a good topical anesthetic applied to the throat and trachea before inserting an intratracheal tube. A mixture of compressed air enriched with oxygen is administered through the intratracheal tube and the patient kept lightly asleep with intermittent methyl hexital and fentanyl. Once the local anesthetic is injected into the scalp only a minimal amount of anesthetic agent is ordinarily required and the cortical EEG usually displays the expected epileptiform activity satisfactorily. Nitrous oxide is avoided or discontinued well before the cortical recording is begun because it tends to obliterate the epileptiform activity in the cortical EEG.

The Opening

The skin incision is marked with a dye and the scalp anesthetized with a long-lasting local anesthetic agent. Dibucaine hydrochloride (Nupercaine®) has been used for many years with excellent results. A 1:1,500 dilution is used for the intracutaneous layer; a maximum of 125 cc is permitted in adults. Another 125 cc of 1:4,000 dilution is used for the subgaleal layer and for the temporal fascia and muscle. One-half cc of epinephrine is added to each 125 cc of the dibucaine solutions unless there is some specific contraindication such as the patient's cardiac status. Because of the recent disappearance of dibucaine from the commercial market, other long-lasting local anesthetic agents are currently being evaluated.

A plastic sheet is placed over the head around the operative area and skin towels are sutured securely in place so they will not be dislodged if the patient moves his head or has a seizure during the operation.

A wide exposure of the cortex is essential in order to map the epileptogenic area as completely and accurately as possible and outline its relationship to the sensorimotor area and, in the dominant hemisphere, to the speech areas. The question-mark type of skin incision introduced by Falconer et al. (1955) gives maximum exposure of the anterior portion of the temporal lobe. On the side dominant for speech the posterior limb is placed at the level of the back of the ear. On the nondominant side it may be placed 1 to 3 cm further posteriorly if the preoperative EEG studies indicate that the epileptogenic area may extend into the posterior temporal region. The medial limb of the incision runs 2 cm lateral to the midline so as to provide a satisfactorily wide base to the skin flap anteriorly. If the epileptogenic area involves the frontal as well as the temporal lobe, the medial limb of the skin incision should be placed at the midline to permit maximal exposure of the frontal as well as the temporal lobe.

If the epileptogenic area is limited to the frontal lobe according to the preoperative EEG studies and the patient's attack pattern, a large C-shaped incision is used with the medial limb placed at the midline and the postero-lateral limb extended downward to the level of the zygoma. The incision extends posteriorly far enough to expose at least the lower portion of the precentral gyrus so it can be identified by electrical stimulation for localization purposes. This incision permits good exposure of the Sylvian region of the anterior portion of the temporal lobe, which is sometimes also actively epileptogenic in patients whose attack patterns and preoperative studies point only to a frontal lobe localization.

When the epileptogenic area involves the central region, a U-shaped incision is used, exposing the Rolandic and adjacent regions as needed. The exposure should permit extension of the cortical resection into the frontal or parietal lobe as indicated by the cortical EEG recording.

A C-shaped incision exposing the posterior third of the cerebral hemisphere is used in patients with parietal or occipital epileptogenic areas, again exposing enough of the sensorimotor strip to provide adequate localization.

The skin and muscle are reflected as a single layer and a free bone flap removed, since this gives a more complete exposure of the cortex with less discomfort to the patient than the use of a hinged bone flap. When the temporal lobe or the anterior third of the hemisphere is to be exposed, burr holes are first placed just above and below the sphenoid ridge and connected by ronguering the bone between, anesthetizing the nerves along the middle meningeal vessels by injecting the local anesthetic into the dura with a short 25-gauge hypodermic needle. This makes it possible to put in the other burr holes or use the craniotome and raise the bone flap without discomfort to the patient. The temporal incision through the bone is made as low as possible so as to avoid a cosmetically undesirable depression in this region postoperatively. In patients with temporal lobe epilepsy, bone is ronguered from the anterior and inferior margins of the middle fossa exposure so as to expose the cortex of the temporal lobe as completely as possible.

Cortical EEG Recording

After meticulous hemostasis, the dura is opened widely, exposing the cortex as completely as the bony opening permits. The cortical electrode holder is then attached to the skull. The recording system used at the Montreal Neurological Institute for the past 15 years consists of 16 electrodes providing for 12 channels of cortico-cortical linkage arranged in four rows of three channels each (Fig. 2). A master switch on the EEG machine in the operating room gallery permits recording in both a horizontal and vertical grid without moving the electrodes

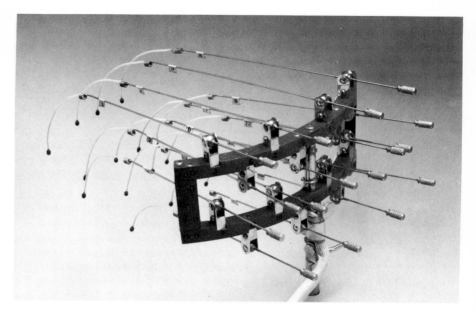

FIG. 2. Cortical EEG electrode assembly consisting of four rows of four electrodes each. The vertical bars of the frame contain plug-in electrode contacts which permit the use of flexible wire electrodes instead of the surface electrodes at the ends of each row. The vertical bars also contain a plug-in contact for a reference electrode which may be clipped to the edge of the skull to permit monopolar as well as bipolar recording montages.

and also provides for monopolar as well as cortex-to-cortex linkages. Plug-in contacts at the ends of each row of electrodes permit the use of up to eight flexible wire electrodes instead of the ordinary electrodes. These flexible wire electrodes can easily be slid underneath the temporal or frontal lobes or along the falx to record from the medial surface of the cerebral hemisphere.

The master switch at the EEG machine also permits the use of two blunt-tipped needle depth electrodes with four recording contacts, 1 cm apart, on each needle (Fig. 3). These needle electrodes are employed in patients with temporal lobe epilepsy and are inserted by hand into the second temporal gyrus so that the bottom contact of the anterior depth electrode is in the amygdaloid nucleus and the bottom contact of the posterior one is in the hippocampus. The superficial contacts are in the surface gray matter. The next deeper contacts record from the circuminsular cortex at the midportion of the insula in the case of the anterior electrode and from the gray matter in the depths of Heschl's gyri in the case of the posterior electrode.

The surface electrode sites yielding epileptiform activity are marked by small tickets bearing letters, and the location and nature of the abnormal wave forms are dictated to a secretary in the gallery (Penfield and Erickson, 1941; Penfield and Jasper, 1954).

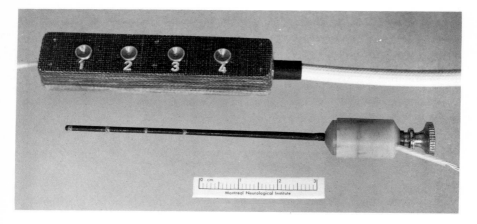

FIG. 3. Blunt-tipped needle depth electrode with stimulation contact points for each of the electrodes on the needle shaft. Indigo carmine is injected through the needle at the end of the recording and stimulation procedure so the electrode tract can be identified during the temporal lobectomy and the approximate location of each recording contact noted in the dictated operation report.

Cortical Stimulation

After the cortical electrical activity has been adequately sampled, the central region is identified by electrical stimulation. In order to facilitate stimulation of the depth electrode contacts, a unipolar stimulating electrode is ordinarily used. The parameters of the stimulating current are not critical, but a 2-msec square wave pulse at a frequency of 60/sec has been proven by usage to provide reliable responses with minimum input of energy and with minimum risk of inducing undesired seizures. For convenience, a unidirectional square wave pulse has been used. The safeguards against undesirable electrolytic effects at the electrode contact provided by biphasic stimulating pulses (Lilly et al., 1955) are relatively unimportant in these stimulations because the metal-tissue interface where the electrolytic changes take place is at the pia-arachnoid surface and not the cortex, and because the number of stimulations is limited.

The cortical stimulation is started with a subthreshold intensity, 1 V or ½ mA, and increased by ½ V or ½ mA increments until motor or sensory responses are obtained. These are marked by small numbered tickets and the nature of the response is dictated to a secretary in the gallery. Unless the epileptogenic area and the proposed cortical excision require detailed mapping of the central region, three or four positive responses from each of the two central convolutions provide accurate identification of the fissure of Rolando and the pre- and postcentral gyri.

In the dominant hemisphere the frontal, parietal, and temporal speech areas are stimulated while the patient is carrying out verbal tasks such as counting, saying the days of the week, and naming objects. Aphasic speech interference responses positively identify convolutions that are essential for speech, but the failure to interfere with verbal tasks by stimulation does not guarantee that the area being stimulated is unimportant for speech functions. A negative response to cortical stimulation does not carry the same validity as a positive response.

Cortical EEG recording is carried out during the stimulation procedure and any stimulation points yielding electrical afterdischarges are also marked with numbered tickets. The maximum stimulation strength employed ordinarily does not exceed the threshold intensity for eliciting sensory or motor responses in the central region by more than 2 to 3 V in order to minimize the risk of producing physiologic seizures unrelated to the patient's habitual seizure problem.

After the motor, sensory, and speech areas have been identified as completely as required, stimulation of the epileptogenic area, including the depth electrode contacts in the case of temporal lobe epilepsy, is carried out, again increasing the stimulation intensity by ½ V or ½ mA increments in an effort to reproduce the patient's habitual aura. This is often not possible, but afterdischarges without clinical accompaniment are frequently produced. The patient is asked to carry out verbal and motor tasks during the afterdischarges to determine whether or not the afterdischarge represents a clinical or only an electrographic seizure. The significance of the latter in planning the extent of the cortical excision awaits further analysis of accummulated data. Stimulation in an effort to produce the patient's aura is ordinarily abandoned if this has not been successful with current intensities of 2 to 3 V, above the threshold for sensory or motor responses in the central region.

Cortical Resection

After completion of the cortical EEG and stimulation procedures, the brain is photographed and the lettered and numbered ticket sites noted on a standard brain diagram to aid in later study of the brain photographs. The area of the cortex to be excised is decided on based on the cortical EEG findings, preoperative EEG studies, and the patient's attack pattern or patterns, and is outlined by placing a white thread on the brain, following sulci as far as possible. The rest of the exposed surface of the brain is covered with a thin plastic sheet to prevent it from drying during the cortical resection. The pia-arachnoid over the convolutions at the periphery of the area to be excised is coagulated and incised and the incision carried down into the underlying white matter with a small bore suction. The cortical incision is carried around the periphery of the area in this fashion, gradually deepened through the white matter, and the block of brain tissue is removed. Larger arteries are clipped as well as coagulated. These clips provide useful markers in the postoperative X-rays to indicate the size and area of the excision as well as to safeguard against postoperative hemorrhage. Areas of marked gliosis sometimes need to be cut with a small scissors if use of the suction tip moves the brain rather than cutting through the tissue. The less movement of the brain there is during the excision, the less the postoperative edema and ultimate gliosis due to the surgical procedure.

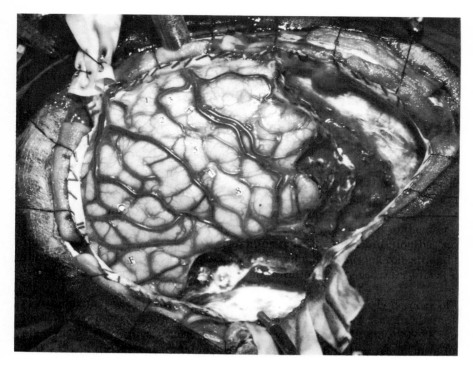

FIG. 4. Right frontal and temporal lobectomy with the cortical excision following sulci and leaving untraumatized convolutional banks at the edge of the removal wherever possible.

After the bulk of the specimen is removed, the cortex at the periphery is gently sucked away from the pial walls of the remaining convolutions, making every effort to avoid traumatizing or retracting these remaining convolutional surfaces (Fig. 4). Bleeding from these pial banks is usually minimal and is controlled by gentle packing with small moist pledgets of cotton rather than by coagulation so as to leave behind an absolute minimum of gliosis and scarring in the gyri surrounding the area of the excision.

Postexcision Cortical EEG Recording

The electrode holder is reattached to the skull and the electrodes placed on the brain, suitably arranged to record the electrical activity from the area surrounding the excision. If a significant amount of spiking persists in an area that could be removed with reasonable safety, further cortical removal and a second postexcision cortical EEG recording are carried out. One, two, or three such additional excisions are often made before a satisfactorily clear EEG record is obtained or the effort to achieve this abandoned. The appropriate anticonvulsant medication is then added to the intravenous setup.

Closure

Meticulous hemostasis in the removal cavity is essential. The dura is sutured completely, leaving a 1-cm opening beneath the temporal muscle into which a Penrose drain is inserted. The peripheral end of the drain is brought out through a posterior burr hole and a stab wound in the scalp 1 cm behind the scalp incision. An ample and secure head dressing is applied. Seizures are relatively common in the early postoperative period and may dislodge a poorly fashioned dressing. The drain is removed when the dressing is changed on the first postoperative day.

POSTOPERATIVE CARE

Early Postoperative Care

Anticonvulsant medication is given intravenously until the patient starts taking oral fluids, usually 12 to 18 hours after leaving the operating suite. The daily fluid requirement, limited to 1,500 cc, is also given intravenously the first day. Most patients are ready to take the required fluids orally on the second postoperative day, but occasionally it is necessary to continue the intravenous fluids throughout the second, and, rarely, third postoperative day. Fluid intake is restricted to 1,500 cc per day for the first 4 to 5 days.

Cortisone or dexamethasone is continued at a high level for the first 3 to 4 postoperative days and is then tapered off progressively over the ensuing week.

Seizures are common during the first 7 to 10 days but are not necessarily significant in regard to the ultimate result. Conversely, freedom from attacks during the early postoperative period does not necessarily indicate that the patient will ultimately achieve a satisfactory reduction in seizure tendency. These early postoperative attacks are usually minor focal seizures, sometimes like the patient's habitual preoperative attacks, sometimes different and clearly arising in adjacent cortical areas, so-called neighborhood attacks. Rarely, the seizures are frequent and severe enough to require parenteral phenobarbital or paraldehyde, oral or rectal. The occurrence of early postoperative seizures of this severity has been markedly reduced since the routine use of cortisone was started in 1958 (Rasmussen and Gulati, 1962).

Most patients are ready to start getting out of bed and to become ambulatory progressively by the third or fourth postoperative day.

Late Postoperative Care

It is important for the patient to remain on a realistic dose of anticonvulsant medication until time proves the seizure tendency to be satisfactorily reduced. It is our practice to put all patients on a daily dose of 300 mg of diphenylhydantoin (Dilantin®) and 120 mg of phenobarbital unless some other anticonvulsant regimen has been proven preoperatively to be more effective or more suitable.

If the patient has no attacks and no warnings of an attack during the first postoperative year, and if the EEG is then reasonably free of epileptic activity, the diphenylhydantoin dosage is reduced to 200 mg per day for the second postoperative year. If there have been a few attacks or auras, the original dosage schedule is maintained until 2 seizure-free years have elapsed. If the patient remains seizure-free, the diphenylhydantoin dosage is reduced to 100 mg per day for the third postoperative year and then stopped. The phenobarbital dosage is then reduced progressively at yearly intervals.

If a seizure recurs as the medication is reduced, the dosage is restored to the original levels and reduced again only after at least a 2-year seizure-free interval has elapsed.

SURGICAL RISKS AND COMPLICATIONS

Cortical resections, controlled by cortical electrographic recording and stimulation, are lengthy operations, but carry a low mortality rate. There have been two postoperative deaths in 820 consecutive operations in patients with nontumoral epileptogenic lesions carried out since 1957, an operative mortality rate of 0.2% for the past 15 years. Thirteen other postoperative deaths, occurring in the earlier years of the series, bring the overall operative mortality rate, covering 1,497 operations in 1,359 patients and spanning a period of 45 years (1928 to January 1, 1974) to 1.0%.

One of the two deaths of the past 15 years occurred in a 2-year-old child as a result of a complication of a tracheostomy tube inserted because of postoperative laryngeal stridor. The second death, in a young retarded adult male, was due to sensitivity to intravenous tetracycline administered for a severe postoperative bronchopneumonia.

In the temporal lobe series there have been no operative deaths in just over 700 operations carried out from 1950 to the end of 1973.

In earlier years, a persistent hemiparesis of variable severity and permanence followed temporal lobectomy in a small percentage of patients (Penfield, Lende, and Rasmussen, 1961). Since the importance of avoiding manipulation or retraction of the middle cerebral artery branches on the insula was appreciated and we learned that removal of insular cortex was not necessary (Silfvenius, Gloor, and Rasmussen, 1964), this complication has been avoided and it has not occurred in over 500 consecutive temporal lobectomies carried out at the Montreal Neurological Institute since 1958.

In cortical excisions above the fissure of Sylvius, the incidence of persistent hemiparesis and/or dysphasia as an operative complication is approximately one half of 1%, unless the epileptogenic area involves mainly the sensorimotor region itself. When this is the case, it is sometimes necessary to take a calculated risk of producing some weakness in the arm or leg, or more frequently, of increasing a preexisting weakness, in patients with particularly severe or frequent Jacksonian seizures.

A partial or complete upper quandrantic homonymous hemianopsia may be produced by temporal lobectomy with increasing frequency as the line of excision moves posterior to the level of the fissure of Rolando at the Sylvian fissure (Marino and Rasmussen, 1968). This upper quadrantic defect, however, is rarely noticed by the patient and does not constitute a significant handicap when it does occur. However, when particular care is taken to preserve the white matter lateral to the temporal horn of the ventricle, it is usually possible to avoid producing this upper quadrantic visual field defect even in temporal lobe removals extending as far as 7 to 8 cm from the anterior end of the middle fossa.

On rare occasions, it is worth producing a complete homonymous hemianopsia if this is necessary to eradicate a large epileptogenic area in the posterior third of the hemisphere which is producing particularly severe and intractable seizures. This decision usually arises in patients with infantile type hemiplegia who are hemispherectomy candidates. If such a patient has a preserved visual field and if the principal EEG abnormality is anterior to the occipital lobe, only the anterior two thirds of the hemisphere is removed, as a rule, sparing the occipital lobe and posterior portions of the parietal and temporal lobes in order to preserve the homonymous visual field. In a few instances, however, persistence of seizures has made it necessary to complete the hemispherectomy later on and to sacrifice the contralateral homonymous field in order to stop the seizures.

Milner, in her psychological investigation on the localization of highly intellectual functions, has identified subtle deficits produced by cortical epileptogenic lesions and by excisions of various regions of the brain, but these are rarely of clinical significance (Milner, 1954 to 1968; Corkin, Milner, and Rasmussen, 1970). An exception is the production of a serious global memory deficit by removal of a temporal lobe, including the hippocampal region, in a patient whose *opposite* hippocampus is nonfunctioning (Scoville and Milner, 1957). This complication, which has occurred in three patients after unilateral temporal lobectomy and has been reported in detail by Penfield and Milner (1958), has subsequently been avoided by carrying out special memory tests in all potential temporal lobectomy patients who have either EEG, X-ray, or psychological evidence of damage to both temporal lobes. These memory tests are carried out as part of the Wada intracarotid Amytal speech test and have clearly identified those patients in whom the hippocampal region of one temporal lobe is not dispensable as far as memory functions are concerned (Milner, Branch, and Rasmussen, 1962).

An elevated temperature, apparently due to an irritating effect of the breakdown products of blood, occurs in many patients following cortical resections for epilepsy, particularly with the larger removals (Finlayson and Penfield, 1941; Jackson, 1949). There is usually surprisingly little headache, stiff neck, or other discomfort despite temperature elevations that may go as high as 103 to 104°F. The white cell count in the blood may be normal or moderately elevated with less polymorphonuclear preponderance than would be expected with a septic cause. The cerebrospinal fluid shows a pleocytosis ranging from several hundred to several thousand, with less preponderance of polymorphonuclear cells than would be expected with a bacterial meningitis with a similar cell count. The lumbar puncture pressure is usually normal or only slightly elevated. This aseptic meningeal reaction does not require any specific treatment and clears up progressively over 10 to 20 days.

RESULTS

A total of 1,267 patients had undergone cortical excision for nontumoral epileptogenic lesions up to the end of 1971 at the Montreal Neurological Institute. Twenty-two patients who died during the first 2 postoperative years and 85 patients who have less than 2 years' follow-up data have been deleted from this analysis of results along with the 15 patients who died in the early postoperative period (Fig. 5).

In the follow-up analysis and studies, a persisting clinical seizure tendency is roughly quantitated as auras, minor attacks, or major attacks. An episode is classified as an aura if it consists only of a sensory phenomenon without a motor manifestation and if it does not interrupt the patient's mental activity or contact with the environment and cannot be detected by an observer. It is classified as a minor attack if it is detectable by an observer or interrupts thinking or contact with the environment but does not result in falling or a generalized convulsion. Even a single jerk of a shoulder, lasting a fraction of a second, or an epigastric sensation associated with a few seconds of mental confusion, amnesia, or loss of

Results of Cortical Excision for Focal Epilepsy

Patients with non-tumoral lesions operated upon 1928 through 1971

Seizure free since discharge	237 pts. (21%)	416 pts. (36%)	736 pts. (64%)	1145 pts. with follow-up data of 2-41 yrs.
Became seizure free after some early attacks	179 pts. (15%)			
Free 3 or more years then rare or occasional attacks	122 pts. (11%)	320 pts. (28%)		
Marked reduction of seizure tendency	198 pts. (17%)			
Moderated or less reduction of seizure tendency	409 pts. (36%)			median 10 yrs.

Inadequate follow-up data 85 pts.
Deaths in first 2 years   22 pts.
Postoperative deaths   15 pts.

Total   1267 pts.

FIG. 5.

contact with the environment is classified as a minor attack. A patient who has only auras, as defined above, is considered seizure-free in this follow-up analysis, since the social impact of these brief sensory episodes is not significantly greater than the presence of persistent spiking in the EEG.

There are thus 1,145 patients with satisfactory follow-up data of 2 to 41 years' duration, with a median follow-up period of 10 years. Two hundred and thirty-seven patients (21%) have had no attacks since discharge from the hospital and another 179 patients (15%) have become and remained seizure-free after having had a few attacks during the early postoperative months or years. Thus, 416 patients (36%) have become and remained seizure-free. One hundred and twenty-two patients (11%) have had rare or occasional attacks after being seizure-free for periods ranging from 3 to 20 years. One hundred ninety-eight (17%) have had only up to 1 to 2% as many attacks as preoperatively. Thus 320 patients (28%) have had a marked but not quite complete reduction of seizure tendency. Added to the seizure-free group, this results in 736 patients (64%) who have had a complete or nearly complete reduction of seizure tendency.

The remaining 409 patients (36%) have had a variable reduction: some have had only 5 to 10% as many attacks compared with the preoperative rate, many have had a 40 to 60% reduction, and a few, little or no reduction.

The patients in this series have been classified into both anatomic and etiologic groups for further follow-up analysis. The results in the anatomic groups are given in Chapters 10 and 11, but the key figures may be summarized here. A complete or nearly complete reduction of seizure tendency resulted in the temporal lobe group in 71%, in the frontal lobe group in 59%, in the parietal group in 62%, in the central group in 61%, in the small occipital group in 67%, and in the group with large destructive brain lesions in 68%.

The results were comparable when these patients were separated into etiologic groups based on the presumed cause of the original brain injury. A complete or nearly complete reduction of seizure tendency resulted in 72% of the birth trauma and anoxia group, 68% of the posttraumatic group, 70% of the postinflammatory group, and in 58% of the group of unknown etiology (Rasmussen, 1974).

Our data thus indicate that the effectiveness of cortical resection in reducing seizure tendency is correlated with the completeness of removal of the epileptogenic cortex rather than with the location of the epileptogenic area or the nature of the lesion or injury responsible for the original brain damage.

REFERENCES

Corkin, C., Milner, B., and Rasmussen, T. (1970): Somatosensory thresholds—Contrasting effects of postcentral gyrus and posterior parietal-lobe excisions. *Arch. Neurol.,* 22:41–58.

Falconer, M. A., Hill, D., Meyer, A., Mitchell, W., and Pond, D. A. (1955): Treatment of temporal lobe epilepsy by temporal lobectomy. *Lancet,* 1:827–835.

Finlayson, A. J., and Penfield, W. (1941): Acute postoperative aseptic leptomeningitis: Review of cases and discussion of pathogenesis. *Arch. Neurol. Psychiatry,* 46:250–274.

Foerster, O. (1925): Zur Pathogenese und chirurgischen Behandlung der Epilepsie. *Zentralbl. Chir.,* 52:531–549.

Foerster, O. (1926): Zur operativen Behandlung der Epilepsie. *Dtsch. Z. Nervenh.,* 89:137–147.

Foerster, O., and Penfield, W. (1930*a*): Der Narbenzug am und im Gehirn bei traumatischer epilepsie in seiner Bedentung für das Zustandekommen der Anfälle und für die Therapeutische Bekämpfung derselben. *Z. Ges. Neurol. Psychiatr.,* 125:475–572.

Foerster, O., and Penfield, W. (1930*b*): The structural basis of traumatic epilepsy and results of radical operation. *Brain,* 53:99–120.

Horsley, V. (1886): Brain surgery. *Brit. Med. J.,* 2:670–675.

Horsley, V. (1892): The origin and seat of epileptic disturbance. *Brit. Med. J.,* 1:693–696.

Horsley, V. (1909): The function of the so-called motor area of the brain. Linaere Lecture. *Brit. Med. J.,* 2:125–132.

Jackson, I. J. (1949): Aseptic hemogenic meningitis. *Arch. Neurol. Psychiatry,* 62:572–589.

Krause, F. (1909–1912): *Surgery of the Brain and Spinal Cord Based on Personal Experience.* Translated by H. Hambold and M. Thorek. Rebman Co., New York, Vols. 1:282 pp., 2:283–819 pp., 3:820–1201 pp.

Lilly, J. C., Alvord, E. C., Jr., and Galkin, T. W. (1955): Brief non-injurious electric waveform for stimulation of the brain. *Science,* 121:468–469.

Marino, R., and Rasmussen, T. (1968): Visual field changes after temporal lobectomy in man. *Neurology,* 18:825–835.

Marshall, C. (1951): Surgery of epilepsy and motor disorders. In: *A History of Neurological Surgery,* edited by A. E. Walker, pp. 288–300. Williams and Wilkins, Baltimore.

Milner, B. (1954): Intellectual functions of the temporal lobe. *Psychol. Bull.,* 51:42–62.

Milner, B. (1958): Psychological defects produced by temporal lobe excision. *Res. Publ. Assoc. Res. Nerv. Ment. Dis.,* 36:244–257.

Milner, B. (1964): Some effects of frontal lobectomy in man. In: *The Frontal Granular Cortex and Behaviour,* edited by J. M. Warren and K. Akert. McGraw-Hill, New York.

Milner, B. (1965): Visually-guided maze learning in man: Effects of bilateral hippocampal, bilateral frontal and unilateral cerebral lesions. *Neuropsychologia,* 3:317–338.

Milner, B. (1968): Visual recognition and recall after right temporal lobe excision in man. *Neuropsychologia,* 6:191–209.

Milner, B., Branch, C., and Rasmussen, T. (1962): Study of short term memory after intracarotid injection of sodium amytal. *Trans. Am. Neurol. Assoc.,* 87:224–226.

Penfield, W. (1930): The radical treatment of traumatic epilepsy and its rationale. *Can. Med. Assoc. J.,* 23:189–197.

Penfield, W. (1936): Epilepsy and surgical therapy. *Arch. Neurol. Psychiatry,* 36:449–484.

Penfield, W. (1939): The epilepsies: With a note of radical therapy. *N. Engl. J. Med.,* 221:209–218.

Penfield, W. (1949): Epileptic manifestations of cortical and supracortical discharge. *Electroencephalogr. Clin. Neurophysiol.,* 1:3–10.

Penfield, W. (1951): The clinical classification of the epilepsies with notes on surgical therapy. *IVth International Congress on Neurology, Comptes Rendus,* 3:435–449. Masson, Paris.

Penfield, W., and Baldwin, M. (1952): Temporal lobe seizures and technique of subtotal temporal lobectomy. *Ann. Surg.,* 136:625–634.

Penfield, W., and Erickson, T. C. (1941): *Epilepsy and Cerebral Localization.* Charles C Thomas, Springfield, Ill.

Penfield, W., and Flanigin, H. (1950): Surgical therapy of temporal lobe seizures. *Arch. Neurol. Psychiatry,* 64:491–500.

Penfield, W., and Gage, L. (1933): Cerebral localization of epileptic manifestations. *Arch. Neurol. Psychiatry,* 30:709–727.

Penfield, W., and Jasper, H. H. (1940): Electroencephalography in focal epilepsy. *Trans. Am. Neurol. Assoc.,* 66:209–211.

Penfield, W., and Jasper, H. H. (1954): *Epilepsy and the Functional Anatomy of the Human Brain.* Little, Brown, Boston.

Penfield, W., and Kristiansen, K. (1951): *Epileptic Seizure Patterns.* Charles C Thomas, Springfield, Ill.

Penfield, W., Lende, R. A., and Rasmussen, T. (1961): Manipulation hemiplegia, an untoward complication in the surgery of epilepsy. *J. Neurosurg.,* 18:760–776.

Penfield, W., and Milner, B. (1958): Memory deficit produced by bilateral lesions in the hippocampal zone. *Arch. Neurol. Psychiatry,* 79:457–497.

Penfield, W., and Paine, K. (1955): Results of surgical treatment of epileptic seizures. *Can. Med. Assoc. J.,* 73:515–531.

Penfield, W., and Steelman, H. (1947): The treatment of focal epilepsy with cortical excison. *Am. Surg.,* 126:740–762.

Rasmussen, T. (1963): Surgical therapy of frontal lobe epilepsy. *Epilepsia,* 4:181–198.

Rasmussen, T. (1964): Traitement chirurgical de l'epilepsie. *Neurochirurgie,* 10:471–476.

Rasmussen, T. (1969): The neurosurgical treatment of focal epilepsy. In: *Modern Problems of Pharmacopsychiatry, Vol. 4: Epilepsy, Recent Views on its Therapy, Diagnosis, and Treatment,* edited by E. Niedermeyer. S. Karger, Basel.

Rasmussen, T. (1969): The role of surgery in the treatment of focal epilepsy. In: *Clin. Neurosurg.,* Vol. 16, pp. 288–311.

Rasmussen, T. (1969): Surgical aspects of post-traumatic epilepsy. In: *Late Effects of Head Injury,* edited by W. F. Caveness and A. E. Walker. Charles C Thomas, Springfield, Ill., pp. 277–305.

Rasmussen, T. (1974): Cortical excision for medically refractory epilepsy. In: *The Natural History and Management of Epilepsy,* edited by P. Harris and C. Maudsley. Churchill Livingston *(in press).*

Rasmussen, T., and Branch, C. (1962): Temporal lobe epilepsy: Indications for and results of surgical therapy. *Postgrad. Med. J.,* 31:9–14.

Rasmussen, T., and Gossman, H. (1963): Epilepsy due to gross destructive brain lesions. *Neurology,* 13:659–669.

Rasmussen, T., and Gulati, D. R. (1962): Cortisone in the treatment of postoperative cerebral edema. *J. Neurosurg.,* 19:535–544.

Rasmussen, T., and Jasper, H. H. (1958): Temporal lobe epilepsy: Indication for operation and surgical technique. In: *Temporal Lobe Epilepsy,* edited by M. Baldwin and P. Bailey, Charles C Thomas, Springfield, Ill., pp. 440–460.

Rasmussen, T., Mathieson, G., and Leblanc, F. (1972): Surgical therapy of typical and a forme fruste variety of the Sturge-Weber syndrome. *Schweiz. Arch. Neurol., Neurochir. Psychiatr.,* 111:393–409.

Rasmussen, T., and McCann, W. (1968): Clinical studies of patients with focal epilepsy due to "chronic encephalitis." *Trans. Am. Neurol. Assoc.,* 93:89–94.

Scoville, W. B., and Milner, B. (1957): Loss of recent memory after bilateral hippocampal lesions. *Neurol. Neurosurg. Psychiatry,* 20:11–21.

Silfvenius, H., Gloor, P., and Rasmussen, T. (1964): Evaluation of insular ablation in surgical treatment of temporal lobe epilepsy. *Epilepsia,* 5:307–320.

Starr, M. A. (1893): *Brain Surgery.* William Wood, New York, pp. 19–113.

Advances in Neurology, Vol. 8, edited by D. P. Purpura, J. K. Penry, and R. D. Walter. Raven Press, New York © 1975.

8
Surgery of Temporal Lobe Epilepsy

J. M. Van Buren, C. Ajmone-Marsan, N. Mutsuga, and D. Sadowsky

INTRODUCTION

In the field of focal seizure disorders suitable for surgical treatment, epilepsy originating from temporal lobe structures has emerged as the most prevalent type (Penfield and Jasper, 1954). Although a high percentage of patients affected by such a disorder can be controlled by medication (Currie, Heathfield, Henson, and Scott, 1971), a significant residual remain who are resistant to available drug therapy (McNaughton, 1954; Gibbs, 1954; Strobos, 1959; Frantzen, 1961; Hedenstroem and Schorsch, 1963; Rodin, 1968). It is with this group that we deal in the present chapter. The problems rest, in essence, on the identification and selection of individuals who can be expected to benefit from surgical removal of the temporal lobe.

MATERIAL FOR STUDY AND METHODS

General Evaluation of the Material

This study is based on a group of 143 patients operated on over a 15-yr period (1954–1969). All had electrographic evidence of a potentially epileptogenic process within the temporal region. All of these patients have undergone craniotomy, and in 127 of them an excision of temporal structures was carried out. A total of 124 patients have been available for postoperative follow-up of at least 3 yr, and most of the analyses to be presented and discussed are based on these patients.

As an anamnestic study, the material from the patient charts was transcribed to data sheets by the present investigators and reduced to approximately 800 entries on standard IBM punch cards. In view of the relatively small number of cases, manual work with the data printout sheets proved to be the most practical means of analysis and correlation of the data.

The headings included in the study are given in Appendix #1 and have drawn upon forms employed elsewhere (Rodin, 1968).

Radiologic examination included plain skull X-rays in all patients, fractional pneumoencephalography in all except case #160, and carotid arteriography with or without examination of the posterior circulation in over 70% of the cases.

The technique of EEG examination was standard, using a minimum of 21 electrodes applied according to the International System. Basal leads were used in 92% of the cases. The routine examination included hyperventilation, photic stimulation, and sleep. In 63 patients (51%), a Metrazol activation test was also performed. Chronically implanted electrodes were used in 17 patients who later came to operation. (Five of these patients are not included in this series because of no excision or insufficient follow-up period.)

As a rule the preoperative workup consisted of a minimum of three (exceptionally two) records, but in the large majority of patients between four and over 15 tracings were obtained through a period of 1 month to several years prior to the operation (see Table 5).

The electrographic localization of the epileptogenic process was based on the overall impression derived from all preoperative tracings and was, in all cases, dependent on the presence of typical, clearly epileptiform interictal abnormalities. In a considerable number of cases localization and lateralization were additionally confirmed by the occurrence of (spontaneous or induced) electrographic ictal episodes.

Clinical-EEG Evaluation

Since the EEG findings appeared in every case, as opposed to the rather meager findings on physical and radiological examination, particular attention was paid to reducing this material to a form suitable for the evaluation of the postoperative results and such that it could be correlated with scores representing the clinical results of temporal resection.

EEG Scoring

In each patient all of the preoperative records have been evaluated for presence or absence of clearly epileptiform abnormalities and classified respectively as positive or negative records. The same procedure was followed for all of the tracings obtained in the postoperative period and the percentages of positive records in the two periods were determined. The EEG scoring was based on the ratio of the percentages of positive tracings between the post- and the preoperative period. A ratio of zero indicates that all postoperative records are negative; a ratio of $> 0 < 1$ suggests some improvement; a ratio of 1 indicates no change and $>$ 1 a deterioration. In practice, all cases have been eventually subdivided into five main groups of progressively less satisfactory EEG results (see Table 7B) according to the ratios of 0 (very good), 0.01–0.25 (good), 0.26–0.50 (fair), 0.51–0.75 (poor), and > 0.75 (very poor). The individual members of each group can also be displayed in a chronological, postoperative follow-up, with the indication of positivity and/or negativity of EEG tracings in each year (but this form of display—analogous to that shown in Table 8—is not included here for reasons of space).

Clinical Scoring

Evaluation of each patient was carried out first on a yearly basis in the postoperative period with a single rating of 1 (no seizures[1]), 2 (seizure incidence significantly decreased), 3 (seizures unchanged), or 4 (seizure incidence increased). These yearly ratings were then added, and the total divided by the number of follow-up years provides the global score for the clinical results in each patient. As shown in Table 7A, all patients were then subdivided into five main groups of results on the basis of this score: 1 (seizure-free), 1.01–1.39 (very rare seizures), 1.40–1.79 (rare seizures), 1.80–1.99 (moderate improvement), and 2 and over (no changes). It should be noted that this scoring is conservative inasmuch as the results are considered satisfactory only in patients with global scores of less than 2, in spite of the fact that a 2 in any given postoperative year stands for a decrease in incidence of seizures. Furthermore, a patient must have been entirely seizure-free for *at least* 1 year, sometime in his follow-up period, in order not to be included in the group of postoperative failures, and even a seizure-free year might not be sufficient if the seizures were unchanged or the conditions had deteriorated in another year. In other similar studies, the occasional occurrence of seizures in the early postoperative period is generally disregarded if the patient becomes subsequently seizure-free, and the case is considered a total success. With the present scoring system, the same case could only be included in the group of considerable improvement since his scoring would be > 1. This method of scoring also takes into account the length of the follow-up period. Thus, for instance, a patient with a 5-year follow-up (and yearly ratings of 1,1,2,2,1) will have a global score of 1.4 and be included in the group of "rare seizures," whereas another patient with a 6-year follow-up (and yearly ratings of 1,2,2,1,1,1) will fall into the group of "very rare seizures" (score of 1.33). These global scores can be integrated by the presentation of the clinical results in a chronological way. This form of display (see Table 8) shows the actual duration of the follow-up period in each case, the corresponding global scores and EEG ratios and the distribution of years with or without seizures (plus and minus signs) throughout this period.

CLINICAL FEATURES OF TEMPORAL LOBE EPILEPSY

Various data related to the temporal lobe epilepsy group are displayed in Tables 1–4. Table 1 shows the age group distribution, age average and range of the

---

[1] "Seizures" in our nomenclature indicate an ictal episode characterized by loss of consciousness without regard to other phenomena. Thus it includes psychomotor seizures (automatisms) and generalized convulsions unless otherwise indicated. Seizures would also include focal motor attacks which did not appear in the present series. Sensory or psychic aura, however, were not considered seizures although their epileptic character is obvious. For example, a patient is considered free of seizures after temporal lobectomy in the absence of psychomotor attacks and generalized fits even though the epigastric aura might reoccur occasionally. Of the 24 patients without any post-temporal lobectomy seizures (see Table 8), five retained the epigastric aura (cases 147, 074, 088, 142, 005), two an aura of general body sensation (cases 067, 100), and one an aura of choking sensation (case 132).

TABLE 1. *Age, seizure onset, and seizure duration*

Age at seizure onset (yr)	1–5	6–10	11–15	16–25	>25
%	25.0	26.6	17.7	17.7	12.9
Seizure duration (yr)	1–10	11–20	>20		
%	29.0	37.9	33.1		
Age at surgery (yr)	Up to 20	21–30	31–40	>40	
%	20.1	38.8	28.2	12.9	

Seizure duration ($N = 141$): median 15; average 16; range 1–43. EEG temporal unilateral, $N = 88$: median 15.5; average 16.4; range 1–43. EEG temporal bilateral, $N = 53$: median 13.5; average 15.5; range 3–42.
Age at surgery ($N = 124$): median 29; average 29.2; range 11–57.
Seizure duration and age are at the time of the first operation.

TABLE 2. *Anamnestic data (N = 124)*

Variable	N	%
History of febrile convulsions	31	25
at 0–2 yr	23	18.5
at >2 yr	8	6.5
History of head trauma (with unconsciousness and/or skull fracture)	28	22.5
Family history positive	19[a]	15.3
History of maternal labor complications	16[b]	13
History of CNS infections	11	8.9

[a] History of seizure disorder: positive paternal side (5), maternal side (8), both sides (1), siblings (5).
[b] Forceps (9), cesarean (2), breech (1), delayed (2), cord wrapped around neck (1), manual rotation (1).

patient population at the time of surgery, age of seizure onset, and duration of the seizure disorder.

Anamnestic data with possible relationship to seizures of temporal lobe origin were generally negative. The positive data and their relatively low incidence in the population under study are shown in Table 2.

Temporal Lobe Seizure Pattern

The type of aura and ictal patterns characterizing the patient population under study is shown in Table 3. Among the auras, the feeling of an epigastric-abdominal sensation was rather common, having been reported by about half of the patients. Only less than 10% of all patients denied the occurrence of any immediately preictal phenomenon. Among the seizure patterns, automatisms of various types were clearly predominant either as the only form of seizure (24%) or in association with other motor ictal phenomena. This characteristic form of ictal

TABLE 3. *Aura and ictal patterns in 124 patients[a]*

	N	%
Aura		
Epigastric-abdominal	54	43.5
Oropharyngeal	19	15.3
Cephalic	24	19.4
Feelings of fear	20	16.1
Déjà vu—jamais vu	13	10.5
Visual[b]	21	16.9
Auditory[b]	17	13.7
Olfactory-taste	17	13.7
Vestibular	21	16.9
None	12	9.7
Ictal Pattern		
Akinetic with loss of posture	24	19.4
Akinetic without loss of posture	34	27.4
Automatisms (with chewing, swallowing, etc.)	51	41.1
Automatisms (gestural, etc.)	42	33.9
No automatism	34	27.4
Only automatism	30	24.2
Automatism + tonic posture(s)	11	8.9
Head and eyes adversive	10	8.1
Clonic motor phenomena, unilateral	11	8.9
No generalized convulsions (regardless of medication)	62	50.0

[a] More than one type of aura and/or ictal pattern may coexist in some patients.
[b] Includes crude, elementary sensations as well as illusions and/or more complex hallucinations.

manifestation, however, had never been present in over 25% of our patients in spite of the electrographic evidence of temporal lobe involvement. Generalized, grand mal convulsions have never been reported in half of the patients of this study.

Autonomic phenomena are probably a constant feature of psychomotor attacks although reported in relatively few of the present series (40/124 cases or 32%). Of the 43 phenomena reported in the 40 cases, the following incidence was observed: pallor (17), flushing (7), desire to urinate (5), salivation (5), pupillary dilatation (3), and miscellaneous features (11). Close observation of these patients during spontaneous or induced attacks suggested a wider range of autonomic fluctuations (Van Buren, 1958, 1961, 1963; Van Buren and Ajmone-Marsan, 1960) than in, for example, petit mal seizures (Mirsky and Van Buren, 1965). The autonomic sequence in an ictal episode was found to have a remarkable stereotypy from seizure to seizure and patient to patient and is exemplified in Fig. 1.

Various forms of psychiatric disturbances were present in about 40% of the cases and nine of these (plus another four patients) were mentally retarded as well (see Table 4).

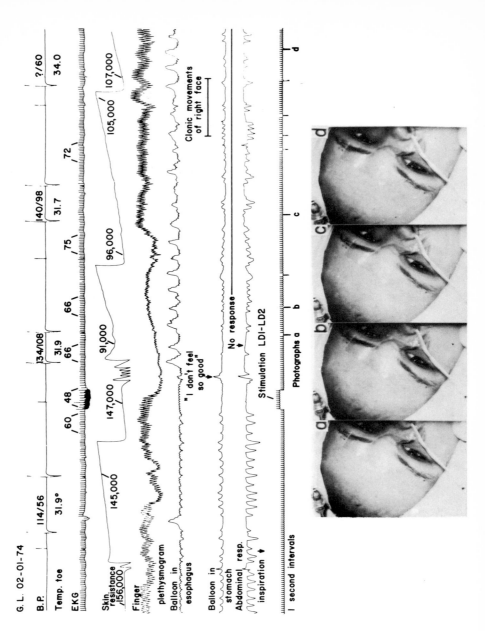

FIG. 1. Autonomic changes associated with an ictal episode of automatism induced by electrical stimulation of the amygdala in a patient affected by temporal lobe seizures. Stimulation (4 mA, diphasic pulses at 60/sec) was carried out through electrodes (LD1-LD2) placed 10 mm anterior and 5 mm above the antero-inferior extremity of the temporal horn. At the onset of expiratory apnea, the patient was questioned and her reply is noted on the record. She swallowed once in the sample before stimulation and the wave of esophageal peristalsis is shown. Note the regularity of esophageal peristalsis before and during the automatism. The size of pupils in photographs *a* and *b* is 4 mm, in *c* and *d* 3 mm. Skin resistance is in ohms. Note the sudden warming of the pad of the great toe late in the automatism (from Van Buren, 1961).

TABLE 4. *Mental retardation, psychiatric disorders, and personality problems in preoperative period (N = 124)*

Disorder	N	
Poor emotional control	17	
Depression	7	
Personality problems	7	
Destructive or assaultive behavior	6	
Suicidal attempts	4	
Schizophrenic reactions	2	
Hypochondriasis	2	
Obsessive compulsive syndrome	2	
Deviant sexual behavior	1	
Severe memory disturbance	1	
Total	49	(39.5%)
Mental retardation	4 (+9)[a]	(10.5%)
No disturbances	71 (+4)	(57.3%; 60.5%)

[a] Mental retardation present also in one case each of depression, schizophrenic reaction, deviant sexual behavior, and violent behavior; in three cases of personality problems; and in two cases of poor emotional control.

Neurological Signs

Thirteen of 124 cases had a hemiparesis, six of these with atrophy of the limbs and two with hemisensory defects. All of these signs were on the side opposite to the EEG lateralization and surgery. In general, however, the clinical examination of the temporal lobe epileptics was not particularly useful either in lateralizing or localizing the lesion.

The postoperative clinical score for this group was 1.7 (see Table 7). Since the average clinical score of the entire series was also 1.7, it appeared that major motor and sensory signs did not necessarily indicate a bad prognosis.

X-ray Features

X-ray findings, including contrast studies, seldom provide useful localizing or lateralizing information in the field of seizure disorders. They are obviously needed, however, to rule out expanding lesions.

On the plain skull films of the 124 patients, the findings were as follows: elevation of petrous ridge on one side (15); unilateral intracranial calcification (7); unilateral flattening of the cranial convexity (6); and unilateral thickening of the cranial convexity (4). The majority of the lateralizing signs on the plain skull films were congruent with the remainder of the evidence. In four instances these findings were on the side opposite to the clinical and EEG lateralization and the side of temporal lobectomy. Elevation of the petrous ridge was implicated twice in these "false" lateralizations and cranial thickening and flattening each once. Except for one case (#230) lacking improvement, the average postoperative score in the remaining three cases was 1.6 (see Table 7).

The pneumoencephalogram provided positive evidence in 50 of 124 cases. Ventricular dilatations of more or less focal character were seen in 47 individuals. Seventeen cases had unilateral dilatation of the temporal horn, seven had frontotemporal enlargement, and 18 had nontemporal enlargements of varying degrees and extent. In 13 cases the lateralization indicated by the EEG and pneumoencephalogram did not agree, and in 12 cases the EEG lateralization was picked for surgery. In these cases the average clinical result was 1.8 (see Table 7).

Arteriography in 88 cases proved to be generally uninformative. Only two cases showed minor arterial displacements, one of which was not confirmed by the air study. Although no vascular malformations were detected by this method, we feel that arteriography should be routinely included in any preoperative evaluation. The unexpected finding of a vascular malformation of any size with craniotomy under local anesthesia would require closing and the postponement of the operation to a later date, after further studies. In addition, the angiographic patterns, particularly the variable venous patterns, at times provide useful information in planning the resection (and this information is also needed if depth electrodes are to be inserted).

Since the clinical follow-up scores for cases with demonstrable radiographic abnormalities were approximately the same as for the group as a whole (1.7), the presence of these findings did not appear to bear upon the prognosis.

Electroencephalographic Findings

As already described in one of the preceding sections, the EEG records showing clearly epileptiform abnormalities were classified as "positive." As shown in Table 5B (see also Ajmone-Marsan and Zivin, 1970), the incidence of such records would vary in different patients; epileptiform discharges in all of their preoperative tracings (100% positive records) were found in over half of the present patient population. All cases had evidence of epileptiform involvement of temporal lobe structures; in some the EEG abnormalities were strictly unilateral while in others they were bilateral and independent with either right- or left-sided predominance.[2] For some patients the epileptiform discharges were clearly limited to the temporal region whereas in others there was evidence of additional extratemporal (suprasylvian) involvement; the temporal discharges could be strictly localized to the antero-inferior portions of the lobe or spread to involve (in some cases predominantly) its posterior portions, etc. According to these and other localizing criteria, the patients have been subdivided into a number of subgroups, as described in Table 5C. The purpose of this classification

---

[2] It is of interest that in this series of patients there was no relationship between the duration of seizure disorder and the incidence of bilateral temporal abnormalities. This finding, shown in Table 1, is at variance with the data of Gupta, Dharampaul, Pathak, and Singh (1973).

TABLE 5. *EEG data*

A. Number of preoperative EEG tracings per patient ($N = 124$)

No. of records:	2–3	4–5	6–7	8–9	10–12	13–15	>15
No. of patients:	19	43	33	12	7	5	5

B. Percent of preoperative tracings with epileptiform abnormalities ($N = 114$)[a]

Percent + records:	Up to 25	26–50	51–75	76–99	100
No. of patients:	1	9	18	23	63
%	0.9	7.9	15.8	20.2	55.3

C. Localization of epileptiform discharges

	N	%
Temporal unilateral	78	62.9
Temporal bilateral	46	37.1
Left, or predominantly left temporal	48	38.7
Right, or predominantly right temporal	76	61.3
Temporal, also suprasylvian	45	36.3
only temporofrontal	20	16.1
temporo-extra-frontal	10	8.1
Also posterior temporal	36	29.0
Maximum mid-posterior temporal	18	14.5
Maximum ant.-inferior-mesial temporal	72	63.2[b]
No involvement of inferior-mesial temporal	28	24.6[b]
Temp. unilateral, maximum ant.-inf.-mesial, no posterotemporal, no suprasylvian	35	30.7[b]
Temporal unilateral, no posterotemporal	61	49.2
Temporal unilateral, also posterotemporal	17	13.7
Temporal bilateral, also suprasylvian	15	12.1
Temporal bilateral, also posterotemporal	19	15.3
Temporal bilateral, no posterotemporal, no suprasylvian	15	12.1

D. Number of postoperative tracings per patient ($N = 124$)

No. of records:	3	4–5	6–7	8–9	10–12	13–15	>15
No. of patients:	6	22	25	22	20	14	15

[a] Exclusive of patients with only two preoperative tracings and of three patients with inadequate postoperative EEG follow-up.
[b] Percent based on 114 patients in whom nasopharyngeal leads were used.

was to correlate the localizing criteria with the results of surgical excision in the hope of better defining the most (or least) favorable electrographic criteria in the selection of candidates for this type of treatment.

CRITERIA FOR SELECTION OF SURGICAL CANDIDATES

In the selection of the most favorable candidates for surgical therapy and in deciding on the suitability of an epileptic individual for focal cerebral resection, the not infrequent complexities of the lateralization and localization of the epileptogenic process obviously play an important role. However, before embarking on the time-consuming series of studies required for this determination, a reasonable assessment of the medical intractability of the seizures and their impact on the patient's present life and future must be established. Although perhaps appearing a cut-and-dried matter, this decision requires extensive consultation of the surgeon with his medical colleagues, the patient, and his family, as well as the hospital social service department and the social welfare facilities in the patient's home town.

Medication

Since surgical therapy should be considered only when the course of medication has proven inadequate, the decision as to when seizures are indeed intractable to medication becomes a very important one. Unfortunately, there are no simple criteria since several variables inevitably occur in combination. The type, dosage, and duration of medication and the combination of medications must be considered in relationship to how these affect the socioeconomic status of the patient. Thus, if occasional seizures remain on dosages just short of those producing toxic symptoms, obviously medication is not successful. Yet, on the other hand, if the individual is able to function in a fashion reasonably acceptable to himself and his associates, this medication must be considered as successful in returning the individual to a useful situation. Thus the patient's evaluation of his own condition must be considered. Whereas some individuals will accept and adjust fairly well to the occasional seizure, others find any abnormality intolerable.

In recent years, the advent of direct determination of the serum levels of antiepileptic medication has provided a further index by which medication can be adjusted. When these facilities are available they may be of great assistance. However, not infrequently, accepted "therapeutic levels" cannot be reached without provoking many complaints of unpleasant side effects. There is also the occasional patient who is either unwilling or unable to persist in taking his medication on a sufficiently regular basis to achieve the projected blood levels. After repeatedly reemphasizing the need for regular medication, one may be faced with either abandoning the patient or undertaking surgical treatment in the hope of alleviating an otherwise disastrous socioeconomic situation.

The selection of medication for temporal lobe seizures remains arbitrary. Our present schedule is to administer primidone, diphenylhydantoin, and phenobarbital in sufficient quantities to achieve blood levels, respectively, of 0.5 to 1.0, 1.0 to 2.0, and 2.0 to 4.0 mg%, if these can be tolerated. This commonly amounts to divided daily oral doses of 750 mg primidone, 300 mg diphenylhydantoin, and 90 mg phenobarbital, although higher doses are often employed.

As is well known, different types of seizures may show differing therapeutic thresholds to medication. Thus it is not uncommon to find that in the case of a patient with both generalized and psychomotor attacks full medication will totally suppress or considerably decrease the incidence of the former but have little effect upon the latter type of seizures (see McNaughton, 1954; Rodin, 1968).

Socioeconomic Factors

In attempting to find a place in society and acceptance by his associates, the patient with temporal lobe epilepsy not only must face the difficulties associated with his seizures but frequently is also burdened by disabling emotional and personality problems. The precise incidence of the latter disorders is still a matter of dispute and figures differ in different patient populations. Some authors do not feel that temporal lobe epileptics, in comparison with epileptics in general, have a particular predilection to psychopathic or personality disorders (Small, Milstein, and Stevens, 1962; Mignone, Donnelly, and Sadowsky, 1970), whereas according to Taylor and Falconer (1968) only 13% of 100 temporal epileptics subjected to temporal lobectomy could be defined as psychiatrically normal. Hill (1959) also noted a high incidence of personality disorders with temporal lobe epilepsy. The relationship of this form of seizure disorder with schizophrenia and schizoid states has been much discussed (Panet-Raymond, 1958; Serafetinides and Falconer, 1962; Small et al., 1962; Scott, 1968; Taylor and Falconer, 1968).

The most common feature has been interictal personality problems related to aggressiveness, irritability, and depression often associated with paranoid trends (Serafetinides and Falconer, 1962; Serafetinides, 1965; Knox, 1968—see also Table 4). Such difficulties may well prevent employment even in the absence of the epileptic disorder. The advisability of an early operation, with view to cure of the seizure disorder before behavior patterns have become fixed, has been advocated by Serafetinides (1965). Certainly the struggle required for the transition from a life of chronic invalidism to the responsibilities of a competent person is best undertaken during the early years.

The second behavioral alteration is that of the ictal automatism itself. The fumbling, random behavior of an individual no longer in contact with his environment may well be frightening to the uninitiated and may prevent employment. In addition, well-intentioned attempts to restrain the patient in a psychomotor attack may result in strong resistance or, rarely, in a directed assault. Years of handling psychomotor attacks on an open surgical ward, however, has taught us that the staff and other patients have nothing to fear from these seizures. These attacks are characterized by a duration of only a few minutes. Ictal episodes of unusually long duration (up to 1 hr according to Knox, 1968) are exceptional in our experience.

Postictal psychotic states, however, may last for hours to days and, as opposed to the psychomotor attack, may not be accompanied by complete amnesia. The behavior is usually well coordinated, gives evidence of planning, and the patient will respond to those about him, though often in an inappropriate fashion. The ideation often has an aggressive paranoid coloration. Active restraint may be needed and resistance to this may be active and effective. Although the frequency with which temporal epileptic patients commit aggressive acts with homicidal potential is grossly exaggerated in most discussions of the subject, it is probable that the true (very rare) instances of such behavior occur when the patient is in this condition.

It should be realized, however, that the dividing line between the true psychotic and postictal psychosis often cannot be drawn at the moment of observation and only the past history and the seizure-related nature of the postictal psychosis will, at times, help in making the differential diagnosis (see Scott, 1968). Even these distinctions may be blurred in the occasional case of a psychotic patient who indeed also suffers of temporal lobe seizures (Knox, 1968; Gunn and Fenton, 1971).

In terms of operative indication, the ictal and postictal features of the temporal lobe seizure may be expected to respond to proper operative treatment. Interictal personality problems are generally more refractory to surgical therapy, in spite of some reports to the contrary (Preston and Atack, 1964; Serafetinides, 1965; Taylor and Falconer, 1968; Hierons, 1971).

POSTOPERATIVE RESULTS

The evaluation of the results of treatment in the field of seizure disorders is generally difficult as there is no fully satisfactory method for such an evaluation and for an objective presentation of the results. This is particularly true for the large group of cases in which the treatment was neither a total success nor a total failure. Such cases appear to be improved, but the definition of "improvement" and the evaluation of its type and degree are often subjective and are based on variable and generally empirical criteria. It is practically impossible to present the results in a reliable and quantitative form, and, as a consequence, it becomes very difficult to compare them in the different studies carried out in various centers throughout the world. The reasons for this situation are implicit in the nature of the seizure disorder itself and the capriciousness of its manifestations.

The method selected for the presentation of results in this study (see section on "Material for Study and Methods") represents an attempt: (1) to evaluate clinical and electroencephalographic results, both separately and in association; (2) to provide both a global, overall result and a "chronological" evaluation throughout each postoperative year of follow-up which is, unavoidably, nonuniform; and (3) to present these results in a quantitative form so as to increase the accuracy of evaluation and, hopefully, permit a comparison with other similar studies.

Complications and Mortality

Early in the series of 143 cases there were two mortalities associated with subdural hemorrhage and a single late death from hepatitis related to blood transfusion given at the time of surgery.

Complications of note consisted of two cases of aseptic meningitis, three cases of dysphasia lasting over 6 weeks, and two instances of hemiparesis. All of these eventually cleared. In addition, there were two cases of serious psychiatric decompensation and one instance of memory deterioration following surgery.

Due to the nature of the operative incision (see Appendix 2), nearly all patients had paresis of the frontalis muscle on the side of operation but this did not provoke complaints. Nearly all of the "total" resections (see footnote 3) had varying degrees of upper quadrantanopias (see Van Buren and Baldwin, 1958). Curiously, we have never had a patient spontaneously mention this defect although the latter may be readily demonstrated by confrontation examination. This may be related to a less extensive functional utilization and retinal representation of this portion of the visual field (Van Buren, 1963).

Pathology of the Temporal Resections

Due to the surgical technique, which usually removed the medial structures by subpial suction after removing the lateral temporal mass, the pathological specimen has generally been limited to portions of the latter. Thus we are not in a position to comment on the pathology of mesial temporal sclerosis which has been reported in detail by others (Meyer, Falconer, and Beck, 1954; Haberland, 1958; Falconer, 1967, 1972).

The listing of the various gross pathological diagnoses is provided in Table 6. The high proportion of specimens showing gliosis was probably related to the use of metallic staining methods in most specimens. The most characteristic change was fibrous transformation of the protoplasmic astrocytes within the lower cortical layers, often associated with an increased density of the normal subpial population of fibrous astrocytes. The group labeled "encephalopathy" was somewhat heterogeneous but in general consisted of perivascular accumulations of pigment-filled macrophages and/or inflammatory cells. Fat stains often showed perivascular fat and occasionally intraneuronal accumulations of material staining as lipid. Of the more specific lesions, nine small vessel or capillary angiomas were encountered (none of these had appeared on the preoperative arteriograms). The four benign gliomas were: two astrocytomas (follow-up 10 and 17 years), one ganglioglioma (follow-up 8 years), and one mixed glioma

TABLE 6. *Pathologic diagnosis*

Diagnosis	N	%
No pathological findings	31	24
Gliosis	67	53
Encephalopathy	15	12
Microangioma	9	7
Tumor		4
Astrocytoma	2	
Ependymoastrocytoma	1	
Ganglioglioma	1	
Glioblastoma	1	
Total	127	100

(ependymoastrocytoma—follow-up 8 years). None of these was suspected prior to operation, and none of the patients since has shown evidence of an expanding lesion. The single glioblastoma was not suspected on contrast studies nor at the initial surgical exploration, but no resection was carried out at that time. Two years later, progressive signs prompted reexploration and partial resection of the tumor. The postoperative survival was 3 years. Worth noting is the fact that no obvious pathology was found in one-fourth of the surgical specimens.

Seizure Control by Surgery

The results of surgical control of seizure are summarized in Table 7, utilizing the evaluation scoring methods described in Section II. The clinical data shown in A indicate 21% of the patients with total recovery, 46% with considerable

TABLE 7. *Temporal lobe excision: Postoperative results*

Results		All resections		"Total" resections[a]		"Partial" resections[a]	
		N	%	N	%	N	%
A. Clinical Score[b]							
1	(Seizure-free)	26	21	24	31.6	2	4
1.01–1.39	(Very rare seizures)	17	14	14	18.4	3	6
1.40–1.79	(Rare seizures)	24	19	16	21.1	8	17
1.80–1.99	(Moderate improvement)	16	13	7	9.2	9	19
≥ 2	(No improvement)	41	33	15	19.7	26	54
		(124)		(76)		(48)	
B. EEG Ratio % positive post/preop. tracings[b]							
0	(Very good)	20	17.5	15	22.1	5	11
.01–.25	(Good)	10	8.8	6	8.8	4	9
.26–.50	(Fair)	14	12.3	12	17.6	1	2
.51–.75	(Poor)	27	23.7	17	25.0	11	24
> .75	(Very poor)	43	37.7	18	26.5	25	54
		(114)[c]		(68)		(46)	

C. Correlations between clinical and EEG postoperative data[b]

EEG	Clin.	1	−1.39	−1.79	−1.99	≥ 2	Total
	0	11	2	3	2	2	20
	−.25	2	5	1	—	2	10
	−.50	6	3	3	—	2	14
	−.75	6	4	4	6	7	27
	> .75	1	2	8	7	25	43
	Total	26	16	19	15	38	114[c]

[a] See text footnote 3.
[b] Clinical scores and EEG ratios as per explanation in Methods.
[c] Excluding 10 patients with an inadequate number of pre- or postoperative EEG tracings to permit a reliable comparison.

improvement, and 33% with no significant changes from their preoperative conditions. These data are from all 124 members of the patient population who had undergone a surgical excision of variable type and extent. If, however, the patients are subdivided into two main subgroups of "total" excision (76 cases) and of "partial" excision (48 cases),[3] the trend of the results shows a considerable difference (Table 7A). Indeed, about 33% of the patients with "total" excision became totally seizure-free and only 20% can be considered therapeutic failures, whereas among the cases with "partial" excision, the failures amount to over 50% and total successes decrease to less than 5%.

These results can also be evaluated in a chronological display of the individual patients such as in Table 8 which includes the 76 cases with "total" excision. This form of display allows a more objective evaluation of the actual postoperative course in each case and is particularly useful for assessing those results which have been scored as neither total successes (Table 8 top group, clinical score: 1) nor total failures (bottom group, clinical score: 2 and > 2). Thus one can see that in addition to the 24 patients with perfect scores, six patients of those with scores of 1.01 to 1.39 had a few seizures in the postoperative year I and/or II but have been subsequently seizure-free for the entire follow-up period (6 to 10 or > 10 years). On the other hand, in six other patients in the two groups of "very rare" and "rare" seizures which had remained seizure-free in the first 4 or 5 years postoperatively, seizures have begun to reappear later on, as the follow-up was prolonged.

The data displayed in Table 8 also provide information on the number of cases which become seizure-free in the first postoperative year and on those which remain so at each subsequent year of follow-up. This information is graphically displayed in Fig. 2, both for the total population and for the cases with "total" surgical excision. The percentages of seizure-free patients in each follow-up year are based on N's which become progressively smaller due to the progressive loss of patients as the follow-up period gets longer (and it is reasonable to presume that patients who are doing well might tend to be less eager to avail themselves of reexamination than those who are doing poorly). In spite of this unavoidable bias, the graphs clearly show that the incidence of surgical successes is much higher at shorter than at longer periods of follow-up. These same data would seem to suggest not only that short periods of postoperative follow-up (3 years or less) are rather meaningless for a reliable assessment of surgical results, but that, actually, even with longer follow-ups, one may seldom be able to state with complete certainty that the treatment has indeed been fully successful. On the

---

[3] "Total" excision included all three temporal gyri (exposing the insula) as well as the fusiform and hippocampal gyri. It included the medial structures (hippocampus, amygdala, and uncus). Of the 76 operative reports and drawings, 10 lacked specific mention of removal of the hippocampus. "Partial" excision varied from gyrectomies to excisions sparing one or more temporal gyri. Medial removals in the 48 cases of "partial" excision were as follows: amygdala alone, seven cases; uncus and amygdala, four cases; uncus, amygdala, and hippocampus, one case; amygdala and hippocampus, two cases.

TEMPORAL LOBE EPILEPSY

TABLE 8. *Presence (+) or absence (−) of seizures throughout the entire postoperative follow-up period* [a]

Case no.	Postoperative year						>X	Clinical score	EEG ratio
	I	II	III	IV	V	VI–X			
084	−	−	−	−	−	−−−−−−	−−−−−−−	1	.75
090	−	−	−	−	−	−−−−−−	−−−−−−−−	1	.50
145	−	−	−	−	−	−−−−−−	−−−−−−−	1	0
207	−	−	−	−	−	−−−−−−	−−−−−−−	1	0
147	−	−	−	−	−	−−−−−−	−	1	.75
024	−	−	−	−	−	−−−−−−		1	.50
240	−	−	−	−	−	−−−−−−		1	.50
132	−	−	−	−	−	−−−−−		1	.25
148	−	−	−	−	−	−−−−−		1	.50
046	−	−	−	−	−	−−−−		1	0
067	−	−	−	−	−	−−−		1	.75
028	−	−	−	−	−	−−−		1	.50
074	−	−	−	−	−	−−−		1	.50
021	−	−	−	−	−	−		1	0
075	−	−	−	−	−	−		1	0
088	−	−	−	−	−	−		1	0
142	−	−	−	−	−			1	.25
146	−	−	−	−	−			1	0
005	−	−	−	−	−			1	.75
049	−	−	−	−	−			1	.75
077	−	−	−	−	−			1	0
100	−	−	−	−	−			1	1.00
184	−	−	−	−	−			1	0
239	−	−	−	−	−			1	0
072	+	+	−	−	−	−−−−−+	−−−−−−−	1.18	.75
124	−	+	−	−	−	−−−−−−	−−−−−−	1.07	.75
082	+	−	−	−	−	−−−−−−	−−−−−	1.13	.75
071	+	+	−	−	−	−−−++−	−−−−	1.20	.50
143	−	−	−	−	−	−−−−−+	++	1.25	1.00
126	−	+	−	−	−	−−−−−−		1.10	.50
136	+	+	−	−	−	−−−−−−		1.20	.75
051	−	−	−	−	−	−+++		1.33	1.00
004	+	−	−	−	−	−−−−−		1.17	.25
102	+	−	+	−	−	−−−−		1.21	.25
031	+	−	−	+	−	−+−		1.38	.75
157	−	−	−	−	−	+−−		1.12	0
032	+	−	−	−	−	−		1.17	.25
053	−	−	−	−	+	+		1.33	.50
034	+	−	−	−	−	−−−−−+	++++++	1.50	.50
042	−	−	−	+	+	+−+++	++++++	1.75	.75
041	−	−	−	?	+	++++++	+++++	1.64	.75
016	+	+	+	+	+	+−−−−	−−−−−	1.78	.50
025	+	+	+	+	+	++−−−	−	1.64	1.00
152	−	−	−	+	+	+++++	+	1.73	1.00
116	−	−	−	−	+	+++++		1.60	.50
050	−	+	+	+	+	+−−−−		1.70	.75
109	−	+	−	+	+	++++		1.78	.75
209	+	+	+	+	+	−−−−−		1.55	.75
054	+	−	−	−	−	−++		1.50	.50

TABLE 8 Continued

Case no.	I	II	III	IV	V	VI–X	>X	Clinical score	EEG ratio
052	+	+	−	−	+	++		1.71	1.00
111	−	−	+	+	+	++		1.72	0
013	−	−	−	−	+	+		1.50	0
159	−	−	−	+	+			1.40	1.00
022	−	+	−	+				1.50	0
037	+	+	−	+	+	+++++	++++++	1.94	.75
040	−	−	−	?	?	?????	++++++	1.81	>1.00
047	+	−	−	+	+	+++++	++++++	1.87	.75
072	−	+	+	+	+	+++++	++++++	1.93	.50
008	−	+	+	+	+	+++++	++	1.92	1.00
009	−	+	+	+	+	+++++	+	1.91	>1.00
057	−	+	+	+	+			1.80	0
093	+	+	+	+	+	+++++	++++++	2.00	1.00
104	+	+	+	+	+	+++++	++++++	2.72	>1.00
030	+	+	+	+	+	+++++	++++	3.00	1.00
007	+	+	+	+	+	+++++		2.00	.75
060	+	+	+	+	+	+	+	2.85	1.00
014	−	+	+	+	+			4.00	>1.00
099	+	+	+	+	+			2.00	.75
113	+	+	+	+	+			2.80	.50
101	+	+	+	+	+			2.00	0
164	+	+	+	+	+			2.00	1.00
230	+	+	+	+				3.00	1.00
259	−	+	?	+				2.00	1.00
153	+	+	+	+				2.25	1.00
195	+	+	+	+				2.00	.25

[a] Data are from each individual patient in which a "total" surgical excision was carried out. Year I refers to the year of operation. The patients are arranged into five subgroups of progressively poorer therapeutic results according to their clinical scores (see text and Table 7A), and the length of the follow-up period. The actual individual scores as well as the corresponding EEG ratios (see text and Table 7B) are provided in the two columns on the right.

other hand, it should be kept in mind that the descending slope of the two graphs of Fig. 2 is strongly influenced by the inclusion in the *N* of *all* patients available at any given year of follow-up (i.e., both of seizure-free patients and of patients with seizures in the preceding years). Thus, the graphs simply provide a general indication of the absolute incidence of seizure-free patients, in the overall population and for the cases with satisfactory excision, at different postoperative periods. Yet, even if one takes into consideration *only* the cases which are seizure-free in the first postoperative year and throughout the length of the follow-up period, one notes a 25 to 30% decrease of such cases in the second year, and then a 10 to 15% progressive decrease at each subsequent year. In conclusion, it seems safe to state that of those patients who have been seizure-free for 5 continuous years, at least 90% have a very high probability to remain seizure-free permanently.

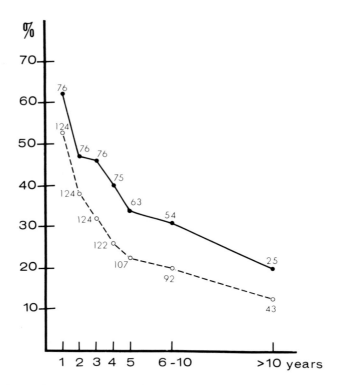

FIG. 2. Graphic display of the incidence of seizure-free patients at various years in the postoperative follow-up period. The figures represent the number of patients available for follow-up at any given year. The plotted percentages of seizure-free cases are based on these numbers. Open circles, all population; filled circles, patients with "total" excision.

Of the 120 temporal resections in which measurements of the length of the resection[4] were available, the average "total" resection (see footnote 3) was 6.2 cm on the right and 4.8 cm on the left. Similarly, the average "partial" resection was 4.5 cm on the right and 3.9 cm on the left. The right and left clinical scores of these cases (Table 7) were, respectively, 1.66 and 1.81, suggesting a slightly better clinical result associated with the larger right-sided resections. (The degree of medial removal was essentially similar on both sides.) This difference, however, did not prove to be statistically significant.

In 12 cases later coming to temporal lobectomy, depth electrodes were inserted to assist in localizing the epileptic process. Ten of 12 had nearly equal bitemporal epileptiform abnormalities, whereas the remaining two cases showed unilateral temporal and extratemporal involvement of nearly equal degree. The implanta-

---

[4] These measurements were made from the anterior margin of the amputated second temporal gyrus to the most anterior extremity of the temporal fossa.

tions (Van Buren, Ajmone-Marsan, and Mutsuga; *in preparation*) consisted of a multiport needle electrode directed to the medial temporal structures about the tip of the temporal horn and multiport epidural electrodes inserted through the same burr hole (usually over the second temporal gyrus) and passing anterior and posterior to the burr hole. We have not employed the large numbers of electrode contacts advocated by others (Bancaud, Talairach, Bonis, Schaub, Szikla, Morel, and Bordas-Ferer, 1965) nor inserted electrodes in areas lacking some evidence of electrographic abnormality on the scalp recordings. In this group of 12, four cases were rendered seizure-free (three off medication, average follow-up 6.5 years—range 4 to 10 years). Four patients had seizure-free periods after operation ranging from 2 to 5 years, then the reappearance of rare attacks (average follow-up 6.6 years). The last four patients had no significant improvement.

Of the total 143 patients in whom craniotomies were performed, 15 had no excision of cerebral structures. None of these patients became seizure-free (i.e., none had a clinical score of 1) and 14 had a score of > 2. Only one had a score of 1.3 (being seizure-free for 4 of 5 years of postoperative follow-up).

Patients who underwent more than one operation (with excision) have been included in the main group of 124 cases, their postoperative follow-up being based on the years after the last operation. In two, of 16 such cases, the second excision resulted in total disappearance of seizures while in all of the others their clinical scores showed no significant differences following the first and the second excision.

Socioeconomic and Psychiatric Results

The preceding analysis on "clinical" results has been exclusively limited to the main target of surgical therapy, i.e., the management of seizures. As mentioned before, however, about 40% of the patients in this series had also some form of psychiatric disorder and/or personality problem in addition to their seizures (see Table 4). After surgical treatment the psychiatric abnormality was abolished in about 33% of the patients, it remained unaffected in 14 patients (about 30%), and persisted under a different form in the remaining 18 patients (37.5%). It should also be pointed out, however, that of the 75 subjects with no psychiatric disorder in their preoperative period, 17 (about 23%) developed some form of psychiatric abnormality in their postoperative period. Thus, the overall incidence of cases with such abnormality remained almost exactly equal (40%) in both pre- and postoperative stages. The type of temporal lobe excision (whether total or partial) did not seem to have any significant bearing on its effects (or lack thereof) on the psychiatric syndrome.

Due to the severity of their seizure disorder (and/or to coexisting psychiatric or personality problems), the large majority (95%) of the patients in this series were impaired in their capacity to perform proficiently in their profession, to hold steady jobs, or to be usefully employed in areas requiring a certain amount of

TABLE 9. *Work impairment*

	Degree of impairment (rating)				
	None (1)	Minimal (2)		Moderate (4)	Unable to work (5)
Preoperative period (N = 109)[a]					
No. of patients	5	40	28	24	12
%	4.5	36.5	26	22	11
Postoperative period (N = 119)[a]					
No. of patients	36	41	17	13	12
%	30	34.5	14	11	10

Effects of surgical treatment on work impairment

Ratio pre/postop.[b] (N = 102)[a]	5–4	3–2	1.7–1.5	1.3–1.2	1	.75	.67–.50	.2
No. of patients	7	29	13	5	35[c]	4	8	1
	←――――― Improvement ―――――→				No change	←――― Deterioration ―――→		

[a] N represents the number of patients for whom the specific information was available.
[b] See text for explanation.
[c] Excluding three cases with no impairment in either the pre- or postoperative period and including five patients with rating 5 and five patients with rating 4 in the preoperative period.

responsibility. This diminished efficiency in work capacity manifested itself in various degrees of severity (Table 9). Table 9 also shows how the surgical excision for the treatment of seizures had an indirect, beneficial effect on the work capacity of a considerable portion of the patient population. Thus, in the postoperative period 30% of the patients had no obvious impairment compared to less than 5% before surgery. In an attempt to evaluate more effectively the degree of such changes, each patient was rated along an arbitrary scale of 1 to 5 (as indicated in Table 9) according to the severity of their work impairment in both pre- and postoperative periods. The ratio of these two ratings provides a relatively faithful index of the extent of improvement (if any) in the work capacities of each patient. A ratio of 5 indicates that a subject, totally unable to work before surgery, shows no detectable impairment in the postoperative period; ratios of $< 5 > 1$ indicate progressively lesser degrees of improvement, whereas a ratio of 1 is equivalent to no appreciable changes from the preoperative conditions. The results of this analysis, given in Table 9, show some improvement in over 50% of the cases, no change in 36%, and deterioration in over 12%. These figures are from the entire population of patients in which the specific information was available and includes cases with either total or partial excision. Almost exactly similar percentages are obtained, however, if this analysis is limited to the group of cases with total temporal lobe excision.

Electroencephalographic Results

All patients had an EEG postoperative follow-up which included a large number of examinations (see Table 5D). These were generally spread out on a yearly basis with at least one but more often several tracings obtained in each subsequent year of the follow-up period. The method of evaluating the electrographic data is based on a comparison between pre- and postoperative EEG findings and has been described in the section on "Material." The results of this comparison are summarized in Table 7B and refer to both the entire population and the two groups of patients with total excision and with partial removal of the temporal lobe.

The EEG data were generally consistent with the clinical results, although striking discrepancies could be noted in several cases. The correlations between clinical and EEG postoperative results (in the overall population) are presented in Table 7C. Of the patients with perfect clinical results, about 50% also tend to have a decrease of epileptiform activity in their EEGs and 42.5% show a total disappearance of such an activity. Similarly, of those patients who can be considered therapeutic failures (score of over 2), only 5% have a complete normalization of their EEG, and 67% show either no changes in the amount of epileptiform discharges or an increase in positive tracings. Additional considerations on the effects of surgery on the EEG and the overall significance of such changes are offered in the following section.

DISCUSSION

Surgical Results of Temporal Lobectomy for Epilepsy

Table 10 shows the results of surgical therapy in different series of patients affected by temporal lobe seizures, as reported by various authors. The percentages of "cure" in such a table may not be taken entirely on face value. Criteria of evaluation and particularly the duration of follow-up must be taken into consideration. The short minimal follow-up period (6 months to 1 year) of many studies renders their final results suspect in view of our results and those of the Montreal series (Rasmussen, 1974, *personal communication*) indicating late recurrence of attacks in a certain proportion of cases.

As is apparent from our findings (see Table 7) and from the findings summarized in Table 10, the results of surgery in temporal lobe epilepsy are *totally* satisfactory in only a relatively small portion of the population. Even when the excision had been considered to be fairly complete, only about 33% of the cases turned out to be perfect clinical results, and there are still a 20% of total failures. It would therefore be of great practical usefulness if it were possible to improve the screening of patients and to select those which are most likely to benefit from the surgical treatment. For this purpose an attempt was made to correlate the postoperative clinical results with a number of anamnestic, clinical, and EEG variables characterizing the patient population in the preoperative period. Some of these variables are outlined in Tables 1–4. Such correlative studies carried out for more than 50 variables have been negative in the large majority, or the few instances of positive trends did not pass a test of statistical significance. Thus we could find no valid criteria to determine the most favorable cases and the best candidates for surgical treatment among patients affected by a seizure disorder of temporal lobe origin. In fact, the lack of any significant correlation would also seem to indicate that the postoperative results are not unfavorably affected by such factors as, for instance, a positive family history of seizures (see also Anderman, Metrakos, and Rasmussen, 1972), a history of CNS infections, and the age of seizure onset (possibly, patients with seizure onset at an early age seem to score slightly better than those with a late onset). Similarly negative have been the correlations between the pathological observations (presence and type or absence) and the postoperative effects on the seizure disorder.

Also somewhat unexpected was the finding that certain features of the EEG localization (see Table 5) have little bearing on the outcome of surgery. For instance, one would have anticipated a more favorable prognosis for those patients with an exclusively unilateral temporal involvement and with epileptiform discharges strictly limited to the anterior-inferior portions of one temporal lobe, yet these cases showed no particularly high incidence of total clinical successes nor a significantly low incidence of clinical failures in comparison with data of the overall population. In fact, the incidence of failures and successes in these patients is very similar to that of patients with (1) EEG evidence of bitemporal

TABLE 10. Results of temporal lobectomy for epilepsy

Reference[a]	Duration of follow-up	No. of cases		Seizure-free	Seizures improved	Seizures unchanged	Remarks
Bailey (1961)	5 yr	60	PM	18[b] 30%	23 38%	19 32%	2 seizure-free & off
			GM	28[b] 56%	5 10%	17 34%	medication; 1 death
Bloom et al. (1960)	1–10 yr, av. 4.4	29	BiT	7 24%	—21–76%—		
		33	UniT	21 64%	—12–36%—		
Brown et al. (1956)	5 mo–5 yr	25		12 50%			1 death
DeVet (1972)	2+ yr	40		18 45%	18 45%	4 10%	2/40 deaths
Fasano and Broggi (1957)	3+ yr	36		6 17%			
French (1958)	2–7 yr	25		12 48%			1/25 death
Green et al. (1957)	1½–8½ yr	38		15 40%	15 40%	8 20%	
Guillaume and Mazars (1956)	½–7 yr,	110		72 65%	20 18%	17 16%	
	5–7 yr	36		23 64%	9 25%	4 11%	
Kachaev (1961)	4 yr	33		8 24%	15 45%	8 24%	2/33 deaths
Maspes and Marossero (1954)	7 mo–2 yr	26		14 54%	8 31%	4 15%	
Mathai and Chandy (1970)	1–5 yr	24		8 33%	11 46%	11 46%	
Morris (1956)	3–9 yr, av. 5 yr	36		15 42%	16 44%	5 14%	
Northfield (1966)	1–11 yr	58		18 32%	28 48%	12 20%	
Paillas et al. (1953)	½–4 yr	29		9			
Penfield and Flanigin (1950)	1–10 yr	65		35 54%	17 26%	13 20%	1.5% death rate
Taylor and Falconer (1968)	2–12 yr	100		42 42%	42 42%	16 16%	
Rasmussen and Branch (1962)	1–25 yr, av. 5 yr	389		168 43%	97 25%	124 32%	1.6% death rate
Rasmussen, T. (1974)[c]	2–38 yr, av. 11 yr	629		256 41%	177 28%	196 31%	0.4% death rate

[a] Full references are given following main list of references for this chapter. Due to lack of uniformity and substantial variations in the assessment of the results and the presentation of the various reports among the different authors, the data summarized in this table should be considered as approximate.

[b] "Greatly improved."

[c] Personal communication.

PM = psychomotor seizures; GM = grand mal; BiT = bitemporal; UniT = unitemporal.

independent involvement with lateral preponderance, (2) evidence of additional extratemporal abnormalities, or (3) epileptiform discharges predominantly localized over the mid-posterior portions of the temporal lobe(s). Thus, at least in our series of cases, these apparently complicating EEG features do not seem to have represented a particularly negative factor in the determination of the surgical outcome.

Prognostic Value of the Postoperative EEG

The preceding data on the clinical and EEG results of surgical treatment of temporal lobe seizures and especially those illustrated in Tables 7C and 8 and in Fig. 2 have shown that the longer the follow-up period, the more valid and reliable is the assessment of the results themselves, and that there might be considerable discrepancies between the clinical results and the postoperative EEG findings. For instance, we have found in our series nine patients with an EEG score of 0 (i.e., all postoperative records negative) but with clinical scores of either over 1 (i.e., rare or considerably decreased, but persisting seizures) or over 2 (seizure disorder unchanged). In addition, there were 15 patients who can be considered as total therapeutic successes while some (or all) of their postoperative records have continued to show clearly epileptiform discharges.

Whereas a full clinical recovery is obviously more important to the patient than the positivity or negativity of an EEG examination, it is also true that a very long seizure-free follow-up period is always necessary before one can conclude that the clinical recovery is indeed permanent and complete. In view of this, the presence or absence of seizures and their association with either positivity or negativity of the EEG should not be visualized simply as puzzling examples of meaningless discrepancies (or of expected consistencies). Rather, the association of these two sets of data in the early postoperative period could be utilized for practical purposes of prognostic significance. In fact, the data presented in Table 11 indicate that the type of early postoperative EEG permits one to predict with relatively greater accuracy whether surgery has been a clinical success or a failure. At year 1 this prediction is less certain, but after the first 2 postoperative years the prognosis becomes more reliable. Indeed, only 7% of the patients with positive records will be and will remain totally seizure-free, whereas when the records show absence of epileptiform discharges in the first 2 years, only 13% of the cases will turn out to be total clinical failures.

The occurrence—or absence—of seizures in the early postoperative period seems to have an even greater prognostic significance. Thus, of the patients who continue to have seizures in the first 2 years, about 80% will be clinical failures; of those who have no seizures in this same postoperative period, more than 55% will remain totally seizure-free. As shown in Table 11, the prognosis becomes even more reliable if *both* EEG and clinical data in the first 1 or 2 postoperative years are taken into consideration. Whereas the presence or absence of seizures in the early postoperative stage seems to have a slightly stronger prognostic value

TABLE 11. *Early postoperative follow-up: Prognostic value of seizures and EEG*[a]

Clinical score[b] (N = 124)		1	1.01–1.39	1.40–1.79	1.80–1.99	≥2
First postop. year	N					
EEG +, Seizure +	35	(—)	(14.3)	(11.4)	(—)	(74.4)
Seizure +	58	(—)	(15.5)	(13.8)	(5–1)	(65.5)
Seizure +, EEG −	21	(—)	(19)	(14.3)	(14.3)	(52.5)
EEG +	66	(16.7)	(12.1)	(18.2)	(12.1)	(41)
EEG −	54	(27.8)	(14.8)	(22.2)	(14.8)	(20.2)
Seizure −, EEG +	30	(36.8)	(10)	(23.2)	(26.6)	(3.4)
Seizure −	66	(39.4)	(12.1)	(24.2)	(19.7)	(4.5)
Seizure −, EEG −	33	(45.5)	(12.1)	(27.2)	(15.1)	(—)
First 2 postop. years	N					
EEG +, Seizure +	27	(—)	(7.4)	(11.1)	(—)	(81.5)
Seizure +	48	(—)	(8.3)	(10.4)	(2)	(79)
Seizure +, EEG −	9	(—)	(22)	(11)	(11)	(55.5)
EEG +	41	(7.3)	(9.8)	(17)	(9.8)	(56)
Seizure −, EEG +	10	(30)	(20)	(30)	(20)	(—)
EEG −	38	(34.3)	(15.8)	(29)	(7.8)	(13.2)
Seizure −	47	(55.5)	(8.5)	(23.4)	(10.6)	(—)
Seizure −, EEG −	18	(72.5)	(—)	(27.5)	(—)	(—)

[a] The + and − refer, respectively, to the presence or absence of EEG epileptiform abnormalities and of seizures.
[b] See text and Table 7.
Figures in parentheses refer to percentages.

than the EEG data of the same period, the latter tend to reinforce or, alternatively, weaken the trend suggested by the clinical findings. Thus, for instance, the presence of seizures in the first year is indicative of a very poor prognosis if associated with a positivity of the EEG (about 75% of total failures), but the prognosis is slightly better if the EEG is negative (about 50% of total failures). Similarly, the favorable prognostic significance of an absence of seizures in the first 2 postoperative years (see above) decreases if the EEG is positive (30% of total successes) but markedly increases if the EEG is negative (72.5% of total successes).

SUMMARY

1. This study is based on 143 patients who underwent surgical treatment for the relief of temporal lobe seizures. A number of pre- and postoperative data have been analyzed and correlated in the 124 cases that could be followed for at least 3 years after surgery.

2. The anamnestic data provided little hint as to the origin of the temporal lobe seizures, except for history of febrile convulsions and head trauma (with unconsciousness and/or skull fracture) which appeared, respectively, in about a quarter of the patients.

3. The age of onset of seizures was about equally divided between the intervals

below and above 10 years of age. There was no significant difference in the length of seizure duration between patients with independent bitemporal and those with clearly unilateral epileptiform EEG activity; actually the average duration was slightly longer in the latter group.

4. The most common auras were related to trunkal sensation (epigastric, cephalic, oropharyngeal). Ten percent of the patients reported no aura. Typical "psychomotor" seizures (i.e., automatisms) were also lacking in somewhat less than one-third of the patients.

5. Forty percent of the patients had significant personality and/or psychiatric problems with poor emotional control being the most common symptom. This was associated with mental retardation in 10% of the patients.

6. An attempt has been made to evaluate and present both clinical and electrographic results of surgical treatment in a quantitative form and in relation to the duration of the postoperative follow-up period. The overall results showed 21% total abolition of seizures, 46% considerable improvement, and 33% unchanged. Mortality and serious morbidity were less than 2%. These results can be compared with those reported in other studies.

7. The cure and improvement rate in seizures was significantly higher with "total" than with "partial" resection (e.g., cure rate of 32 versus 4%), and this seemed more related to removal of the medial structures of the temporal lobe than to the extent of the lateral removal.

8. Although about one-third of the patients with personality or psychiatric abnormalities showed alleviation of their symptoms after surgical treatments, about one-fifth of the patients in whom symptoms of this type were not recorded preoperatively had note of them in the postoperative follow-up.

9. After surgical treatment, improvement in work capacity occurred in 50% of the cases, no change in 36%, and deterioration in 12%. No differences were noted between the total and partial resection groups, suggesting that factors other than solely seizure control played a part.

10. The combination of temporal and extratemporal or bitemporal epileptiform EEG abnormalities with unilateral preponderance did not appear to offer a poorer prognosis for seizure control with temporal resection than did the pure unitemporal foci.

11. Twenty-one cases in the series showed some degree of seizure reappearance postoperatively, after a few to many years of freedom from seizures. Thus, short follow-up intervals (3 years or less) have little value in the study of seizure therapy. A minimum of 5 years would seem to be necessary for a more accurate assessment of surgical results. On the other hand, combining the postoperative clinical seizure rate and the EEG findings at the first 1 or 2 years of follow-up may prove of reasonable prognostic value. Thus, absence of seizures for 2 years with negative EEGs indicates a probably eventual cure rate of 72.5% which decreases to 30% if the EEGs remain positive. Similarly, the presence of early post-hospitalization seizures and positive EEGs indicate the 75% likelihood of total failure, which becomes a 50% failure rate if the EEGs are negative.

ACKNOWLEDGMENTS

The authors would like to point out the significant contributions of the late Dr. Maitland Baldwin to the present study. Dr. Baldwin established the study of the surgical treatment of epilepsy at the National Institute of Neurological Diseases and Blindness in 1953 and personally undertook the surgery of the majority of the early cases. The senior author's contribution to the series came somewhat later. Some further cases were added by Drs. Ayub Ommaya, Choh-luh Li, George Ojemann, and Edward Laskowski over the years.

APPENDIX 1

PREOPERATIVE STUDY
Seizure Etiology, Precipitation, Arrest, Frequency,

Medication, Socioeconomic Factors

1–3 Card-set number
4–6 Patient number
7–8 Age when first seen
  9 Sex
10 Handedness
11 Left-handedness in family
12–25 Etiology
    12 Family history
    13–14 Pregnancy of mother
        with patient
    15–18 Labor and delivery
    19–23 Labor complications
    20–23 Birth weight
    24 Abnormality at birth
    25 Developmental milestones
26–31 Neurological history
    26 Neurological defect from
       birth
    27 First febrile convulsions
    28–29 Head injury
    30 Infections of CNS
    31 Electroconvulsive therapy
32–33 Age of onset of present
    seizure problem
34–36 Modifying factors
    34–35 Precipitating factors
    36 Arresting factors
37–44 Seizure frequency—Average fit
    frequency on best medication
    37 Generalized convulsions
    38 Seizures with
      unconsciousness without
      general convulsions
    39 Remission of generalized
      convulsions
    40 Remission of seizures with

      unconsciousness without
      general convulsions
Maximum fit frequency regardless of
medication
    41 Generalized convulsions
    42 Seizures with
      unconsciousness without
      general convulsions
Seizure clusters in one day
    43 Generalized convulsions
    44 Seizures with
      unconsciousness without
      general convulsions
45–50 Medication
    45 Were one or more drugs
      taken at an adequate level?
    46 Was the average fit
      frequency on adequate
      medication?
    47 Adequate trial (over 3 mos.,
      one or more, at accepted
      dosage)
Inadequate trial (less than 3 mos.
trial and/or less than accepted
dosage)
    49 Drugs
    50 Side reactions
51–64 Socioeconomic factors
    51 Mental retardation
    52–53 Psychiatric abnormality
    54–58 Behavior
      54 Relationships with parents
      55 Decreased personal relations
        in adolescence
      56 Socialization at present
      57 Devoutness

58 Use of alcohol
59 Amount of schooling
60 Average grades
61 Level of occupation

62 Degree of work impairment
63 Jobs held in last 3 years
64 Current employment in relation
   to education

Aura

1–3 Card-set number
4–6 Patient number
7–30 Aura
   7–8 Sensory—Type
   9–18 Sensory—Location
   19 Motor—Type
   20–21 Motor—Location
   22 Olfactory

23 Taste
24 Visual—Location
25 Auditory
26 Vestibular
27 Speech
28–29 Psychic change
30 Autonomic change
Repeat 3 times

Ictus, Neurological and Radiological Examinations

1–3 Card-set number
4–6 Patient number
7–12 **Ictus** (with amnesia)
   7–8 Motor—Type
   9–10 Motor—Location
   11–12 Postictal state
Repeat 3 times
25–53 **Neurological exam**
   25 Mental retardation
   26 Behavior disorder
   27 Severe neurosis or psychosis
   28–29 Fine finger movement
   30–31 Weakness—Arm
   32–33 Weakness—Leg
   34–35 Atrophy—Arm and/or
     leg
   36–37 Cortical sensation
     loss—Arm/hand
   38–39 Cortical sensation
     loss—Leg/foot
   40–41 Touch, pain, temperature
     loss—Arm/hand
   42–43 Touch, pain, temperature
     loss—Leg/foot

44–47 Deep tendon reflexes
48–53 Other neurological signs
Radiological findings
54–60 Plain skull film
   54 Thickening of skull—Side
   55 Flattening of convexity (on
     comparison of sides)
   56–57 Intracranial calcification
     (exclude pineal,
     petroclinoid ligament,
     etc.)
   58–59 Sinus enlargement (on
     comparison of sides)
   60 Petrous ridge elevation—Side
61–70 Pneumoencephalogram—
   Ventriculogram
   61 Quality of study
   62–63 Subarachnoid
     space—Dilatation
   64–65 Ventricular
     space—Dilatation
   66–67 Ventricular
     space—Compression
   68–69 Porencephalic cavities
   70 Midline shift—Direction

1–3 Card-set number
4–6 Patient number
7–20 Arteriogram (carotid)
    7–9 Vessel displaced
    10–12 Direction of displacement
       (lateral)

13–15 Direction of displacement
       (vertical)
16–18 Direction of displacement
       (sagittal)
19–20 Vascular malformation

EEG

1–3 Card-set number
4–6 Patient number
7–8 Age (at time of first EEG)
9 Sex
10–75 EEG data
    10–17 Number of records
    10–11 Preop.—Scalp
    12–13 Preop.—Implant
    14–15 Postop.
18–19 Follow-up period before first
    operation
    20–26 No. of records with
       epileptiform discharges
    20–21 Scalp—positive
    22–23 Scalp—negative
    24–26 % positive (scalp &
       implant)
27–30 Presence of epileptiform
    discharges
    27 At rest

28 HV
29 Sleep
30 Metrazol
31–32 Ictal episode(s)
33–34 Epileptiform
    discharges—Distribution
35–36 EEG localization
39–62 Localization (scalp EEG
    electrodes)
63 Implanted electrodes (type & site)
64 Implanted
    electrodes—Lateralization
65–66 Implanted
    electrodes—Localization
67 EEG diagnostic conclusion (based
    on)
68–69 Temporal
70–71 Temporal & suprasylvian
72–73 Suprasylvian (± infrasylvian)
74–75 Other

OPERATION AND ECoG

1–3 Card-set number
4–6 Patient number
7–31 Operation—Repeat for each
    operation
    7–12 Date of operation
    13–14 Years from seizure
       onset to operation or
       last operation
    15–16 Age at operation
    17 Operator
    18–19 Anesthesia
    20 Side of excision

Location and extent of removal
    21 First temporal thru
       hippocampal gyri
    22 Medial temporal
    23 Lateral temporal sparing
       one or more gyri
    24 Frontal lobe
    25 Parietal
    26 Occipital
    27 Combined removals
    28–29 Complications up to 3
       mos. postop.

30–31 Pathology
32–45 ECoG
    32–33 ECoG pre-excision
    34 Localization
    35–36 Region(s) involved
        (temporal)
    37–38 Region(s) involved
        (temporal &
        suprasylvian)

39 Region(s) involved:
    temporal quadrants
40–41 Region(s) involved:
    suprasylvian
42 Electrical stimulation
43–44 Electrical stimulation
    (ADs)
45 ECoG post-excision (final)

POSTOPERATIVE STUDY
Seizure Frequency, Medication, Socioeconomic Factors

1–3 Card-set number
4–6 Patient number
7–9 Duration of follow-up (from operation to next operation or most recent examination)
10–25 Interim effect on overall seizure frequency on year to year basis
26 Effect on seizure activity at last follow-up as compared with preop. status
27–30 Major postop. seizure remission (longest remission over 3 mos.)
    27 Time of appearance of remission
    28–30 Duration of remission
31 Altered postop. seizure pattern
Modifying factors
32 Menses
33 Precipitating factors
34 Arresting factors
35–47 Postoperative medication
    35 Stopped postoperatively
    36–38 Interval between last operation
    39–41 Interval between cessation of medication & last examination
42–43 Postoperative medication
44–45 Adequate trial (over 3 mos. one or more at accepted dosage)
46–47 Inadequate trial (less than 3 mos. trial and/or less than accepted dosage)
48–60 Socioeconomic effect of surgery
48 Mental retardation
49–50 Postop. psychiatric symptoms
52 Socialization at present
53 Devoutness
54 Use of alcohol
55–56 Postop. school history
57–60 Postop. work record
General follow-up summary
61 Seizure frequency
62 Seizure type
63 Medication
64 Neurologic examination
65–66 Socioeconomic situation
66 Work situation

Aura

Repeat of Preoperative Study—Aura

Ictus and Neurological Examination

Repeat of Preoperative Study—Ictus & Neuro Exam

EEG

1–3 Card-set number
4–6 Patient number
7 Postop. study—I operation (date)
8 Other operation (II)
9 Other operation (III)
12–67 EEG postop. findings
    12–16 After first operation: 1st
        year (date)
    12–13 No. of records positive
    14–15 No. of records negative
    16 Same as preop.
    17 Compatible re. localization
    18 Compatible re. lateralization
    19 Different from preop.

20–67 Same as #12–19, repeated for
    up to over 10th year
68–73 Total number of records
    68–69 Total no. after I
        operation
    70–71 Total no. after II
        operation
    72–73 Total no. after last
        operation
74–79 Follow-up period (years)
    74–75 After I operation
    76–77 After II operation
    78–79 After last operation

APPENDIX 2

THE TECHNIQUE OF TEMPORAL RESECTION

Anesthesia

Although the use of general anesthesia has been advocated by some (see below), we continue to use local anesthesia for practically all epileptic excisions since its several advantages seem well worth the slight increase in time and effort entailed in its use (Penfield and Jasper, 1954).

As with all procedures of this type, the confidence inspired by daily contact of the surgeon with the patient, and particularly by a step-by-step review of the procedure during the preoperative period, is essential. The two painful periods, that of infiltration of the local anesthesia and that at the time of separation of the dura from the bone as the bone flap is outlined with burr holes and raised, should be pointed out. Having two definite periods of recognized discomfort rather than an indefinite and generally threatening prospect of "surgery" often provides the patient with a more positive outlook upon the procedure.

Skin preparation is started 2 to 3 days before surgery with a close clip and inspection of the scalp, followed by daily scrubs with a surgical detergent. Decision is made at this time as to whether to withdraw antiepileptic medication or not. In general, this is done 48 hr before surgery in order to provide the maximal positive evidence on the electrocorticogram (ECoG).[5] The decision, however, may be modified if withdrawal of medication during the preoperative workup occasioned serious seizure difficulties within 48 hr.

In recent years we have found it useful to give 50 to 100 mg of chlorpromazine intramuscularly 1 hr before taking the patient to the operating room. The dosage should be tested several days before surgery as there are sufficient individual variations in response to this drug to make dosage based solely upon weight unreliable. Under ward conditions the proper dosage leaves the patient quiet and drowsing in bed but rousable and capable of performing tests (object naming and definition, mathematical problems, etc.) appropriate to his unsedated level of intelligence.

Difficulties with hypotension or cardiac irregularities possibly attending the use of epinephrine in the local anesthetic in conjunction with chlorpromazine have not presented a practical problem. The anesthetist, however, should be warned about giving additional drugs—in particular (for recording purposes), barbiturates or diazepam. If restlessness is encountered later in the procedure, additional chlorpromazine in 4-mg increments intravenously may be useful. This should be used judiciously, however, as certain patients show a tendency toward cumulative effects, manifesting themselves in the latter part of the procedure, and for several hours thereafter, in the form of pupil constriction and a deep somnolence from which the patient can only be aroused with difficulty.

Chlorpromazine used in this fashion does not appear to interfere with epileptiform activity on the ECoG. Occasional spindling and slow activity may appear in relation to periods of spontaneous sleep, easily eliminated by talking to the patient. The drug has proved useful in dispelling the anxiety attending the occasionally painful procedure under local anesthesia and in particular the suffering compounded of fatigue and inevitable minor discomforts of being restrained in the same position for many hours.

We have continued the use of dibucaine hydrochloride USP (Penfield and Jasper, 1954) for local anesthesia and have found it more satisfactory than shorter-acting agents since, once "set," reinfiltration is rarely necessary. This is prepared as 100 ml of the 1:1,500 solution with 0.5 mg of epinephrine and a similar amount of the 1:4,000 solution with a similar amount of epinephrine.

After skin preparation and outlining of the skin flap, the 1:1,500 dibucaine solution is injected in the subgaleal space in a circumferential fashion forming

---

[5] ECoG technique, evaluation of the ECoG data and their significance as a surgical guide have been discussed in a recent publication (Ajmone-Marsan and O'Connor, 1973; see also Ajmone-Marsan and Baldwin, 1958). These data are also reported elsewhere in this volume.

a continuous weal 5 to 8 mm high 2 to 3 cm outside of the line of incision. Particular care should be taken to anesthetize about the base of the ear and to have the weal extend some 2 cm below the zygoma and forward to just behind the frontal ramus of the zygoma to provide an area for drape sutures. Lastly, the zygomatic arch is palpated with the needle tip, and approximately 30 cc of dibucaine is instilled deep in the temporalis muscle just above the arch from just anterior to the tragus to the frontal process of the zygoma. Sensory nerves apparently accompany vascular bundles deep in the temporalis muscle and can cause much pain if not attended to.

This initial infiltration of some 80 cc of solution is the most painful part of the procedure. This can be minimized by working slowly anteriorly and posteriorly from weals made just above the base of the ear and outside the mid portion of the incision superiorly.

Following the above circumferential infiltration, 1:4,000 dibucaine is injected with the needle point touching bone following the line of incision with again particular attention to the deep temporal muscle just above the zygoma. Usually 50 to 60 cc of this solution is used in this maneuver.[6]

The adhesive plastic field drape and field towels held by sutures are then applied. Care should be taken to expose the zygomatic arch in the inferior margin of the exposure. To obviate the possibility of the patient's fingers sliding up under the drape to the field, sutures should be closely spaced on the preauricular and frontal areas. A light strap about the patient's free arm permitting him to reach his nose (but not above) may be useful. Drapes around the face should be supported on special bars or malleable supports to provide the patient a clear view of the anesthetist and permit ready access to the nose and mouth.

It should be pointed out that the matter of anesthesia, although subject to differing opinions, is largely decided on the basis of what is desired during the procedure. If the patient's cooperation and an ECoG unmarred by anesthetic agents is desired, one must obviously use local anesthesia with the possible addition of a small amount of tranquilizer. Blind nasal intubation, in the late stages of the operation, as carried out by Pasquet (see Penfield and Jasper, 1954) is an ideal procedure if done skillfully, but in our experience few anesthetists will attempt it under the mechanical restrictions inherent to our operating setup.

On the other hand, if the decision regarding temporal lobectomy is made prior to surgery (Falconer, 1967) and a "standard" removal is contemplated, ECoG no longer determines the extent of the excision, and speech damage is obviated by leaving the first temporal gyrus intact. In this case, general anesthesia provides a quicker procedure which is less burdensome for both the surgeon and patient. It has yet to be demonstrated that excisions designed on the basis of extended ECoG studies show a superior cure rate to a "standard" excision, providing the medial structures in the temporal lobe are removed in both cases.

---

[6] It is generally considered unwise to exceed a total dose of 100 mg of dibucaine hydrochloride USP in an adult.

The combination of a light, general anesthesia (nitrous oxide–pentothal or nitrous oxide–halothane) as advocated under some conditions by Penfield and Jasper (1954) and Stepien, Szpiro, Zurkowska, and Gralinska (1969) has proved to be less than satisfactory in our hands, resulting in frequent "negative" ECoG examinations and at times, if the anesthetic is discontinued on the table to "improve" the tracing, in a confused and combative patient out of vocal control by the attendants.

On occasion we have used light endotracheal anesthesia for the opening, then have permitted the patient to awaken while paralyzed with succinyl choline with the endotracheal tube in place. With the field block to prevent pain from the incision, the patients have reported no particular discomfort or anxiety despite the presence of the endotracheal tube and the cortical recording may show little evidence of drug effect. We have come to use this method less as experience with the chlorpromazine–local combination was gained.

The Exposure and Intraoperative Examination

The two major surgical approaches are those of Penfield [Penfield and Baldwin, 1953 (Fig. 3); Penfield, Lende, and Rasmussen, 1961 (Fig. 4)] and Falconer [1971 (Fig. 5)]. Our personal preference has been for the Penfield exposure which seems somewhat more convenient for use with local anesthesia, in spite of the paresis of the ipsilateral frontalis muscle which appears in most cases with such a procedure.

With local anesthesia, pain is frequently encountered over the middle meningeal artery in the temporal fossa and is apt to be particularly troublesome with placement of the burr hole at the pterional point at the junction of the frontal and temporal lobes. Patties soaked in 1:1,500 dibucaine and placed on the dura through the burr holes while attention is turned to other parts of the opening will often alleviate pain on later manipulation of the sensitive regions of the dura. Once the bone flap is turned back on its peduncle of temporal muscle, the dura is sutured to the boney margins and opened to expose the brain.

ECoG is carried out followed by cortical stimulation (see Ajmone-Marsan and O'Connor, 1973). The lower margin of the motor strip and the temporal representation of speech, if the procedure is carried out upon the dominant hemisphere, are mapped. Although an apparatus permitting observation of speech latency (Fedio and Van Buren, 1974) affords more precise information, a selection of common objects presented in cadence with the stimulation is adequate to map the temporal and opercular speech representations. Occasionally, reproducible speech arrests from stimulation are found as far forward as 2 to 3 cm from the anterior extremity of the temporal fossa. Assuming this to be a displacement of the cortical representation owing to "epileptic facilitation," we have resected cortex bearing these responses (providing the speech representation was also encountered in its more usual position posteriorly, which has been the rule to date) without detriment to the patient. In general, up to 5 cm of the first temporal

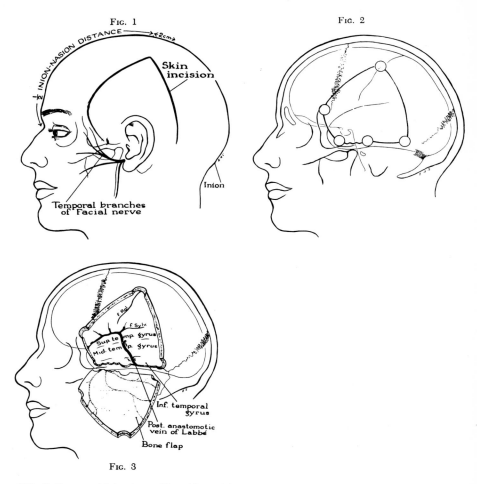

FIG. 3. Temporal lobectomy. The skin and bony opening after Penfield and Baldwin (1953).

convolution (measured from the tip of the temporal fossa) and slightly more of the second and third convolutions can be resected without producing a permanent dysphasic defect.[7] At times, however, sylvian arteries emerge from the fissure

---

[7] Rasmussen *(personal communication)* has recently pointed out the importance of the position of the central fissure at the sylvian fissure as an indicator of the plane of the anterior margin of the temporal cortical speech area. He points out this is of importance in two instances. In the case of a very atrophic temporal lobe, the level of the central fissure may be only 4 cm or less from the end of the middle fossa. In this case he would not carry out a 5 cm removal under general or even under local anesthesia unless, under the latter circumstances, cortical stimulation indicated a posterior position of the temporal speech area. The second instance is when the fissure of Rolando is unusually far posterior, sometimes as far as 6½ cm from the end of the middle fossa. He reports never having seen any permanent speech deficits from removals carried back to the fissure of Rolando in such patients.

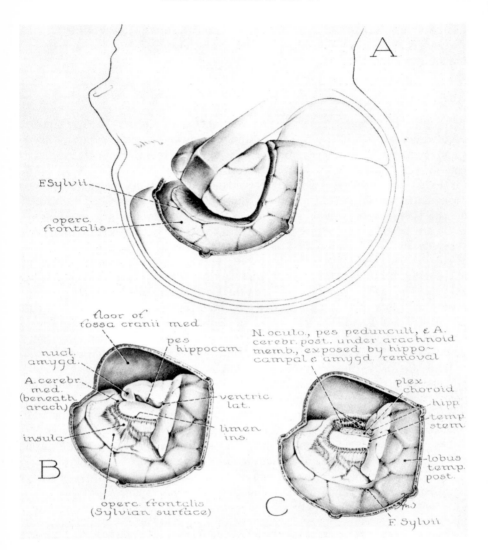

FIG. 4. Temporary lobectomy. The brain excision after Penfield et al. (1961).

quite far anteriorly, loop over the first temporal gyrus and run posteriorly to supply speech cortex. These vessels must be recognized and scrupulously spared even in the event that the cortex beneath them must be removed by subpial suction.

Once the area for removal has been decided upon on the basis of gross inspection, ECoG findings, and stimulation results, the proposed line of resection is outlined with a white thread laid on the cortex and the field is photographed. This, together with a routine operative sketch on the standard brain map designed by Penfield and Jasper (1954, p. 768), provides an accurate record of the procedure and is particularly useful should the area have to be reapproached for revision at a later date.

Temporal Excision

The steps in temporal resection are well shown in Figs. 3–5. Fine bipolar coagulating forceps and magnification are useful adjuncts as the exposure must extend medially to expose the oculomotor nerve, cerebral peduncle, and the posterior cerebral artery for the removal of the medial structures.

If the first temporal gyrus is to be removed (as is our custom), the pia-arachnoid is coagulated and incised in midgyrus, then the incision is extended anteriorly and the posterior margin of the excision is outlined by an incision running downward toward the floor of the temporal fossa. The cortex of the temporal operculum can be carefully lifted off the insula and middle cerebral vessels with the suction until the inferior portion of the semicircular sulcus of the insula is encountered. From here the incision transects the temporal stem and enters the ventricle. The incision may be extended through the medial portion of the hippocampus so that this structure is included with the operative specimen (Crandall, Walter, and Rand, 1963; Falconer and Serafetinides, 1963; Falconer, 1971) or the excision may reach the floor of the temporal fossa lateral to the hippocampus as advocated by Penfield et al. (1961) and Walker (1967). We have preferred the latter approach, removing the hippocampus, amygdala, and uncus by a subpial dissection, leaving the pia-arachnoid membrane intact over the tentorial opening and sparing the vital structures medial to it. This offers the advantage, when using local anesthesia, of not having to separate the arachnoid from the sensitive tentorial margin which often has small venous attachments. The latter readily respond to coagulation (or suture of an oxycel pledget over the dural orifice if it is large), but these manipulations can be carried out only after producing local anesthesia of the tentorial margin by dibucaine-soaked patties or using dibucaine injected through the dural covering of the gasserian ganglion. In some individuals, manipulation of the choroid plexus or venous sinuses entering the dura on the anterior or inferior aspects of the temporal lobe is acutely painful and this can be well handled by the trigeminal ganglion block as soon as the posterior line of temporal incision is brought down to the floor of the middle fossa (third stage of Falconer's excision; Fig. 5).

Whenever the conditions permit it, we carry out a post-excision ECoG. The usefulness and value of this procedure has been discussed elsewhere (Ajmone-Marsan and O'Connor, 1973). The prognostic significance of residual epileptiform activity and, in particular, of that arising from the insula is still debatable. Although insular resection is technically feasible (Guillaume and Mazars, 1949; Penfield and Jasper, 1954), the complication rate incident upon manipulation of the middle cerebral vessels is high (Penfield et al., 1961), and in at least one study (Silfvenius, Gloor, and Rasmussen, 1964) the retention or removal of an insular

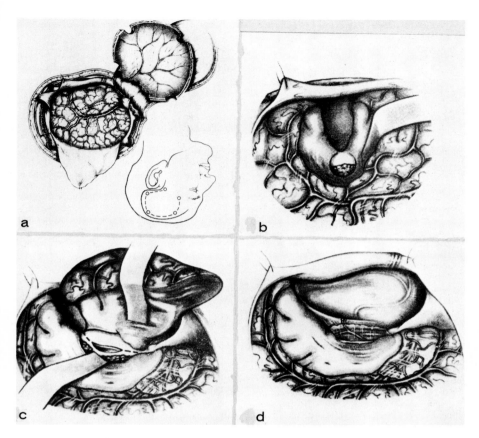

FIG. 5. Temporal lobectomy. The exposure and resection after Falconer (1971). *b*, Exposure of the temporal horn; *c*, the line of incision through the hippocampus; and *d*, the field following removal of the temporal lobe.

focus did not appear to affect the final outcome of the case. In several of our patients, seizures have not reappeared in spite of the presence of epileptiform activity in the insular cortex after the main temporal excision, but their epigastric aura has persisted.

REFERENCES

Ajmone-Marsan, C., and Baldwin, M. (1958): Electrocorticography. In: *Temporal Lobe Epilepsy,* edited by M. Baldwin and P. Bailey. Charles C Thomas, Springfield, Ill.

Ajmone-Marsan, C., and O'Connor, M. (1973): Electrocorticography. In: *Handbook of Electroencephalography and Clinical Neurophysiology,* Vol. 10, Part C, edited by A. Remond. Elsevier, Amsterdam.

Ajmone-Marsan, C., and Zivin, L. W. S. (1970): Factors related to the occurrence of typical paroxysmal abnormalities in the EEG records of epileptic patients. *Epilepsia,* 11:361–381.

Anderman, J., Metrakos, D., and Rasmussen, T. B. (1972): The relationship of genetic factors to surgical outcome in patients operated for focal epilepsy. *Electroencephalogr. Clin. Neurophysiol.,* 33:452.

Bancaud, J., Talairach, J., Bonis, A., Schaub, C., Szikla, G., Morel, P., and Bordas-Ferer, M. (1965): *La Stéréo-Électroencéphalographie dans l'Épilepsie.* Masson, Paris.

Crandall, P. H., Walter, R. D., and Rand, R. W. (1963): Clinical applications of studies on stereotactically implanted electrodes in temporal-lobe epilepsy. *J. Neurosurg.,* 20:827–840.

Currie, S., Heathfield, K. W. G., Henson, R. A., and Scott, D. F. (1971): Clinical course and prognosis of temporal lobe epilepsy. A survery of 666 patients. *Brain,* 94:173–190.

Falconer, M. A. (1967): Surgical treatment of temporal lobe epilepsy. *NZ Med. J.,* 66:539–542.

Falconer, M. A. (1971): Genetic and retarded aetiological factors in temporal lobe epilepsy. A review. *Epilepsia,* 12:13–31.

Falconer, M. A. (1972): Temporal lobe epilepsy in children and its surgical treatment. *Med. J. Aust.,* 1:1117–1121.

Falconer, M. A., and Serafetinides, E. A. (1963): A follow-up study of surgery in temporal lobe epilepsy. *J. Neurol. Neurosurg. Psychiatry,* 26:154–165.

Fedio, P., and Van Buren, J. M. (1974): Memory deficits during electrical stimulation of the speech cortex in conscious man. *Brain Lang.,* 1:29–42.

Frantzen, E. (1961): An analysis of the result of treatment in epileptics under ambulatory supervision. *Epilepsia,* 2:207–214.

Gibbs, F. A. (1954): Diagnosis and prognosis of different types of epilepsy. *Cincinnati J. Med.,* 35:409–412.

Guillaume, J., and Mazars, G. (1949): Technique de résection de l'insula dans les épilepsies insulaires. *Rev. Neurol. (Paris),* 81:900–903.

Gunn, J., and Fenton, G. (1971): Epilepsy, automatism and crime. *Lancet,* 1:1173–1176.

Gupta, P. C., Dharampaul Pathak, S. N., and Singh, B. (1973): Secondary epileptogenic EEG focus in temporal lobe epilepsy. *Epilepsia,* 14:423–426.

Haberland, C. (1958): Histological studies in temporal lobe epilepsy based on biopsy materials. *Psychiatr. Neurol. (Basel),* 135:12–29.

Hedenstroem, I., and Schorsch, G. (1963): Ueber therapieresistente Epileptiker. *Arch. Psychiatr. Nervenkr.,* 204:579–588.

Hierons, R. (1971): Impotence in temporal lobe lesions. *J. Neuro-Visc. Rel. (Vienna),* Suppl. 10:-477–481.

Hill, D. (1959): The difficult epileptic and his social environment. *Trans. Assoc. Industr. Med. Offrs.,* 9:46–50.

Knox, S. J. (1968): Epileptic automatism and violence. *Med. Sci. Law,* 8:96–104.

McNaughton, F. (1954): Observation on diagnosis and medical treatment. In: *Epilepsy and the Functional Anatomy of the Brain,* edited by W. Penfield and H. Jasper. Little, Brown, Boston.

Meyer, A., Falconer, M. A., and Beck, E. (1954): Pathological findings in temporal lobe epilepsy. *J. Neurol. Neurosurg. Psychiatry,* 17:276–285.

Mignone, R. J., Donnelly, E. F., and Sadowsky, D. (1970): Psychological and neurological comparisons of psychomotor and non-psychomotor epileptic patients. *Epilepsia,* 11:345–359.

Mirsky, A. F., and Van Buren, J. M. (1965): On the nature of the "absence" in centrencephalic epilepsy: A study of some behavioral electroencephalographic and autonomic factors. *Electroencephalogr. Clin. Neurophysiol.,* 18:334–348.

Panet-Raymond, J. (1958): Constatations électroencéphalographiques de nature épileptique dans 2200 examens de patients psychiatriques. *Can. Psychiatr. Assoc. J.,* 3:29–37.

Penfield, W., and Baldwin, M. (1953): Temporal lobe seizures and the technic of subtemporal lobectomy. *Trans. Am. Surg. Assoc.,* 70:288–297.

Penfield, W., and Jasper, H., editors (1954): *Epilepsy and the Functional Anatomy of the Human Brain.* Little, Brown, Boston.

Penfield, W., Lende, R. A., and Rasmussen, T. (1961): Manipulation hemiplegia. An untoward complication in the surgery of focal epilepsy. *J. Neurosurg.,* 18:760–776.

Preston, D. N., and Atack, E. A. (1964): Temporal lobe epilepsy. A clinical study of 47 cases. *Can. Med. Assoc. J.,* 90:1256–1259.

Rodin, E. A. (1968): *The Prognosis of Patients with Epilepsy.* Charles C Thomas, Springfield, Ill.

Scott, D. F. (1968): Psychiatric aspects of epilepsy. *Postgrad. Med. J.,* 44:319–326.

Serafetinides, E. A. (1965): Aggressiveness in temporal lobe epileptics and its relation to cerebral dysfunction and environmental factors. *Epilepsia,* 6:33–42.

Serafetinides, E. A., and Falconer, M. A. (1962): The effects of temporal lobectomy in epileptic patients with psychosis. *J. Ment. Sci. (Lond.)* 108:584–593.

Silfvenius, H., Gloor, P., and Rasmussen, T. (1964): Evaluation of insular ablation in surgical treatment of temporal lobe epilepsy. *Epilepsia,* 5:307–320.

Small, J. G., Milstein, V., and Stevens, J. R. (1962): Are psychomotor epileptics different? *Arch. Neurol.,* 7:187–194.

Stepien, L., Szpiro Zurkowska, A., and Gralinska, K. (1969): The technique of temporal lobectomy and hemispherectomy. *Neurol. Neurochir. Pol.,* 19:179–184 (in Polish).

Strobos, R. R. J. (1959): Prognosis in convulsive disorders. *Arch. Neurol.,* 1:216–225.

Taylor, D. C., and Falconer, M. A. (1968): Clinical, socioeconomic and psychological changes after temporal lobectomy for epilepsy. *Br. J. Psychiatry,* 114:1247–1261.

Van Buren, J. M. (1958): Some autonomic concomitants of ictal automatism. *Brain,* 81:505–528.

Van Buren, J. M. (1961): Sensory, motor and autonomic effects of mesial temporal stimulation in man. *J. Neurosurg.,* 18:273–288.

Van Buren, J. M. (1963): The abdominal aura. A study of abdominal sensations occurring in epilepsy and produced by depth stimulation. *Electroencephalogr. Clin. Neurophysiol.,* 15:1–19.

Van Buren, J. M., and Ajmone-Marsan, C. (1960): A correlation of autonomic and EEG components in temporal lobe epilepsy. *Arch. Neurol.,* 3:683–703.

Van Buren, J. M., Ajmone-Marsan, C., and Mutsuga, N. (1974): Temporal lobe seizures with additional foci treated by resection *(in preparation.)*

Van Buren, J. M., and Baldwin, M. (1958): The architecture of the optic radiation in the temporal lobe of man. *Brain,* 81:15–40.

Walker, A. E. (1967). Temporal lobectomy. *J. Neurosurg.,* 26:642–649.

TABLE 10 REFERENCES

Bailey, P. (1961): Surgical treatment of psychomotor epilepsy: Five year follow-up. *South. Med. J.,* 54:299–301.

Bloom, D., Jasper, H., and Rasmussen, T. (1960): Surgical therapy in patients with temporal lobe seizures and bilateral EEG abnormality. *Epilepsia,* 1:351–365.

Brown, J. A., French, L. A., Ogle, W. S., and Jahnson, S. (1956): Temporal lobe epilepsy; Its clinical manifestations and surgical treatment. A preliminary report I. *Medicine (Baltimore),* 35:425–459.

DeVet, A. C. (1972): Temporal epilepsy, e.g. psychomotor epilepsy. Experiences and present day conceptions. *Schweiz. Arch. Neurol. Neurochir. Psychiatr.,* 111:453–461.

Fasano, V. A., and Broggi, G. (1954): Studio delle modificazioni del linguaggio in dieci casi di lobectomia temporale per epilessia. *Chirurgia (Bucur.),* 9:235–237.

French, L. A. (1958): Resection of the temporal lobe in patients with convulsive disorders. *Minn. Med.,* 41:373–375.

Green, J. R., Steelman, H. F., Duisberg, R. E. H., McGrath, W. B., and Wick, S. (1957): The surgical and rehabilitation results of radical temporal lobectomy in the treatment of psychomotor epilepsy. In: *Proceedings of the Fourth International Congress of Electro-Encephalography and Clinical Neurophysiology and Eighth Meeting of the International League Against Epilepsy,* Brussels, July 21–28. Excerpta Medica, Amsterdam.

Guillaume, J., and Mazars, G. (1956): Indications et résultats du traitement chirurgical des épilepsies temporales. *Sem. Hôp. Paris,* 32:2013–2018.

Kachaev, V. L. (1961): Neurological disorders in focal epilepsy treated by surgical methods (Russian). *Zh. Nevropatol. Psikhiatr.,* 61:1328–1331.

Maspes, P. E., and Marossero, F. (1954): L'epilessia temporale ed il suo trattamento chirugico. *Chirurgia (Bucur.),* 9:171–217.

Mathai, K. V., and Chandy, J. (1969): Temporal lobectomy for temporal lobe epilepsy. *Int. Congr. Ser.* #193, pp. 65–66. Excerpta Medica, Amsterdam.

Morris, A. A. (1956): Temporal lobectomy with removal of uncus, hippocampus and amygdala. Results of psychomotor epilepsy three to nine years after operation. *Arch. Neurol. Psychiatry,* 76:479–496.

Northfield, D. W. C. (1966): The place of surgery in controlling epilepsy. In: *Second Symposium on Advanced Medicine,* edited by J. R. Trounce. Pitman, London, pp. 161–165.

Paillas, J. E., Gastaut, H., Bonnal, J., and Vigouroux, R. (1953): Corrélations anatomo-électro-cliniques dans l'épilepsie temporale; à propos des résultats obtenus chez 38 opérés. *Rev. Neurol. (Paris),* 88:568–574.

Penfield, W., and Flanigin, H. (1950): Surgical therapy of temporal lobe seizures. *Arch. Neurol. Psychiatry,* 64:491–500.

Rasmussen, T., and Branch, C. (1962): Temporal lobe epilepsy. Indications for and results of surgical therapy. *Postgrad. Med.,* 31:9–14.

Advances in Neurology, Vol. 8, edited by D. P.
Purpura, J. K. Penry, and R. D. Walter. Raven
Press, New York © 1975.

9
Surgery of Frontal Lobe Epilepsy

Theodore Rasmussen

ETIOLOGY

Epileptogenic lesions largely limited to the frontal lobe in front of the sensorimotor strip are second in frequency to temporal lobe epileptogenic lesions in the anatomic classification. Three hundred and forty-six patients with seizures involving primarily the frontal lobe have been operated on at the Montreal Neurological Institute from 1928 to the end of 1973 (Fig. 1). Neoplasms were present in 97 patients and arteriovenous malformations in 5, the total, 102 patients, constituting 29% of the total frontal lobe series. In most of these 102 patients the diagnosis of a space-occupying or vascular lesion was made preoperatively, but the surgical procedure was carried out as a seizure operation because the patients' primary problem was seizures rather than increased intracranial pressure or advancing neurologic deficit. In about a fifth of these patients, however, the lesion was not disclosed preoperatively despite complete and sometimes repeated radiologic investigations, and the diagnosis was made only at operation.

The remaining 244 patients exhibited cicatricial lesions of various etiology and are the primary focus of this chapter. In 110 patients (45%), postnatal trauma was the presumed cause of the original brain injury. Birth trauma and postinflammatory brain scarring were the causes in 11% and 12%, respectively. The eti-

Etiology of Frontal Lobe Epilepsy

Patients operated upon from 1928 through 1973

Non-Tumoral Lesions				
Birth trauma or anoxia	27 pts. (11% of non-tumoral lesions)			
Postnatal trauma	110 pts. (45% "	"	"	)
Postinflammatory brain scarring	30 pts. (12% "	"	"	)
Miscellaneous	26 pts. (11% "	"	"	)
Unknown	51 pts. (21% "	"	"	)
	244 pts. (100%)			
Tumors	97 pts.	29% of total series		
Arteriovenous malformations	5 pts.			
Total	**346 pts.**			

FIG. 1.

Montreal Neurological Institute Reprint No. 1171.

ology was classified as unknown in 51 patients (21%), often because more than one potential cause for the brain injury was present and neither the history, radiologic findings, nor the operative findings clearly indicated which was responsible for the epileptogenic lesion. The remaining 26 patients (11%) exhibited a variety of miscellaneous lesions such as tuberous sclerosis, pial angiomatosis of the Sturge-Weber variety, hamartomas, scarring from previous craniotomies for intracerebral hematoma or brain tumor removal or for excision of vascular malformations, encephalopathy, etc.

ATTACK PATTERNS

Generalized convulsive seizures, as opposed to partial seizures, are relatively more frequent in frontal lobe epilepsy than in seizures arising in other cortical areas. There are usually some lateralizing phenomena at the onset of some of the attacks which provide clues that the patient's seizure problem is a focal one rather than idiopathic or primary epilepsy, but these signs may be brief and easily missed if the onset of the attack is not witnessed by an accurate and knowledgeable observer. In addition, these lateralizing signs may be absent in a significant proportion of any individual patient's attacks.

In general, frontal lobe attacks begin in one of six ways (Penfield and Kristiansen, 1951; Penfield and Jasper, 1954; Rasmussen, 1963):

(1) Immediate unconsciousness followed by a generalized tonic–clonic convulsion with minimal or no lateralizing or localizing signs.

(2) Immediate unconsciousness associated with initial turning of the head and eyes, and sometimes the body, to the opposite side and promptly followed by a generalized convulsion. This unconscious contraversive pattern points to an origin in the anterior third or fourth of the frontal lobe of the side the patient turns away from.

(3) Initial turning of the head and eyes away from the side of the lesion with preserved consciousness and conscious contraversive attacks. The attack may stop at this point and last only 5 to 20 sec, but usually it continues with loss of consciousness and a generalized convulsion. These attacks usually arise from the convexity of the intermediate frontal region.

(4) Posturing movement of the body with tonic elevation of the contralateral arm, downward extension of the ipsilateral arm, and turning of head away from the side of the lesion as though looking at the upraised hand. This pattern represents a discharging lesion on the medial aspect of the intermediate frontal region in the vicinity of the supplementary motor area.

(5) A vague sensation in the head or in the body generally, which the patients find difficult to describe, usually calling it a "feeling" or "dizziness" (which is clearly not vertigo) or a "flush" or "weak feeling." The attack may stop at this point and last only a few seconds, in which case it is classified as an aura. The discharge may continue and cause a brief arrest of activity, confused thinking and staring, without motor activity. This minor attack may resemble a true petit

mal absence attack, even to experienced observers. More frequently, the aura is quickly followed by a generalized convulsive seizure with or without lateralizing features at the onset.

(6) Some sudden alteration in thought processes classified as "forced thinking" by Penfield and described by the patients in various ways, "forced to think about something," "my thoughts suddenly became fixed," "loss of thought control." As in the previous group, this aura may be the whole attack or it may proceed to a minor attack resembling a petit mal absence or continue on to a generalized major convulsion.

Rarely, seizures arising from the orbital surface of the frontal lobe may be associated with ictal or postictal automatisms and/or autonomic phenomena similar to those characteristically seen in patients with temporal lobe epilepsy (Schneider, Crosby, Bagchi, and Calhoun, 1961; Schneider, Crosby, and Farhat, 1965; Tharp, 1972). Postictal dysphasia indicates that the seizure involved the dominant cerebral hemisphere but does not differentiate between seizures arising close to the frontal speech area and those arising in or near the parieto-temporal speech zones.

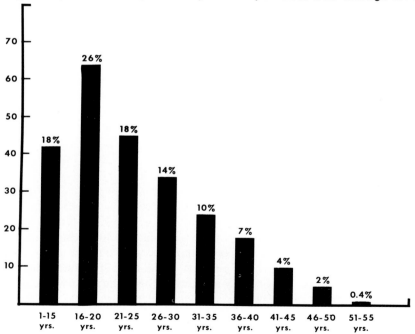

Frontal Lobe Epilepsy
Age at operation-244 patients operated upon from 1929 through 1973

FIG. 2.

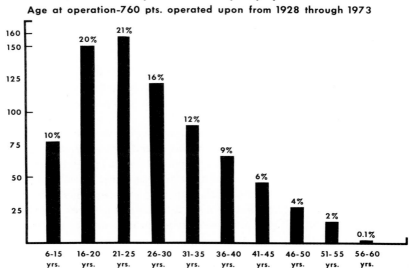

FIG. 3.

While the above attack patterns identify the frontal lobe origin of the seizure discharge, they do not differentiate between a neoplastic, vascular or cicatricial or gliotic lesion as responsible for the seizure.

The age distribution of the patients at time of operation (Fig. 2) was similar to that of the temporal lobe group (Fig. 3) and is in contrast to the age distribution of patients with large destructive lesions or with epileptiform lesions of the central (sensorimotor) region, in whom the presence of some degree of hemiparesis led to operation in childhood in a considerably larger percentage (Chapter 10, Figs. 2 and 8).

EEG INVESTIGATION

Routine Studies

Standard EEG recordings often provide a satisfactory localizing diagnosis by showing well lateralized random spiking more or less confined to the anterior and intermediate frontal regions of one side of the head (Fegersten and Roger, 1961). This epileptiform activity may appear only after the anticonvulsant medications are reduced or withdrawn. Frontal lobe epileptiform discharges are rarely enhanced by sleep.

Not infrequently, frontal lobe epileptogenic lesions produce bursts of bilaterally synchronous spike-and-wave complexes or bilaterally synchronous and symmetrical multiple spike complexes, instead of, or in addition to, localized random sharp waves and spikes. These patterns sometimes show few or no lateralizing features and may closely mimic patterns of idiopathic, centrencephalic, or generalized cortico-reticular epilepsy. When these EEG patterns are associated with some evidence of lateralization in the clinical attack patterns or X-ray studies, special EEG techniques are required to determine whether the patient's seizure problem is a focal one with secondary bilateral synchrony in the EEG, or represents a diffuse or multifocal seizure problem or primary idiopathic epilepsy.

Special Studies

Carotid Amytal-Metrazol EEG Test

The intracarotid Amytal-Metrazol EEG test (Rovit, Gloor, and Rasmussen, 1961; Gloor, Rasmussen, Garretson, and Maroun, 1964; Garretson, Gloor, and Rasmussen, 1966) provides the best available evidence as to whether or not a unilateral cortical focus is actually responsible for the bilaterally synchronous epileptiform EEG activity (see Chapter 5). When both the Amytal and the Metrazol portions of the test point to a predominance of epileptogenicity in the same cerebral hemisphere, a diagnosis of secondary bilateral synchrony is made, encouraging consideration of operation.

The symmetry of the arterial supply to the cerebral hemisphere must be considered, however, in interpreting the test. The test is most accurate in differentiating between secondary and primary bilateral synchrony either if the arterial supply to the brain is symmetrical or if the carotid artery on the side of the presumed pacemaker focus supplies *less* of the brain than the contralateral carotid artery. When the arterial supply of the brain is asymmetrical and the carotid artery on the side of the presumed focus supplies *more* of the brain than the contralateral artery, the test is less accurate in predicting that a satisfactory reduction of seizure tendency will result from frontal lobectomy or cortical resection elsewhere in the hemisphere, apparently showing the predominant epileptogenicity.

If the carotid Amytal-Metrazol EEG test gives the characteristic picture of a primary bilateral synchrony or evidence of independent epileptogenic processes in both cerebral hemispheres, operation is contraindicated unless there is overwhelming evidence from the patient's attack pattern of a consistent localized onset and supporting X-ray evidence of unilateral brain injury of the region indicated by the attack pattern. The test is thus not completely conclusive and must be regarded as an important, but not the sole, element of the diagnostic facets that enter into the decision for or against operation. The test is of lateralizing significance only and usually does not give good localizing evidence within the involved cerebral hemisphere.

The intracarotid Amytal-Metrazol EEG test is a lengthy one, is expensive from the standpoint of the personnel and time involved, and requires patience and good cooperation from the patient. It is not applicable, therefore, to children below the age of 12 to 13.

Lombroso-Erba Pentothal Activation Test

The Lombroso-Erba (1970) Pentothal activation test is a more indirect method of attempting to differentiate between secondary and primary bilateral synchrony in the EEG and diffuse multifocal epileptiform processes which generate bilaterally synchronous epileptiform discharges. It has the advantage, however, of being applicable to children as young as 2 years of age and is a considerably less formidable test from the standpoint of the time and personnel involved (see Chapter 5).

SURGICAL TECHNIQUE

A large C-shaped skin incision is used. The medial limb of the incision is placed at the midline and the posterior limb placed so as to permit exposure of at least part of the precentral gyrus. The medial edge of the bony opening should extend to within 1 cm of the midline to permit access to the medial aspect of the hemisphere. The lateral edge should extend at least to the Sylvian fissure. If the preoperative EEG studies indicate involvement of the fronto-temporal region, the bony opening should extend well down onto the temporal lobe to permit EEG recording both below and above the Sylvian fissure and, if necessary, excision of the anterior temporal region. Flexible wire electrodes are inserted under the frontal lobe and along the falx so as to record the EEG activity from these areas as well as from the convexity of the frontal lobe.

The precentral gyrus is identified by electrical stimulation as required for accurate localization. In the dominant hemisphere the frontal opercular convolutions are stimulated to identify the convolutions concerned with speech. The speech area involves one or two of the first three frontal opercular convolutions, in front of the lower end of the precentral gyrus.

If the patient's attack pattern indicates an anterior frontal localization and if the spiking in the cortical EEG involves only the anterior frontal region, a removal of the anterior quarter or third of the frontal lobe is carried out, removing the cortex of the medial and orbital surfaces as well as the convexity.

If the attack pattern points to the supplementary motor area and the EEG spiking involves primarily the parasagittal region and medial surface of the frontal lobe, the removal should include the medial aspect of the frontal lobe as well as enough of the convexity to include the spiking area. This may necessitate carrying the removal backward close to the precentral gyrus, but it is wise to leave one convolution in front of the motor strip *in situ* at the original removal even though it is issuing spikes, to minimize the risk of hemiparesis. If the postexcision EEG shows this convolution to be still spiking actively, it can be removed by suction safely if exquisite care is taken not to interfere with the circulation to the precentral gyrus or to retract or manipulate its pial bank or produce any movement of the underlying white matter. Constant testing of the patient's hand grips during cortical excision near the precentral gyrus helps to safeguard against hemiparesis.

If the cortical spiking involves the entire frontal lobe a radical frontal lobectomy may be required, including both the medial and orbital surfaces. In the nondominant hemisphere the frontal opercular gyri often need to be removed back to the precentral gyrus, exposing the surface of the insula above the Sylvian fissure. In the dominant hemisphere the frontal opercular convolutions must be carefully preserved, but the orbital cortex can be completely removed, if necessary, in front of the opercular convolutions.

Occasionally, the postexcision EEG shows persistent spiking over the anterior temporal region and further removal of part of the anterior temporal region may be indicated, particularly if automatisms are a consistent part of the attack pattern.

No attempt is made to carry the removal into the frontal horn of the ventricle, but if it is opened into by the removal, the ventricular opening should be temporarily covered with a cotton patty or small dental roll to prevent entrance of blood into the ventricle during the remainder of the operation.

RISKS AND SURGICAL COMPLICATIONS

If the frontal lobe removal is carried out with delicacy and minimal movement and manipulation of the remaining convolutional banks, the risk of hemiparesis is small. The risk increases when it is necessary to carry the removal close to the precentral gyrus, but after the bulk of the frontal specimen is removed, the convolution in front of the precentral gyrus can be gently removed with suction without undue risk if any interference with the circulation to the motor gyrus and any movement or retraction of its exposed pial surface are meticulously avoided, with finger movement and hand grips constantly being tested.

In the dominant hemisphere there is usually a temporary dysphasia for a few days, even when the cortical removal is several centimeters away from the frontal speech area. This speech disturbance disappears as the postoperative cerebral edema recedes. If spiking in the opercular area requires cortical removal near the speech area, the cortex near the speech convolutions should be removed slowly by suction while the patient is constantly carrying out verbal tasks. At least one opercular convolution in front of the furthest anterior gyrus yielding aphasic stimulation responses should be preserved, and the upper margins of the preserved frontal opercular gyri must be carefully protected from injury. If aphasic stimulation responses are not elicited from the frontal opercular gyri in a hemisphere known to be dominant for speech, at least the first three opercular gyri in front of the lower end of the precentral gyri must be carefully preserved. Failure to elicit speech interference by electrical stimulation does not guarantee that the cortex stimulated is not involved in speech function.

There have been no operative deaths in 160 consecutive frontal lobe seizure operations since 1950. There were four operative deaths in the preceding 20 years, yielding an operative mortality rate of 1.5% for the total series, consisting of 277 operations in 244 patients from 1929 through 1973.

The repercussions of these cortical resections on higher intellectual functions are discussed in Chapter 15.

RESULTS

In order to permit a follow-up period of at least 2 years, the effectiveness of cortical excision in reducing the seizure tendency in this series of patients with nontumoral epileptogenic lesions of the frontal lobe is analyzed in the patients operated on up to the end of 1971, a total series of 236 patients (Fig. 4). Seventeen patients with less than 2 years of follow-up data have been deleted from the analysis, along with four patients who died in the early postoperative period and three others who died in the first postoperative year from a progressive encephalopathy found to be responsible for the seizures. The remaining 212 patients have satisfactory follow-up data for periods ranging from 2 to 39 years, with a median follow-up period of 14 years. The follow-up data are complete to date or to the patients' death in 75%.

Twenty-two patients (10%) have had no attacks since leaving the hospital and 28 more (13%) have become and remained seizure-free after having a few attacks in the early postoperative months or years. Thus 50 patients (23%) have become and remained seizure-free.

Twenty-six patients (12%) have had rare or occasional attacks after being

Frontal Lobe Epilepsy - Results of Cortical Excision

Patients with non-tumoral lesions operated upon from 1929 through 1971

Seizure free since discharge	22 pts. (10%)	50 pts. (23%)		
Became seizure free after some early attacks	28 pts. (13%)		118 pts. (55%)	212 pts. with follow-up data of 2-39 yrs.
Free 3 or more years then rare or occasional attacks	26 pts. (12%)	68 pts. (32%)		
Marked reduction of seizure tendency	42 pts. (20%)			
Moderate to no reduction of seizure tendency	94 pts. (44%)			median 14 yrs.

Inadequate follow-up data	17 pts.
Death in first postoperative year from progressive encephalopathy	3 pts.
Postoperative death	4 pts.
Total	**236 pts.**

FIG. 4.

seizure-free for periods ranging from 3 to 20 years. Forty-two patients (20%) have had only up to 1 to 2% as many attacks as preoperatively and are classified as having had a marked reduction in seizure tendency. Thus 68 patients (32%) have had a marked but not quite complete reduction in seizure tendency. Added to the seizure-free group, there are thus 118 patients (55%) of this series of patients whose frontal lobe epilepsy could not be adequately controlled with anticonvulsant medication who have had a complete or nearly complete reduction in seizure tendency following operation.

The remaining 94 patients (44%) have had lesser reductions in seizure tendency. Some have had only 5 to 10% as many attacks as preoperatively, many have had 40 to 60% as many, and a few have had little or no reduction in frequency or severity of attacks.

REFERENCES

Fegersten, L., and Roger, A. (1961): Frontal epileptogenic foci and their clinical correlations. *Electroencephalogr. Clin. Neurophysiol.,* 13:905–913.

Garretson, H., Gloor, P., and Rasmussen, T. (1966): Intracarotid amobarbital and metrazol test for the study of epileptiform discharge in man: A note on its technique. *Electroencephalogr. Clin. Neurophysiol.,* 21:607–610.

Gloor, P., Rasmussen, T., Garretson, H., and Maroun, F. (1964): Fractionized intracarotid metrazol injection: A new diagnostic method in electroencephalography. *Electroencephalogr. Clin. Neurophysiol.,* 17:322–327.

Lombroso, C. T., and Erba, G. (1970): Primary and secondary bilateral synchrony in epilepsy: Clinical and electroencephalographic study. *Arch. Neurol.,* 22:321–334.

Penfield, W., and Jasper, H. (1954): *Epilepsy and the Functional Anatomy of the Human Brain.* Little, Brown, Boston.

Penfield, W., and Kristiansen, K. (1951): *Epileptic Seizure Patterns.* Charles C Thomas, Springfield, Ill.

Rasmussen, T. (1963): Surgical therapy of frontal lobe epilepsy. *Epilepsia,* 4:181–198.

Rovit, R., Gloor, P., and Rasmussen, T. (1961): Intracarotid amytal in epileptic patients: A new test in clinical electroencephalography. *Arch. Neurol.,* 5:606–626.

Schneider, R. C., Crosby, E. C., Bagchi, B. K., and Calhoun, H. D. (1961): Temporal or occipital hallucinations triggered from frontal lesions. *Neurology,* 11:172–179.

Schneider, R. C., Crosby, E. C., and Farhat, S. M. (1965): Extratemporal lesions triggering the temporal lobe syndrome. *J. Neurosurg.,* 22:246–263.

Tharp, B. R. (1972): Orbital frontal seizures. An unique electroencephalographic and clinical syndrome. *Epilepsia,* 13:627–642.

Advances in Neurology, Vol. 8, edited by D. P. Purpura, J. K. Penry, and R. D. Walter. Raven Press, New York © 1975.

10
Surgery for Epilepsy Arising in Regions Other than the Temporal and Frontal Lobes

Theodore Rasmussen

INTRODUCTION

While temporal and frontal lobe epileptic patients constitute a little over 70% of the patients in the Montreal Neurological Institute surgical seizure series, focal epileptic problems of other regions of the brain are also suitable for surgical therapy.

This chapter outlines special aspects of the surgical treatment of epileptic lesions largely limited to the central (sensorimotor), parietal, and occipital regions and those associated with large destructive lesions involving more than one lobe of the brain. Patients have been assigned to these anatomic groups on the basis of the location of the principal epileptic area of the brain as determined by their attack patterns and EEG findings, both preoperative and operative. The classification was clear-cut in most patients and a relatively arbitrary assignment was necessary in only a few instances.

CENTRAL REGION

Etiology

Nearly half of the 135 patients operated on from 1931 through 1973 for epilepsy due to lesions of the central region had tumors or vascular malformations (Fig. 1). This high incidence, in comparison with the other anatomic groups, reflects the increased safety of carrying out maximal permissible removals of tumors and adjacent epileptogenic cortex provided by the use of local anesthetic, cortical stimulation, and cortical EEG recording. Thus a larger percentage of patients with tumors in or near the sensorimotor strip than in other regions of the brain were selected for operation utilizing the surgical seizure techniques instead of the standard brain tumor operative techniques.

The remaining 69 patients had cicatricial lesions of various etiology, as in the frontal lobe group discussed in the preceding chapter.

The etiology was known in the largest group, 28 patients (40%). Birth trauma and postnatal trauma were the presumed etiologic factors in 14 patients (21%), and 13 patients (19%). Postinflammatory brain scarring was responsible in 6 patients (9%), and a variety of miscellaneous lesions (tuberous sclerosis, encephalopathy, etc.) were found in 8 patients (12%).

Montreal Neurological Institute Reprint No. 1170.

Epilepsy of Central (Somatosensory Region)
Etiology

Patients operated upon from 1931 through 1973

Non Tumoral Lesions		
Birth trauma or anoxia	14 pts. (21% of non-tumoral lesions)	
Postnatal trauma	13 pts. (19% " " ")	
Postinflammatory brain scarring	6 pts. (9% " " ")	
Miscellaneous	8 pts. (12% " " ")	
Unknown	28 pts. (40% " " ")	
	69 pts. (100%)	
Tumors	62 pts.	48% of total group
Vascular malformations	3 pts.	

Total 134 pts.

FIG. 1.

Attack Patterns

The seizure patterns were considerably more stereotyped in this group than in the other anatomic groups. In the great majority, the attacks were either somatomotor or somatosensory in type. In some patients a significant proportion of the attacks remained localized and were not associated with loss of consciousness, but in nearly all, a certain proportion of the attacks progressed to generalized convulsive seizures.

Focal status epilepticus and epilepsia partialis continua were particularly common and were sometimes associated with small discrete gliomas in the pre- or postcentral gyri, but in other instances the epileptogenic cortex extended surprisingly widely into the adjacent frontal and/or parietal regions.

The presence of some degree of hemiparesis led to operation early in childhood in a considerably higher percentage of patients in this anatomic subgroup than in the temporal, frontal, and parietal groups (Fig. 2). Thus operation was carried out in the 2- to 15-year age period in 41%, whereas in the temporal lobe series only 10% (Chapter 9, Fig. 3), in the frontal lobe series 18% (Chapter 9, Fig. 2), and in the parietal lobe series 23% (Fig. 5, this chapter) were operated upon during this age period.

EEG Investigation

Standard EEG recording often confirms the central localization of the epileptogenic area. Not infrequently, however, the scalp EEG shows surprisingly little

Central (Sensori-Motor Region) Epilepsy
Age at operation-69 patients operated upon from 1931 through 1973

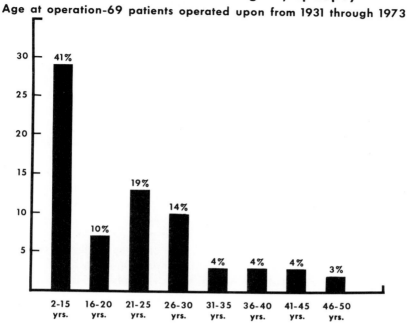

FIG. 2.

interictal epileptiform activity despite the occurrence of frequent seizures. Sometimes even recording an attack fails to show significant abnormality until the record is obscured by muscle artifact. Some of these patients, therefore, must be selected and operated upon on clinical grounds without the blessing of preoperative delineation of the epileptogenic area by the EEG.

Surgical Technique and Risks

A U-shaped skin incision is used, permitting exposure of the central region and the adjacent cortex in front and/or behind as required by the patient's attack pattern and preoperative EEG studies. The sensory and motor areas are mapped in detail so the face, arm, and leg areas are accurately delineated.

The epileptogenic cortex in front of or behind the two central convolutions is first removed in the hope that any spiking in the pre- or postcentral gyrus is secondary to epileptic activity in the adjacent cortex. If the postexcision cortical EEG shows continued spiking from the pre- and/or the postcentral gyri, removal of some of the cortex of these convolutions may be necessary.

The face area of the pre- and postcentral gyri, as defined by threshold electrical stimulation, can be removed with a small bore suction with relatively little risk of hemiparesis if the underlying white matter is moved as little as possible and if the circulation to the remainder of the central convolutions further superiorly is not interfered with. Removal of the face area of the postcentral gyrus results in a decrease of the ability to discriminate between two points over the lower part of the face but no detectable deficit as far as the patient is concerned. Removal of the face area of the precentral gyrus produces a weakness of the contralateral side of the mouth of variable severity and duration. Partial removals of the motor face area usually leave no asymmetry of the face after 3 to 4 weeks have elapsed. Complete removal of the motor face area leaves a persisting minimal or moderate underaction of the contralateral side of the mouth in about half of the patients. In the remaining half the lower facial weakness disappears during the first postoperative month or two.

The face area of the pre- and postcentral gyri can be removed completely in the dominant hemisphere without producing a dysphasia if the adjacent pial banks of the frontal and parietal opercular gyri are not manipulated or traumatized.

The leg area of the postcentral gyrus can be removed with little significant deficit as far as the patient is concerned, although an enduring decrease in appreciation of joint movement and joint discrimination in the foot is produced. Removal of the leg area of the precentral gyrus is rarely advisable unless there is considerable existing leg weakness from the original brain injury responsible for the seizures. On rare occasions, particularly severe and frequent somatomotor attacks have led to resection of the leg area of the precentral gyri, despite the presence of normal motor function preoperatively, after removal of the adjacent cortical regions has failed to stop the attacks. This results in an immediate flaccid paralysis of the leg with, however, a considerable recovery of motor functon during the following few months if the remainder of the pre- and postcentral gyri are intact.

If the motor and sensory function of the arm is normal preoperatively, removal of the pre- or postcentral arm area is rarely indicated and is carried out only if removal of adjacent spiking cortex fails to reduce the seizure tendency adequately in a patient whose seizure tendency is particularly severe and disabling. When the original brain injury or the effects of repeated bouts of focal status epilepticus have produced a significant degree of arm weakness, excision of a portion of the arm area is sometimes indicated and usually results in only a minimal increase in the patient's neurologic deficit which is well worthwhile if the seizure tendency is satisfactorily reduced.

If portions of the pre- and postcentral gyri are to be removed, the cortex is gently removed to the depth of the sulci, gyrus by gyrus, with a small bore suction, carefully preserving the vessels in the adjacent sulci. When the face area is removed it is important to remove the cortex covering the insula and Sylvian fissure. Movement of the underlying white matter must be avoided to prevent damage to axons entering the internal capsule from the arm area.

Results

By the end of 1971, 68 patients had been operated on for nontumoral epilepto-genic lesions of the central region (Fig. 3). There was one postoperative death in 1951 and two deaths in the first postoperative year, one accidental and one due to progressive encephalopathy. These three patients and two others with less than 2 years' follow-up data have been deleted from the following analysis. The remaining 63 patients have been followed for 2 to 38 years, with a median follow-up period of 16 years.

Eleven patients (18%) have had no attacks since discharge from the hospital and another nine patients (14%) have become and remained seizure-free after having had a few attacks in the early postoperative months or years. Thus, 20 patients (31%) have become and remained seizure-free. Eight patients (13%) have had recurrence of rare or occasional attacks after being seizure-free for periods ranging from 3 to 18 years. Another eight patients (13%) have had only up to 1 to 2% as many attacks as preoperatively but have not had prolonged seizure-free periods; they are classified as having a marked reduction of seizure tendency. Therefore, 16 patients (26%) have had a marked but not quite complete reduction in seizure tendency. Added to the seizure-free group, there are thus 36 patients (57%) who have had a complete or nearly complete reduction in seizure tendency following operation. The remaining 27 patients (43%) have had lesser degrees of reduction of seizure tendency.

Epilepsy Due to Central (Sensori-Motor) Region Lesions
Results of Cortical Excision
Patients with non-tumoral lesions operated upon from 1931 through 1971

Seizure free since discharge	11 pts. (18%)	20 pts. (31%)		
Became seizure free after some early attacks	9 pts. (14%)		36 pts. (57%)	63 pts. with follow-up data of 2 - 38 yrs.
Free 3 or more years then rare or occasional attacks	8 pts. (13%)	16 pts. (26%)		
Marked reduction of seizure tendency	8 pts. (13%)			
Moderate or less reduction of seizure tendency	27 pts. (43%)			median 16 yrs.

Inadequate follow-up data	2 pts.
Death in 1st postoperative years	2 pts.
Postoperative death	1 pt.
Total	**68 pts.**

FIG. 3.

PARIETAL REGION

Etiology

One third of the 132 patients operated on from 1930 through 1973 for focal epilepsy due to epileptogenic lesions of the parietal region had tumors or vascular malformations (Fig. 4). The remaining 86 had cicatricial lesions of various etiology. Thirty-five patients (41%) were classified as posttraumatic. Birth trauma

Parietal Lobe Epilepsy-Etiology
Patients operated upon from 1930 through 1973

Non-Tumoral Lesions

Birth trauma or anoxia	21 pts. (24% of non-tumoral lesions)	
Postnatal trauma	35 pts. (41% " " ")	
Postinflammatory brain scarring	7 pts. (8% " " ")	
Miscellaneous	6 pts. (7% " " ")	
Unknown	17 pts. (20% " " ")	
	86 pts. (100%)	
Neoplasms	41 pts. ⎫ 35% of total series	
Vascular malformations	5 pts. ⎭	

Total　132 pts.

FIG. 4.

or anoxia was the presumed cause in 21 patients (24%) and the etiology was unknown in 17 patients (20%). Postinflammatory brain scarring was responsible in 7 patients (8%) and a variety of miscellaneous lesions (e.g., tuberous sclerosis, anesthetic anoxic episode, previous tumor removal) were found in the remaining six patients (7%). The age at operation of these 86 patients is shown in Fig. 5.

Attack Pattern

Nearly half the patients with parietal lobe epilepsy had somatomotor or somatosensory attacks similar to those arising in the central region (see preceding section). Most of the remainder exhibited attacks consisting of unilateral motor or sensory phenomena plus additional features such as dizziness, cephalic sensation, conscious or unconscious contraversion, perceptual illusions, unformed visual hallucinations, mental confusion, epigastric sensation, dysphasia, or automatism. About 10% of the patients failed to show any significant localizing features in their attack patterns as far as could be determined.

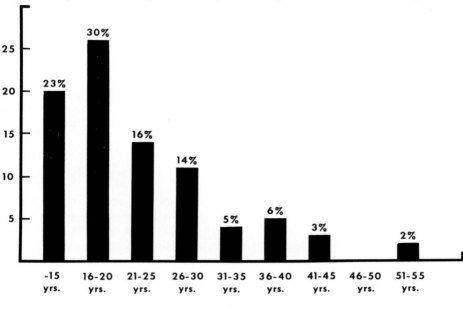

Parietal Lobe Epilepsy

Age at operation-86 patients operated upon from 1929 through 1973

FIG. 5.

EEG Investigation

As with central lesions (see above) standard EEG recording techniques usually confirm the parietal localization of the epileptogenic area and in some cases indicate its extension into the adjacent central, temporal, or occipital area. Bilaterally synchronous epileptiform abnormality is a good deal less frequent than in frontal lobe epilepsy, but occasionally it does occur and may require the special EEG examinations discussed in Chapters 5 and 9.

Surgical Technique and Risks

A C-shaped incision is used, permitting exposure of the parietal region and adjacent portion of the central region for accurate localizaton by identification of the postcentral gyrus and, if necessary, resection of a portion of this convolution. The bone flap should extend to within 1 cm of the midline to permit EEG recording from the medial aspect of the parietal lobe and resection of its medial cortex, if indicated.

If the cortical resection involves only the parietal lobe behind the postcentral gyrus and this convolution is not traumatized, no obvious sensory deficit results

(Corkin, Milner, and Rasmussen, 1964, 1970). The risk of hemiparesis is about ½% with these parietal resections.

Extension of the resection into the parietal opercular area brings with it the risk of producing a contralateral lower quadrantic homonymous hemianopsia unless the underlying white matter is carefully spared. The depth of the sulci in the parietal opercular area sometimes makes it difficult to avoid interfering with the upper portion of the geniculo-calcarine radiations without leaving behind potentially epileptogenic cortex in the depths of the sulci.

In the dominant hemisphere the parietal opercular convolutions must be carefully spared and the convolutions adjacent to the opercular region should be removed only while the patient is constantly carrying out verbal tasks in order to minimize the risk of producing dysphasia.

Results

By the end of 1971, 86 patients had been operated upon for nontumoral epileptogenic lesions of the parietal region (Fig. 6). There was one postoperative death in 1936 and one accidental death 14 months after operation. These two patients and four others with less than 2 years of follow-up data have been deleted from the following analysis. The remaining 80 patients have been followed for 2 to 41 years, with a median follow-up period of 15 years.

Eleven patients (14%) have had no attacks since discharge from the hospital and another 14 patients (18%) have become and remained seizure-free after a few attacks during the early postoperative months or years. Thus, 25 patients (31%) have become and remained seizure-free. Eight patients (10%) have had recurrence of rare or occasional attacks after being seizure-free for periods rang-

Parietal Lobe Epilepsy - Results of Cortical Excision

Patients with non-tumoral lesions operated upon from 1930 through 1971

Seizure free since discharge	11 pts. (14%)	25 pts. (31%)		
Became seizure free after some early attacks	14 pts. (18%)		47 pts. (59%)	80 pts. with follow-up data of 2 - 41 yrs.
Free 3 or more years then rare or occasional attacks	8 pts. (10%)	22 pts. (28%)		
Marked reduction of seizure tendency	14 pts. (18%)			
Moderate to no reduction of seizure tendency	33 pts. (41%)			median 15 yrs.

Inadequate follow-up data	4 pts.
Accidental death 14 mo. postop.	1 pt.
Postoperative death	1 pt.
Total	**86 pts.**

FIG. 6.

ing from 3 to 12 years. Another 14 patients (18%) have had only 1 to 2% as many attacks as preoperatively but have not had prolonged seizure-free periods and are classified as having a marked reduction of seizure tendency. Therefore, 22 patients (28%) have had a marked but not quite complete reduction of seizure tendency. Added to the seizure-free group, there are thus 47 patients, 59% of this series of 80, with parietal lobe epilepsy refractory to medical management who have had a clinically complete or nearly complete reduction of their seizure tendency following operation. The remaining 33 patients (41%) have had lesser reductions of seizure tendency.

OCCIPITAL REGION

Etiology

Epileptiform lesions largely limited to the occipital region are rare, only 25 cases having been operated on between 1931 and 1972. Two patients had gliomas. There were eight patients in whom birth trauma or anoxia was the presumed cause, 35% of the nontumoral group. There was only one patient with post-traumatic epilepsy and three with postinflammatory brain scarring. The cause was unknown in six (26%) and was due to several miscellaneous lesions (encephalopathy, allergic reaction, and pial angiomatosis) in five (22%).

Attack Patterns

These patients' seizures were relatively stereotyped, starting as a rule with unformed visual hallucinations. Blurring of vision frequently followed and was sometimes the initial phenomenon. Contralateral somatosensory and/or somatomotor phenomena with contraversion frequently followed as the seizure progressed, sometimes associated with a vague cephalic or general body sensation. Some of the patients developed perceptual illusions or formed visual and auditory hallucinations soon after the onset of the seizure, indicating spread of the seizure discharge into the adjacent posterior temporal region (Penfield and Perot, 1963).

EEG Investigation

Standard EEG recording generally shows good lateralization of the epileptiform abnormality which is, however, often more widespread over the posterior half or third of the head than the seizure pattern would suggest.

Surgical Techniques and Risks

A C-shaped incision is used, permitting exposure of the occipital and parietal regions up the midline, down to the tentorium laterally and far enough anteriorly to expose the postcentral gyrus for localization purposes. Cortical EEG recording should include use of flexible wire electrodes to record from the medial surface of the occipital and parietal regions and the undersurface of the occipital and posterior temporal regions, as well as from the convexity of the posterior portion of the cerebral hemisphere.

The postcentral gyrus is identified with electrical stimulation for localization purposes. In the dominant hemisphere, the parietotemporal speech area should be identified by electrical stimulation as completely as possible.

If the original injury or lesion has produced a hemianopsia, an occipital lobectomy including the adjacent parietal and posterior temporal region as needed can be carried out with little risk of producing a significant neurologic deficit. In the dominant hemisphere the posterior margin of the parietotemporal opercular area should be widely spared to minimize risk of producing speech deficits. If the cortical excision approaches the parietal speech area too closely a persisting dyslexia may be produced.

If there is no visual field deficit or only a partial one preoperatively, it is wise to spare as much of the calcarine cortex and optic radiations as possible in view of the location and extent of the cortical electrographic epileptiform abnormality.

Results

By the end of 1971, 23 patients had been operated upon for nontumoral epileptogenic lesions of the occipital lobe. There was one postoperative death in 1949 and one death during the first postoperative year of progressive encephalopathy. These two patients and two others with inadequate follow-up data have been deleted from the following analysis. The remaining 19 patients have been followed for 2 to 38 years, with a median follow-up period of 18 years.

Four patients (21%) have had no attacks since discharge from the hospital and one other (5%) became and remained seizure-free for 18 years after one major attack in the third postoperative year. Thus, five patients (26%) have become and remained seizure-free.

Five patients (26%) have had recurrence of one to three minor attacks after being seizure-free for periods of 3 to 19 years. Another three patients (16%) have had only up to 1 to 2% as many attacks as preoperatively but have not had prolonged seizure-free periods and are classified as having a marked reduction of seizure tendency. Therefore, eight patients (42%) have had a marked but not quite complete reduction in seizure tendency. Added to the seizure-free group, there are thus 13 patients (68%) who have had a complete or nearly complete reduction in seizure tendency following operation. The remaining six patients (32%) have had lesser reductions of seizure tendency.

LARGE DESTRUCTIVE BRAIN LESIONS

Etiology

No tumors are included in this anatomic subgroup since tumors involving or damaging more than one lobe of the brain nearly always cause increased intracranial pressure and/or advancing neurologic deficits that preclude surgical treatment directed primarily toward any seizure tendency that might also be present. Large arteriovenous malformations likewise pose primary problems of life and neurologic function so that consideration of any seizure tendency that may also be present must be given a low priority in the surgical handling of the lesion. Patients with large pial angiomatosis of the Sturge-Weber variety have been included, however, as well as those with small discrete vascular malformations that have produced widespread brain damage as a result of intracerebral hemorrhage.

Birth trauma or anoxia was the presumed cause of the epileptogenic lesion in 45% of the 173 patients in this group operated on at the Montreal Neurological Institute from 1930 through 1971 (Fig. 7). Postinflammatory brain scarring was

Large Destructive Epileptogenic Lesions-Etiology

Patients operated upon from 1930 through 1973
(neoplasms and AV malformations excluded)

Birth trauma or anoxia	78 pts. (45%)
Postnatal trauma	23 pts. (13%)
Postinflammatory brain scarring	39 pts. (23%)
Misc.	15 pts. (9%)
Unknown	18 pts. (10%)
Total	**173 pts.**

FIG. 7.

the presumed cause in 39 patients (23%). Twenty-three patients (13%) were classified as posttraumatic and in 18 patients (10%) the etiology was unknown. The remaining 15 patients (9%) exhibited a variety of miscellaneous lesions (e.g., encephalopathy, intracerebral hematoma or brain tumor removal, pial angiomata, anoxic anesthetic complication).

Attack Patterns

As would be anticipated from the nature of the group with large epileptogenic lesions involving varying combinations of brain regions, practically all types of focal and generalized seizure patterns were represented, with many patients exhibiting several diffierent seizure patterns (Rasmussen and Gossman, 1963).

A larger percentage of the patients in this anatomic subgroup came to operation in childhood than in the other subgroups because of the severity of the seizure problem in many instances, and also because the presence of hemiparesis or other neurologic deficits made it practical to carry out radical cortical excisions under general anesthesia without undue risk of adding significantly to the patients'

Epilepsy Associated with Large Destructive Brain Lesions

Age at operation-173 patients operated upon from 1930 through 1973

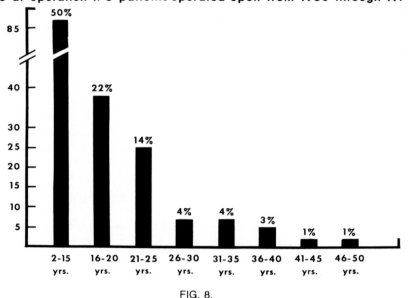

FIG. 8.

existing neurologic deficit. Operation was carried out between the ages of 2 and 15 years in 50% of the patients in this group and during the next decade in another 36% (Fig. 8). Thus, operation was carried out after age 25 in only 13% of these patients.

In comparison with the above age distribution, operation in the temporal lobe series was carried out at ages 16 to 25 in 41% and after age 25 in 49%. In the frontal lobe series, operation was carried out at ages 16 to 25 in 44% and after age 25 in 37%. The age distribution was similar in the parietal series, 46% and 30%, respectively.

EEG Investigation

These patients commonly showed very active and widespread epileptiform activity in standard EEG recordings. Synchronous spread of the epileptiform discharges to the good hemisphere was common. When the destruction in the involved hemisphere was particularly severe and extensive, the voltage of the abnormal discharges was often higher over the good hemisphere, giving the impression on superficial study that it was the more epileptogenic of the two hemispheres. In these cases, however, the background activity is often more abnormal on the side of the major epileptogenic area. This asymmetry of the background activity is a very useful diagnostic sign which should not be overlooked.

Organized, bilaterally synchronous spike-and-wave bursts at 2 to 2.5/sec or bilaterally synchronous polyspike bursts were relatively common and sometimes required use of the intracarotid Amytal-Metrazol and/or Lambroso-Erba Pentothal activation test, as described in Chapters 5 and 9, to obtain evidence that the seizures were in fact arising in the grossly damaged hemisphere.

Surgical Technique and Risks

A wide exposure of most of the hemisphere is required unless the preoperative EEG studies and analysis of the attack patterns indicate that the epileptogenic area is limited to the anterior or posterior half or two thirds of the hemisphere.

Unless the central region has been completely destroyed, it is ordinarily possible to identify the motor area by electrical stimulation even in the presence of a marked and long-standing hemiplegia.

When the original brain injury occurs at birth or during the first few years, speech functions nearly always develop in the other hemisphere, but if there is any doubt on this point the intracarotid Amytal speech test (Wada, 1949; Wada and Rasmussen, 1960; Branch, Milner, and Rasmussen, 1964) must be given preoperatively to permit maximal removal of the epileptogenic area and safeguarding of speech functions.

Many of these patients have long-standing hemiparesis of greater or lesser severity. If there is little or no individual finger movement present and little or no voluntary toe or ankle movement the central region can be removed with little risk of producing a significant increase in the patient's motor or sensory deficit, particularly when the brain injury occurred early in life. When the patient has some individual finger movements, the central (sensorimotor) area should be carefully preserved.

When the epileptiform activity in the preoperative EEG and the cortical EEG examination is largely limited to the anterior half of the head, removal of the frontal and temporal lobes may be required. When the seizure activity is largely limited to the posterior half of the hemisphere and there is a preexisting homonymous hemianopsia, excision of the occipital lobe and variable portions of the parietal and posterior temporal regions may be required. Occasionally, removal of the frontal and parietal lobes with preservation of the parieto-occipital region and temporal lobe is indicated.

Complete Hemispherectomy

When the epileptiform activity involves the whole hemisphere and a maximal hemiplegia is present along with a complete homonymous hemianopsia, removal of the hemisphere peripheral to the corpus striatum and thalamus, introduced by Krynauw (1950), has been the procedure of choice until recently and carries with it the best percentage of good results in reducing the seizure tendency. Complete hemispherectomy is usually carried out in children and is therefore done under light general anesthesia. A large U-shaped skin incision is used to expose as much of the hemisphere as possible. Since the ventricle is always large and the hemisphere atrophic, access to the frontal and occipital poles rarely presents any technical problems.

The removal of the hemisphere is started by exposing the middle cerebral artery at its region and dissecting distally toward the anterior margin of the insula where it is doubly clipped and divided. The temporal lobe is then elevated and the arachnoid over the cerebral peduncle opened and the posterior cerebral artery doubly clipped and divided. The hemisphere is retracted from the falx in the parietal region and the bridging veins to the sagittal sinus coagulated, clipped, and cut. The body of the lateral ventricle is then entered through the cingulate gyrus and the cortical incision carried anteriorly through the cingulate gyrus, coagulating and clipping the branches of the anterior cerebral artery and the bridging veins to the sinus as they are encountered. The anterior cerebral arteries are covered with cottonoid strips as they are exposed to provide maximum protection to the arterial supply to the medial surface of the good hemisphere. At the genu of the corpus callosum the incision is carried downward through the subcallosal gyrus. The foramen of Munro is kept covered with a dental roll or cotton strip on a string to prevent blood from entering the third ventricle.

Attention is then turned to the posterior end of the hemisphere and the cortical incision in the cingulate gyrus is carried posteriorly around the splenium of the corpus callosum and across the medial surface of the occipital lobe. After sectioning the bridging veins of the occipital and posterior temporal regions, the posterior portion of the hemisphere can be gently retracted and the cortical incision extended into the inferior aspect of the temporal region just lateral to the hippocampus and carried forward as far as vision will permit, usually to the posterior aspect of the pes hippocampus. The wall of the ventricle is then incised just lateral to the bulge of the corpus striatum and thalamus. With a fine bore suction in the incision is carried downward through the white matter between the insula and the striatum and thalamus. As the hemisphere is mobilized and gently retracted laterally, the incision in the central white matter is connected with the frontal and temporal ends of the superficial cortical incision and cut through at the fissure of Sylvius at the site of the previously clipped and cut middle cerebral artery.

The hippocampus is then removed completely from its pial bed and remnants of cortex along the original medial cortical excision removed by gentle suction. The choroid plexus is removed completely, clipping as well as coagulating the principal feeding arterioles. A hole at least a centimeter in diameter is made in the septum as a safeguard against sequestration of the remaining lateral ventricle by late cicatricial occulsion of the foramen of Munro of the remaining hemisphere.

The dura is closed completely and a Penrose drain put into the removal cavity and brought out through a separate stab wound in the scalp and sutured to the scalp. The dura is tented up to the bone flap by steel sutures at two points.

Daily lumbar punctures with removal of 15 to 30 cc of cerebrospinal fluid seem to lessen the severity of the postoperative aseptic meningitis that usually follows large cortical removals.

Superficial Cerebral Hemosiderosis

A fourth to a third of hemispherectomized patients who have been followed for more than 5 years develop the syndrome of superficial cerebral hemosiderosis, characterized by insidious onset of neurologic deterioration and evidence of increased intracranial pressure (Oppenheimer and Griffith, 1966; Hughes and Oppenheimer, 1969; Falconer and Wilson, 1969; Wilson, 1970). This results from the gradual accummulation of brown, high-protein- and high-iron-containing fluid in the hemispherectomy cavity, presumably due to the gradual seepage of red cells into the cavity from minor jolts to the head, coughing, etc. (Noetzel, 1940, 1955; Iwanowski and Olszewski, 1960; Tomlinson and Walton, 1964). As a result of the toxic effects of this fluid on the ependyma and leptomeninges, a granular ependymitis develops with gradual occlusion of the acqueduct and sometimes of the foramen of Munro along with thickening of the leptomeninges and microscopic cystic degenerations beneath the ependyma and leptomeninges.

Nine of the 27 hemispherectomized patients at the Montreal Neurological Institute who survived the first postoperative year developed this complication after being neurologically stable for periods of 4½ to 20 years after operation (Rasmussen, 1973). While prompt recognition of this late complication and treatment by a ventriculo-atrial shunt usually restores the patient promptly to his previous state, a delay in its recognition may result in a significant permanent increase in neurologic deficit. In addition, complications of the shunt are frequent and sometimes lethal. Thus five of the above nine patients with this complication have died from the condition or complications of the shunting procedures. The remaining four, after the appropriate shunt was established, have returned to their previous neurologic status and have remained stable since then, 3 months, 3, 5, and 9 years, respectively, after the initial shunt procedure. Two of them, however, have required subsequent shunt revisions.

Subtotal Hemispherectomy

Preservation of a small portion of the hemisphere seems to prevent the development of the above complication. Thus, from 1937 through 1972, 48 patients have had removal of at least three lobes of the brain, but not a complete hemispherectomy. Forty of these have been followed for 4 to 26 years, with a median follow-up period of 10 years, comparable to the hemispherectomy group. None of these have developed this late complication, superficial cerebral hemosiderosis.

Since 1968 it has been our policy, in patients with medically refractory focal epilepsy and infantile hemiplegia who previously would have been considered candidates for complete cerebral hemispherectomy, to preserve a small portion of the least epileptogenic region of the damaged hemisphere. Usually this has meant leaving *in situ* the frontal or occipital pole, occasionally the upper central parasagittal region.

Results

Complete Hemispherectomy

This procedure has been carried out in 29 patients at the Montreal Neurological Institute from 1952 through 1968 (Fig. 9). Two patients died during the first postoperative year of a progressive encephalopathy. The remaining 27 patients have been followed for 5 to 20 years, with a median follow-up period of 11 years.

Thirteen patients (48%) have had no attacks since discharge from the hospital, and another three (11%) have become and remained seizure-free after having a few attacks in the early postoperative months or years. Thus, 16 patients (59%) have become and remained seizure-free. Six patients (22%) have had recurrence of rare or occasional attacks after being seizure-free for 3 to 17 years. Another one patient has had about 1% as many attacks as preoperatively. Therefore, seven patients (26%) have had a marked but not quite complete reduction of seizure tendency. Added to the seizure-free group, there are thus 23 patients (85%) who have had a complete or nearly complete reduction of seizure tendency following the hemispherectomy. The remaining four patients have had about 5 to 15% as many attacks as preoperatively.

Hemispherectomy for Seizures

1952 through 1972

Seizure free since discharge	13 pts. (48%)	16 pts. (59%)	23 pts. (85%)	27 pts. with follow-up data of 5-20 yrs.
Became seizure free after some early attacks	3 pts. (11%)			
Free 3 or more years then rare or occasional attacks	6 pts. (22%)	7 pts. (26%)		
Marked reduction of seizure tendency	1 pt. (4%)			
Moderate or less reduction of seizure tendency	4 pts. (15%)			median 11 yrs.
Died in 1st year of progressive encephalopathy	2 pts.			
Total	**29 pts.**			

FIG. 9.

Subtotal Hemispherectomy

Removal of at least three lobes of the brain, but not a complete hemispherectomy, has been carried out in 48 patients from 1937 through 1972 (Fig. 10). There was one postoperative death in 1957. This patient and seven others with less than 4 years' follow-up data have been deleted to make the follow-up period similar to that of the total hemispherectomy group. The remaining 40 patients have been followed for 4 to 26 years with a median follow-up period of 11 years.

Ten patients (25%) have had no attacks since discharge from the hospital. Eight others (20%) have become and remained seizure-free after having a few attacks in the early postoperative months or years. Thus, 18 patients (45%) have become and remained seizure-free. Five patients (12.5%) have had recurrence of rare or occasional attacks after being seizure-free for 3 to 16 years. Another five have had only up to 1 to 2% as many attacks as preoperatively and are classified as having had a marked reduction in seizure tendency. Thus, 10 patients (25%) have had a marked but not quite complete reduction in seizure tendency. Added to the seizure-free group, there are thus 28 patients (70%) who have had a complete or nearly complete reduction in seizure tendency. The remaining 12 patients (30%) have had lesser reductions of seizure tendency. The majority of these have had 5 to 10% as many attacks as preoperatively, the remainder 80 to 90% as many.

Subtotal Hemispherectomy for Seizures
1937 through 1972

Seizure free since discharge	10 pts. (25%)	18 pts. (45%)	28 pts. (70%)	40 pts. with follow-up data of 4-26 yrs.
Became seizure free after some early attacks	8 pts. (20%)			
Free 3 or more years then rare or occasional attacks	5 pts. (12.5%)	10 pts. (25%)		
Marked reduction of seizure tendency	5 pts. (12.5%)			
Moderate or less reduction of seizure tendency	12 pts. (30%)			median 11 yrs.
Less than 4 yrs. follow-up	7 pts.			
Postoperative death	1 pt.			
Total	**48 pts.**			

FIG. 10.

Lesser Cortical Removals

The remaining 86 patients in this group have had large cortical removals but less than hemispherectomy or subtotal hemispherectomy (Fig. 11). There were four postoperative deaths and one death 11 months after operation from a progressive chronic encephalitis. These five patients and four others with inadequate follow-up data have been deleted from the following analysis, leaving 77 patients with follow-up data of 2 to 31 years duration and a median follow-up period of 11 years.

Eleven patients (14%) have had no attacks since leaving the hospital and another 13 (17%) have become and remained seizure-free after having had a few attacks during the early postoperative months or years. Thus 24 patients (31%) have become and remained seizure-free. Seven patients (9%) have had recurrence of rare or occasional attacks after being seizure-free for periods ranging from 3 to 19 years. Another eight patients (10%) have had only up to 1 to 2% as many attacks as preoperatively but no long seizure-free periods and are classified as having had a marked reduction in seizure tendency. Therefore, 15 patients (19%) have had a marked but not quite complete reduction of seizure tendency. Added to the seizure-free group there are thus 39 patients (50%) who have had a complete or nearly complete reduction of seizure tendency. The remaining 38 patients (49%) have had lesser reductions of seizure tendency.

Epilepsy Due to Large Destructive Non-Tumoral Lesions
(exclusive of patients undergoing total or sub-total hemispherectomy)
Results of Cortical Excision
Patients operated upon from 1930 through 1971

Seizure free since discharge	11 pts. (14%)	24 pts. (31%)		
Became seizure free after some early attacks	13 pts. (17%)		39 pts. (50%)	77 pts. with follow-up data of 2-31 yrs.
Free 3 or more years then rare or occasional attacks	7 pts. (9%)	15 pts. (19%)		
Marked reduction of seizure tendency	8 pts. (10%)			
Moderate or less reduction of seizure tendency	38 pts (49%)			median 11 yrs.

Inadequate follow-up data	4 pts.
Death in 1st postop. yr. due to chronic encephalitis	1 pt.
Postoperative death	4 pts.
Total	**86 pts.**

FIG. 11.

Present Policy

Since 1968 we have not carried out a complete hemispherectomy, but have preserved in each instance a small portion of the least epileptogenic region of the hemisphere. This has usually meant preserving the frontal or occipital pole or the upper central region. Most of these patients have remained seizure-free, or nearly so, and to date it has not been necessary to consider reoperation and removal of the remnant of the hemisphere, although this could easily be done if this remnant produced a significant continuing seizure tendency that was refractory to tolerable doses of anticonvulsant medication. Five of the patients in our complete hemispherectomy series have had the hemisphere removed in two or three stages several years apart and none has developed superficial cerebral hemosiderosis to date.

We have strongly recommended that each of our patients who has had a complete hemispherectomy in the past have a yearly skull X-ray to check on possible displacement of the hemostatic clips. If movement of the clips is detected one can be sure an obstructive hydrocephalus is developing and prompt air studies are indicated to locate the site of the cerebrospinal fluid blockage so that the appropriate shunting procedure can be carried out.

REFERENCES

Branch, C., Milner, B., and Rasmussen, T. (1964): Intracarotid sodium amytal for the lateralization of cerebral speech dominance. *J. Neurosurg.*, 21:399–405.

Corkin, S., Milner, B., and Rasmussen, T. (1964): Effects of different cortical excisions on sensory threshold in man. *Trans. Am. Neurol. Assoc.*, 89:112–116.

Corkin, S., Milner, B., and Rasmussen, T. (1970): Somatosensory thresholds. Contrasting effects of postcentral gyrus and posterior parietal lobe excisions. *Arch. Neurol.*, 22:41–58.

Falconer, M. A., and Wilson, P. J. E. (1969): Complications related to delayed hemorrhage after hemispherectomy. *J. Neurosurg.*, 30:413–426.

Hughes, J. T., and Oppenheimer, D. R. (1969): Superficial siderosis of the central nervous system. A report on nine cases with autopsy. *Acta Neuropathol.*, 13:56–74.

Iwanowski, I., and Olszewski, J. (1960): The effects of subarachnoid injections of iron containing substances on the central nervous system. *J. Neuropath. Exp. Neurol.*, 19:433–448.

Krynauw, R. A. (1950): Infantile hemiplegia treated by removing one cerebral hemisphere. *J. Neurol. Neurosurg. Psychiatry*, 13:243–267.

Noetzel, H. (1940): Diffusion von Blutfarbstoff in der innerne Randzone und äusseren Oberfläche des Zentralnervensystems bei subarachnoidaler Blutung. *Arch. Psychiatr.*, 111:129–138.

Noetzel, H. (1955): Diffusion of iron pigment in the brain. *Excerpt. Med.*, 8:864–845 (abstract 3760, paper read at 2nd International Congress of Neuropathology, London, Sept. 12–17, 1955).

Oppenheimer, D. R., and Griffith, H. B. (1966): Persistent intracranial bleeding as a complication of hemispherectomy. *J. Neurol Neurosurg. Psychiatry*, 29:229–240.

Penfield, W., and Perot, P. (1963): The brain's record of auditory and visual experience—A final summary and discussion. *Brain*, 86:595–696.

Rasmussen, T. (1973): Postoperative superficial hemosiderosis of the brain, its diagnosis, treatment and prevention. *Trans. Am. Neurol. Assoc.*, 98:133–137.

Rasmussen, T., and Gossman, H. (1963): Epilepsy due to gross destructive brain lesions. *Neurology*, 13:659–669.

Tomlinson, B. E., and Walton, J. N. (1964): Superficial hemosiderosis of the central nervous system. *J. Neurol. Neurosurg. Psychiatry*, 27:332–339.

Wilson, P. J. E. (1970): Cerebral hemispherectomy for infantile hemiplegia. A report of 50 cases. *Brain,* 93:147–180.

Wada, J. (1949): A new method for the determination of the side of cerebral speech dominance—A preliminary report on the intracarotid injection of sodium amytal in man. *Igaku to Seibutsugaki (Medicine and Biology),* 14:221–222 (In Japanese).

Wada, J., and Rasmussen, T. (1960): Intracarotid injection of sodium amytal for the lateralization of cerebral speech dominance: Experimental and clinical observations. *J. Neurosurg.,* 17:266–282.

Advances in Neurology, Vol. 8, edited by D. P. Purpura, J. K. Penry, and R. D. Walter. Raven Press, New York © 1975.

11
Surgery of Epilepsy Associated with Brain Tumors

Theodore Rasmussen

DEFINITION OF THE PATIENT POPULATION

Although epilepsy is a common symptom of supratentorial brain tumors, these lesions frequently also cause symptoms and signs of advancing neurologic deficits and increased intracranial pressure, and the symptom, epilepsy, is not the primary focus of treatment. The epilepsy is often the *first* symptom, however, and in slowly growing tumors may be the only symptom for considerable periods of time. The primary focus of this chapter is on the group of patients whose presenting problems, when the patients came for investigation, were seizures, rather than progressive neurologic deficits or signs and symptoms of increased intracranial pressure.

Epilepsy as a Symptom of Brain Tumor

The incidence of epilepsy as a symptom of brain tumors of all varieties and locations has been shown to be of the order of 35% in a number of studies (Sargent, 1921; Dowman and Smith, 1928; Parker, 1930; Furlow and Sachs, 1936; Pederson, 1938; Pilcher and Parker, 1938; Penfield, Erickson, and Tarlov, 1940; Kirstein, 1942; Hoefer, Schlesinger, and Pennes, 1947; White, Liu, and Mixter, 1948; Lund, 1952; Penman and Smith, 1954; Arseni and Petrovici, 1971). When cerebellar and pituitary tumors are excluded, the incidence rises to about 50%.

Analysis of the incidence of seizures in supratentorial tumors shows a direct correlation with chronicity of growth of the neoplasm. Thus, in the Montreal Neurological Institute series reported by Penfield, Erickson, and Tarlov (1940), seizures occurred in 37% of glioblastomas, 70% of astrocytomas, 67% of meningiomas, and 92% of oligodendrogliomas. In 40% of the patients in this series who had seizures secondary to intracranial tumors, recurring seizures were the initial symptoms, and thus these patients originally presented as epileptic problems. Sargent's (1921) data were similar in this regard. Thus a significant percentage of patients with supratentorial brain tumors first present for a variable period of time as seizure problems. Often progressive neurologic deficits and intracranial pressure signs and symptoms soon appear and the correct diagnosis becomes apparent early in the patient's course. In the case of slowly growing tumors, however, seizures may be the only symptom for considerable periods of time. Both air and angiographic X-ray studies and radioactive brain scans may be

---

Montreal Neurological Institute Reprint No. 1172.

normal for several years before the tumor betrays its presence. Thus a brain tumor must be constantly borne in mind as a possible cause of focal epilepsy, particularly when seizures start in adult life and when no evidence of brain atrophy is present in the brain region pointed to by the patient's seizure pattern and EEG abnormality.

Brain Tumor as a Cause of Chronic Epilepsy

Twenty percent of the patients operated on at the Montreal Neurological Institute for focal cerebral seizures were found to have brain tumors, including both neoplastic and a small number of non-neoplastic space-occupying lesions. By the end of 1973 this group consisted of 347 patients (Fig. 1). In most of these

Total Surgical Series-Etiology
Patients operated upon from 1928 through 1973

Non-Tumoral Lesions

Birth trauma or anoxia	379 pts.	(28% of non-tumoral lesions)
Postnatal trauma	294 pts.	(22% " " ")
Postinflammatory brain scarring	202 pts.	(15% " " ")
Miscellaneous	97 pts.	(7% " " ")
Unknown	383 pts.	(28% " " ")
	1355 pts.	(100%)
Tumors	327 pts.	} 20% of total group
Vascular malformations	20 pts.	

Total 1702 pts.

FIG. 1.

patients the presence of a space-occupying or vascular lesion was established by the preoperative studies, but seizure-type operative techniques were employed because seizures were the patients' prime problem rather than advancing neurologic deficit or increased intracranial pressure. In about 10%, however, the presence of a tumor was not suspected until it was disclosed during the operation. This group of 347 patients, of course, represents only a small fraction of the total number of brain tumor patients studied at the MNI during this period who had seizures in addition to signs of progressive neurologic deficit with or without evidence of increased intracranial pressure. Such patients were operated on with standard brain tumor surgical techniques and thus do not appear in this surgical seizure series.

DIAGNOSIS

Clinical

The seizures associated with these various lesions, neoplastic and non-neoplastic masses and vascular malformations, do not differ from those produced by atrophic or cicatricial lesions of the same locations (Penfield and Kristiansen, 1951; Penfield, Jasper, and McNaughton, 1954). Thus, although the nature of the patients' seizure pattern often points to the *location* in the brain of the lesion responsible for the seizures, it does not give any indication as to the *nature* of the lesion. The sole exception to this generalization in our series was the presence of an *initial* olfactory or gustatory aura which usually indicated the presence of a deep-lying indolent glioma in the Sylvian region of one hemisphere rather than a static, cicatricial lesion.

The incidence of brain tumors in patients under treatment for seizures doubtless varies greatly from clinic to clinic, but it has been estimated that intracranial tumors are present in between 5 and 10% of all cases of seizures seen in large general hospital clinics (White, Liu, and Mixter, 1948). In a series of patients studied by Wyke (1959), brain tumors were present in 30% of 1,661 patients with seizures who were selected for study regarding the possible presence of a surgical lesion. Thus the physician caring for patients with seizures must keep an open mind in regard to the etiology of the seizures until definitive investigation and/or the passage of time have proven that the cause of the seizures does not require specific treatment and attention can be concentrated on the treatment of the symptom, the seizures.

The onset of seizures in adult life, with no previous etiologic factors in the earlier history, provides the commonest clue that the patient's seizures might be due to a tumor. Brain injury at birth or early childhood, however, sometimes results in the onset of seizures only after 15 or 20 years or more, and brain tumors occurring in children not infrequently first present as seizure problems, so the age at onset of seizures is not a reliable indicator of the presence or absence of a tumor as the lesion responsible for the seizure tendency.

The development of a progressive neurologic deficit, in addition to the seizures, sooner or later helps to clarify the diagnosis in most patients, but months or years often elapse between the onset of seizures and the appearance of a significant neurologic deficit in the case of slowly growing astrocytomas, oligodendrogliomas, meningiomas, etc. Occasionally, this interval may be as long as 10 to 25 years, and, rarely, even longer. However, various indolent encephalopathies may produce the same picture of slowly progressive neurologic deficit and seizures (Rasmussen, Olszewski, and Lloyd-Smith, 1958; Aguilar and Rasmussen, 1960; Rasmussen and McCann, 1968).

An elevation of the spinal fluid protein to levels between 50 and 100 mg% alerts one to the possible presence of a neoplasm rather than a static cicatricial lesion, but the cerebrospinal fluid (CSF) examination is often normal and the presence of normal CSF findings does not enable one to rule out the presence of a neoplasm. An elevated CSF protein, however, is often found in the presence of a variety of chronic encephalopathic lesions that sometimes present initially as seizure problems. The presence of an elevated spinal fluid protein thus indicates the presence of a progressive destructive lesion or process in the brain, but a normal spinal fluid does *not* enable one to rule out the presence of an expanding or space-occupying lesion in the brain.

Electroencephalography

A progressive change in the EEG abnormality, particularly in the slow-wave band, strongly suggests the presence of a neoplasm or some other progressive degenerative lesion of the brain. The slowly growing gliomas and meningiomas, however, may show surprisingly normal EEG records with little or no evidence of a destructive brain process. The epileptiform abnormality is often less active than one would anticipate from the severity of the patient's seizure problem, but otherwise it resembles the spike or sharp wave forms characteristic of cicatricial or atrophic epileptogenic brain lesions. The EEG is thus not a very efficient tool for ruling out the presence of a neoplasm or other mass lesion in a patient with seizures. Occasionally, the EEG abnormality may mimic closely that of centrencephalic epilepsy, and unless the possibility of an occult neoplasm is recognized, complete investigation of the patient may be omitted or delayed (Tükel and Jasper, 1952).

Radiological and Radioisotopic Studies

A positive radioisotope brain scan provides strong evidence of the presence of a neoplasm and will rarely miss even a slowly growing supratentorial meningioma once it reaches a significant size. Slowly growing gliomas, however, such as indolent astrocytomas and oligodendrogliomas, often exhibit normal brain scans for long periods after the onset of seizures. Thus, a positive brain scan is highly suggestive of the presence of a neoplasm but a negative brain scan does not enable one to rule out the presence of a brain tumor.

There is suggestive early evidence that the recently introduced computerized tomographic EMI scanning technique will be more effective in identifying these indolent gliomas that may masquerade for long periods as ordinary seizure problems, but more experience with this new technique must accumulate before its accuracy in this special group of patients can be properly assessed.

Focal calcification in the skull X-ray also suggests the presence of an indolent neoplasm or vascular malformation, but is occasionally seen in cicatricial brain lesions as well.

Cerebral angiographic studies show some evidence of displacement of vessels in well over half of these patients with seizures due to brain tumor and without evidence of significant neurologic deficit, but tumor stains are rare. As in the case of brain scans, a positive cerebral angiogram gives good evidence of a brain tumor but a negative test does *not* enable one to rule it out with certainty.

The pneumoencephalogram is the most accurate tool in the physician's armamentarium for the investigation of this problem. It provided evidence of an expanding or space-occupying lesion in about 85% of this series of seizure patients harboring brain tumors of various sorts, neoplastic and non-neoplastic. The ventricular distortion is often slight, however, and reference to the clinical and EEG evidence may be necessary to decide whether the pneumoencephalographic asymmetry represents the presence of an expanding or space-occupying lesion in one hemisphere or an atrophic lesion in the other. In the remaining 15% of the patients in this series, the pneumoencephalogram was either normal or showed evidence of an atrophic lesion in the location where a tumor or vascular lesion was subsequently found at operation.

HISTOLOGICAL CLASSIFICATION

Astrocytomas of grade I or II plus a few oligodendrogliomas and other slowly growing gliomas constitute 65% of this series (Fig. 2). The majority of these patients experienced onset of seizures between the ages of 20 and 50, but it is noteworthy that in approximately 20% of these patients with slowly growing gliomas the seizures started during the first and second decades of life. The preoperative duration of seizures in this group of patients ranged from a few months to 31 years, with the median interval being 3 years (Leblanc and Rasmussen, 1973).

The more rapidly growing gliomas—glioblastoma, astroblastoma, anaplastic

Tumoral and Vascular Epileptogenic Lesions

Patients operated upon from 1929 through 1973

Brain Region	Astrocytomas and Other Slowly Growing Gliomas	Glioblastoma and Other Malignant Gliomas	Meningioma and Other Nodular Lesions	AV and Other Vascular Malformations	Total
Temporal	92 pts.	6 pts.	28 pts.	7 pts.	133 pts. (38%)
Frontal	75 pts.	11 pts.	11 pts.	5 pts.	102 pts. (29%)
Central (Sensori Motor)	34 pts.	10 pts.	18 pts.	3 pts.	65 pts. (19%)
Parietal	21 pts.	9 pts.	10 pts.	5 pts.	45 pts. (13%)
Occipital	2 pts.	—	—	—	2 pts. (1%)
Total	224 pts. (65%)	36 pts. (10%)	67 pts. (19%)	20 pts. (6%)	347 pts.

FIG. 2.

mixed gliomas, etc.—constitute 10% of the patients in this series (Fig. 2). Evidence of progressive neurologic deficits appeared early in this group so the preoperative duration of seizures was short, ranging from a few weeks to 6 years, with the median interval being 5 months.

Sixty-seven patients (19%) had meningiomas, hemangiomas, tuberculomas, cholestiatomas, or other non-neoplastic nodular lesions. In the patients with meningiomas, constituting nearly half of this group of 67 patients, the seizures, except in one patient, first appeared in adult life, with a somewhat higher percentage in the older age group that was the case in the previous group of patients with slowly growing gliomas. The preoperative duration of seizures was similar to the indolent glioma group, ranging up to 15 years, with the median interval being 2 years.

In the remainder of this group, with miscellaneous nodular lesions, the preoperative duration of seizures was even longer, with the median duration being 5 years. Onset of seizures occurred in the second, third, and fourth decade of life in most of these patients.

In over half of the 20 patients in this series with arteriovenous malformations or other major vascular malformations of the brain, the seizures appeared in the first decade of life, while in the remainder of the group the seizures appeared in the second, third, or fourth decades.

The temporal lobe was the site of the tumor in 38% and the frontal lobe in 29% (Fig. 2). Nineteen percent were largely confined to the central (sensorimotor) region and 13% were in the parietal region. Only two involved primarily the occipital lobe.

The analysis of the seizure stories of these 347 patients emphasizes the fact that epilepsy is a symptom and not a disease, and points out with great clarity the fact that the type and severity of the seizures as well as the effectiveness of anticonvulsant medication in controlling the seizures are of little help in identifying the nature of the brain lesion responsible for the symptom of epilepsy. Many of these patients were originally diagnosed and treated as ordinary epilepsies. In a significant proportion the original diagnosis was idiopathic or generalized epilepsy, and the conclusion that seizures were actually focal in type was not suspected until a special study of the seizure problem was carried out.

SURGICAL TECHNIQUE

The skin and bone flaps should be fashioned so as to permit identification of the sensorimotor strip by electrical stimulation and thus permit maximal safe removal of the tumor and the adjacent epileptogenic cortex. Cortical EEG recording is carried out in the usual manner, but depth electrodes are not employed because of the risk of producing hemorrhage if the electrode should enter tumor tissue. After the epileptogenic cortex is mapped out as completely as required, the area to be removed is outlined.

In the case of temporal lobe glial tumors in the dominant hemisphere, the incision across the convexity is placed at the level of the Rolandic fissure at its junction with the Sylvian fissure. In the nondominant hemisphere the incision may be placed further posteriorly if required by the location of the surface extent of the tumor or the posterior extent of actively spiking cortex. The removal is carried out with a small bore suction as in an ordinary temporal lobectomy. Tumor tissue, which may be either gelatinous or tough and fibrous, is usually only moderately vascular and can be peeled off the pial bank of the Sylvian fissure in the same fashion as a gliosed cicatricial gyrus. When a glial tumor infiltrates into the white matter beneath the insula it should be cut through with the suction tip or scissors at the level of the lateral and inferior edge of the insula, with an absolute minimum of movement of the tumor-infiltrated white matter extending inward, below the insula. No attempt should be made to remove this tumor-infiltrated white matter extending inward below the insula since this carries great risk of producing hemiplegia. In the dominant hemisphere glial tumor tissue behind the level of the Rolandic fissure should be left in situ, although a discrete tumor-infiltrated hippocampus and hippocampal gyrus may be removed further posteriorly if the posterior temporal convexity is not retracted or manipulated and if the patient is carrying out verbal tasks promptly and correctly.

Gliomas of the insular and Sylvian region are sometimes associated with actively epileptogenic cortex of both the temporal and adjacent portion of the frontal lobe. If the spiking in the frontal opercular and orbital region persists after removal of the temporal lobe and as much of the tumor as is safe, it is often wise to remove the involved portion of the frontal lobe both to improve the likelihood of a satisfactory reduction of seizure tendency and also to provide more complete internal decompression for the residual tumor.

When a glial tumor of the frontal lobe is well anterior and relatively discrete, a radical frontal lobectomy carries with it a good possibility of cure as well as complete reduction of the seizure tendency. More frequently, however, the glioma infiltrates diffusely into the white matter further posteriorly. In this case, the tumor-infiltrated white matter should be cut through well in front of the precentral gyrus and with minimum movement of the underlying brain tissue in order to minimize the risk of producing a hemiplegia. Complete removal of the cortex of the medial and orbital surfaces of the excised portion of the frontal lobe enhances the likelihood of a satisfactory reduction of the seizure tendency.

The glial tumors of the central (sensorimotor) region that produce seizures with little or no hemiparesis tend to be small and discrete with limited invasive tendency. These must be removed with the least possible disturbance of the cortex and white matter of the adjacent portions of the pre- and postcentral gyri, and great care must be used to avoid movement of the underlying white matter leading to the internal capsule. It is ordinarily necessary to cut through the tumor-infiltrated white matter at the base of the tumor with a scissors rather than with the suction tip in order to avoid movement and trauma to the underlying internal capsule.

Gliomas and other intramedullary tumors and the adjacent epileptogenic cortex of the parietal region ordinarily cannot be removed as completely as frontal and temporal intramedullary tumors. As in the case of intermediate frontal lobe intramedullary tumors, the internal capsule must be carefully protected by cutting through the tumor-infiltrated white matter well away from the region of the internal capsule and with as little movement and manipulation of the tissue as possible. In the dominant hemisphere the parietal opercular region must be carefully spared to reduce risk of producing dysphasia.

Postoperative radiation therapy, 5,000 to 5,500 rad tumor dose over a 7- to 8-week period, was ordinarily given to all patients with gliomas unless the tumor was unusually discrete and was removed with at least a 2-cm rim of grossly and histologically normal tissue.

Most of the meningiomas in this series were relatively small and their removal did not pose significant technical surgical problems. After removal of the meningiomas, the adjacent convolutions that had been compressed by the tumor were removed back to normal gyri with undamaged pial banks whenever this was practicable and could be carried out without undue risk of producing a significant neurologic deficit. The same general principles applied to the few cholesteatomas and non-neoplastic tumors such as tuberculomas and chronic abscesses.

Most of the arteriovenous and other vascular malformations in this series could be removed by block dissection and any epileptogenic cortex remaining at the margin of the removal cavity then removed by suction back to undamaged pial surfaces whenever possible. In a few instances, removal of a large arteriovenous malformation was felt to be hazardous and only the epileptogenic cortex adjacent to the malformation was removed. This has resulted in a reasonably satisfactory, although not complete, reduction in seizure tendency.

SURVIVAL AND SEIZURE RESULTS

Astrocytomas and Other Slowly Growing Gliomas

There were 206 patients in this group operated on from 1931 through 1971 (Fig. 3). There were six operative deaths at the primary operation and seven other patients died during the first postoperative year. There were nine patients with inadequate follow-up data. The remaining 184 patients have been followed for periods of 1 to 36 years, with a median follow-up period of 6 years. Ninety-four patients have died; most, but not all, of recurrence of the neoplasm. Ninety-five patients are still living. Sixty-nine patients survived for 10 years or more, 31 for 15 years or more, 17 for 20 years or more, and 2 for 32 and 36 years, respectively.

The results of operation on the seizure tendency in Figs. 3–6 are tabulated for the period up to the time when there was clinical evidence of regrowth of the tumor. This was usually heralded first by recurrence of seizures after seizure-free period of 1 or more years, followed soon after by evidence of progressive neurologic deficit with or without evidence of increased intracranial pressure. Fifty-eight of these patients (31%) were seizure-free, as defined above, after discharge

Astrocytomas and Miscellaneous
Slowly Growing Gliomas

Results of Operation on Seizure Tendency up to Evidence of Tumor Recurrence

(patients operated upon from 1931 through 1971)

No attacks	58 pts. (31%)	80 pts. (43%)	129 pts. (70%)	184 pts. (95 living, 94 dead) data of 1-36 yrs.
Became seizure free	22 pts. (12%)			
Marked reduction in seizure tendency	49 pts. (27%)			
Moderate to no reduction in seizure tendency	55 pts. (30%)			(median 6 yrs.)
Inadequate follow-up data	9 pts.			
Died in 1st postoperative year	7 pts.			
Postoperative death (primary operation)	6 pts.			

Total 206 pts.

FIG. 3.

from the hospital, and another 22 patients (12%) became seizure-free after a few attacks in the early postoperative period. Thus 80 patients (43%) became and remained seizure-free to date, or until there was evidence of tumor recurrence. Another 49 patients (27%) have had only up to 1 to 2% as many attacks as preoperatively. Thus 129 patients (70%) of those who survived the first year experienced a complete or nearly complete reduction in seizure tendency to date or until tumor growth recurred.

Glioblastomas and Malignant Gliomas

There were 35 patients in this group, operated on from 1930 through 1971 (Fig. 4). There were three operative deaths, eight others died during the first postoperative year, and there was inadequate follow-up data in another three patients. The remaining 21 patients lived and were followed for 1 year or more. Eleven died between the first and second anniversary of the operation. Five died during the second postoperative year, 5 in the fourth, one in the fifth and one in the ninth. The one living patient has been seizure-free for 19 years, his incompletely removed left central glioblastoma having remained dormant, presumably as a result of his postoperative radiation therapy. One other patient was seizure-free until his tumor recurred. Seven patients (33%) had only up to 1 to 2% as many attacks as preoperatively. The remaining 12 patients (57%) had lesser reductions of seizure tendency. As would be expected, relief of seizures was considerably less successful than in the previous group, even for the short survival period characteristic of this unfortunate patient population.

Glioblastoma and Malignant Glioma

Results of Operation on Seizure Tendency up to Evidence of Tumor Recurrence
(Patients operated upon from 1930 through 1971)

No attacks	2 pts. (10%)	2 pts. (10 %)	9pts. (43%)	21 pts. (1 living, 20 dead) with follow-up data of 1-19 yrs.
Became seizure free	0			
Marked reduction in seizure tendency	7 pts. (33%)			
Moderate to no reduction of seizure tendency	12 pts. (57%)			(median 1½ yrs.)
Inadequate follow-up data	3 pts.			
Died in 1st postoperative year	8 pts.			
Postoperative death (primary operation)	3 pts.			

Total   35 pts.

FIG. 4.

Meningiomas and Miscellaneous Nodular Lesions

The results of operation in this group of 66 patients with meningiomas, discrete hemangiomas, and miscellaneous non-neoplastic nodular lesions were similar and are combined in Fig. 5. Two patients died in the first postoperative year and there was inadequate follow-up data in another five patients. The remaining 59 patients were followed for periods ranging from 1 to 35 years, with a median follow-up

Meningioma and Miscellaneous Nodular Lesions

Results of Operation on Seizure Tendency
(Patients operated upon from 1929 through 1971)

No attacks	23 pts. (39%)	33 pts. (56 %)	48 pts. (81%)	59 pts. (49 living, 10 dead) with follow-up data of 1-35 yrs.
Became seizure free	10 pts. (17%)			
Marked reduction in seizure tendency	15 pts. (25%)			
Moderate to no reduction in seizure tendency	11 pts. (19%)			(median 11 yrs.)
Inadequate follow-up data	5 pts.			
Died in 1st postoperative year	2 pts.			

Total   66 pts.

FIG. 5.

period of 11 years. Ten patients have died of various causes through the years, while 49 are living.

Twenty-three patients (39%) have had no attacks since leaving the hospital and another 10 patients (17%) have become and remained seizure-free after having a few attacks in the early postoperative period. Thus 33 patients (56%) have become and remained seizure-free. Fifteen patients (25%) have had only up to 1 to 2% as many attacks as preoperatively. Thus 48 patients (81%) experienced a complete or nearly complete reduction of seizure tendency after operation. The remaining 11 patients (19%) had lesser reductions of seizure tendency.

Arteriovenous and Other Major Vascular Malformations

Included in the 20 patients in this group (Fig. 6) are 14 with major arteriovenous malformations and 6 with cavernous angiomatous malformations with bleeding potentialities. Small discrete nodular lesions of possible vascular origin, such as those described by Penfield and Ward (1948) as hemangioma calcificans and discrete solid hemangiomata, are included in the previous group since these lesions did not pose the same technical surgical problems as the major vascular malformations of this group.

There was inadequate follow-up data in two patients. The remaining 18 patients have been followed for periods ranging from 1 to 37 years, with a median follow-up period of 11 years. Five patients (28%) have been seizure-free since discharge from the hospital and five others (28%) have become and remained seizure-free after having a few early attacks. Thus 10 patients (56%) have become and remained seizure-free. Another two patients (11%) have had a marked reduction in seizure tendency, giving a total of 12 patients (67%) with a complete

Arteriovenous Malformation

Results of Operation on Seizure Tendency
(patients operated upon from 1935 through 1971)

No attacks	5 pts. (28%)	10 pts. (56%)		
Became seizure free	5 pts. (28%)		12 pts. (67%)	18 pts. (16 living, 2 dead) with follow-up data of 2-30 yrs.
Marked reduction in seizure tendency	2 pts. (11%)			
Moderate or less reduction in seizure tendency	6 pts. (33%)			(median 11 yrs.)
Inadequate data	2 pts.			

Total 20 pts.

FIG. 6.

or nearly complete reduction of seizure tendency. The remaining six patients (33%) have had lesser reductions of seizure tendency.

SUMMARY

Epilepsy is one of the most common symptoms of brain tumor and in both children and adults may be the only symptom for considerable periods of time, during which the patient presents to the physician as a seizure problem. The nature of the seizures does not enable the physician to determine whether the seizures are due to neoplasm, a non-neoplastic space-occupying lesion, or an area of brain scarring or atrophy. Appropriate radiologic contrast studies and radioisotope brain scans usually, but not always, give proof of the presence of an expanding or space-occupying lesion. Positive evidence may appear only at a second or third investigation 1 or more years after an initial negative study.

A selected series of 347 such patients has been presented and the results on the seizure tendency of surgical removal of the tumoral lesion and surrounding epileptogenic cortex controlled with cortical electrographic and cortical stimulation techniques have been documented. The overall reduction of the seizure tendency in such patients, up to the time of recurrence of neoplastic growth, compares favorably with the results of similar surgical procedures in patients with focal epilepsy due to nontumoral lesions.

REFERENCES

Aguilar, M.-J., and Rasmussen, T. (1960): The role of encephalitis in epilepsy. *Arch. Neurol.*, 2: 663–676.

Arseni, C., and Petrovici, I. N. (1971): Epilepsy in temporal lobe tumors. *Europ. Neurol.*, 5:201–214.

Dowman, C. E., and Smith, W. A. (1928): Intracranial tumors: A review of one hundred verified cases. *Arch. Neurol. Psychiatry*, 20:1312–1329.

Furlow, L. T., and Sachs, E. (1936): The occurrence of convulsions in a series of over seven hundred verified intracranial tumors. *South. Surg.*, 5:179–191.

Hoefer, P., Schlesinger, E. B., and Pennes, H. H. (1947): Seizures in patients with brain tumors. *Res. Publ. Ass. Nerv. Ment. Dis.*, 26:50–58.

Kirstein, L. (1942): Epilepsi bei intrakraniellen expansiven Prozessen. *Acta Med. Scand.*, 110:56–68.

Leblanc, F., and Rasmussen, T. (1973): Cerebral seizures and brain tumors. In: *Handbook of Clinical Neurology*, Vol. 15, edited by P. J. Vinken and G. W. Bruyn. North Holland, Amsterdam.

Lund, M. (1952): Epilepsy in association with intracranial tumor. *Acta Psychiatr. Neurol. Scand.*, Suppl. 81, 149 pp.

Parker, H. (1930): Epileptiform convulsions, incidence of attacks in cases of intracranial tumors. *Arch. Neurol. Psychiatry*, 23:1032–1041.

Pederson, O. (1938): Über epileptische anfälle beim tumor cerebri. Zentralbl. Neurochir. 3:204–214.

Penfield, W., Erickson, T. C., and Tarlov, I. M. (1940): Relation of intracranial tumors and symptomatic epilepsy. *Arch. Neurol. Psychiatry*, 44:300–315.

Penfield, W., Jasper, H., and McNaughton, F. L. (1954): *Epilepsy and the Functional Anatomy of the Human Brain*. Little, Brown, Boston, pp. 785–817.

Penfield, W., and Kristiansen, K. (1951): *Epileptic Seizure Patterns*. Charles C Thomas, Springfield, Ill.

Penfield, W., and Ward, A. A. (1948): Calcifying epileptogenic lesions. *Arch. Neurol. Psychiatry*, 60:20–36.

Penman, J., and Smith, M. C. (1954): Intracranial gliomata: Some clinical, radiological and therapeutic aspects of 298 cases. *Spec. Rep. Ser. Med. Res. Coun. (Lond.)*, 284:1–70.

Pilcher, C., and Parker, E. F. (1938): A study of convulsions associated with verified focal intracranial lesions. *Zentral. Neurochir.,* 3:330–341.

Rasmussen, T., and McCann, W. (1968): Clinical studies of patients with focal epilepsy due to chronic encephalitis. *Trans. Am. Neurol. Assoc.,* 93:89–94.

Rasmussen, T., Olszewski, J., and Lloyd-Smith, D. (1958): Focal seizures due to chronic localized encephalitis. *Neurology,* 8:435–445.

Sargent, P. (1921): Some observations on epilepsy. *Brain,* 44:312–328.

Tükel, K., and Jasper, H. (1952): The electroencephalograms in parasagittal lesions. *EEG Clin. Neurophysiol.,* 4:481–494.

White, J. C., Liu, C. T., and Mixter, W. J. (1948): Focal epilepsy—A statistical study of its causes and the results of surgical treatment. I. Epilepsy secondary to intracranial tumors. *N. Engl. J. Med.,* 238:891–899.

Wyke, B. D. (1959): The cortical control of movement: A contribution to the surgical physiology of seizures. *Epilepsia* (Fourth Series), 1:4–35.

Advances in Neurology, Vol. 8, edited by D. P. Purpura, J. K. Penry, and R. D. Walter. Raven Press, New York © 1975.

12
Stereotactic and Other Procedures for Epilepsy

George A. Ojemann and Arthur A. Ward, Jr.

Stereotactic Procedures

The development of stereotactic surgery in man, that is, techniques for placing a discrete lesion in a particular brain site using radiologically detectable landmarks, has largely been concerned with the treatment of dyskinesias, in particular parkinsonism (Ojemann and Ward, 1973). Once these techniques were developed, however, they were applied to patients with medically intractable seizures. Although the first of these stereotactic procedures in patients with epilepsy was performed more than 20 years ago, there are not as yet generally accepted techniques and target areas for seizure disorders, and stereotactic procedures remain largely experimental efforts for the treatment of patients who cannot be managed medically or do not meet criteria for the usual cortical resection.

Stereotactic procedures for epilepsy fall into two major groups. One group includes procedures in which destruction of a particular subcortical target is thought to result in improvement in a given clinical class of epilepsy; for example, destruction of the centromedian nucleus might benefit patients with epilepsy manifest by grand mal seizures. The second group consists of efforts to identify a specific subcortical focus, or multiple cortical and subcortical foci in a particular patient, with therapeutic benefit to follow stereotactic (or open) destruction of these electrographically identified foci.

A wide variety of theoretical formulations have been developed to explain the choice of a particular therapeutic site for a particular type of epilepsy. A few of these will be mentioned under the appropriate target areas, but in general the evaluation of stereotactic surgery of epilepsy at the present state of knowledge seems best left as an empirical matter: a lesion in a particular location in a particular case of what clinical and electrographic type of epilepsy produces what result, followed how long.

This statement, however, highlights many of the problems in the evaluation of the literature on this subject. There is considerable variability in the location of particular subcortical nuclei about the reference points usually utilized in stereotactic surgery (Van Buren and Borke, 1972). Thus the exact structures destroyed in a given stereotactic lesion are not infrequently a matter of conjecture. Larger targets—such as the amygdala—present a similar problem in terms of how much of the nucleus is included in a lesion. This imprecision in the anatomic correlates of human stereotactic lesions may be of great importance in the analysis of results if it should turn out that in man—as in some experimental animal models of epilepsy—considerably different results may result from subcortical lesions only a few millimeters apart (Kusske, Ojemann, and Ward, 1972). The placement of lesions in multiple subcortical sites in a particular patient makes interpretation even more difficult. The problems of anatomic localization are additive, and yet there is no *a priori* reason to believe that the effects of either simultaneous or serial multiple lesions represent merely the sum of the effects of these lesions singly.

There has been a tendency to reserve stereotactic procedures for especially intractable and complicated seizure problems. Thus the exact clinical classification of the seizure disorder treated with a particular lesion is often difficult to ascertain. The natural history of a seizure disorder is not always known. The transient cessation of chronic seizures on admission to the hospital, or following exposure of the cortex when resection is not undertaken, is a well-known phenomenon. Even patients with intractable seizure disorders may have periods of remission in which they are free, if not of all types of seizures, then at least of one type, particularly grand mal. This must be considered in evaluating the results of stereotactic procedures. Long-term follow-up seems essential in these cases, but is not always reported. This problem becomes all the more crucial when there is a diminution but not cessation of seizures following a procedure, especially if the change is from a very high to only a relatively high rate. The criteria often used for evaluating resections of epileptic foci—cessation or near-cessation (less than one seizure per year) of seizures 6 months or more postoperatively—also seem appropriate to the evaluation of stereotactic procedures.

The risks of stereotactic procedures generally are relatively low compared with other brain operations as long as the procedure is carried out in normotensive patients. Because uncontrolled hypertension increases the risk of hemorrhage at the lesion site, we consider it a contraindication for such an operation. Risks of stereotactic surgery also include those associated with inaccurate lesion placement and with unwanted changes in function associated with properly placed lesions, such as the apparent overlap in dominant ventrolateral thalamus of areas where lesions are associated with transient aphasia and improvement in dyskinesias. The nature of these risks for the very large experience with stereotactic surgery in dyskinesias has been dealt with elsewhere (Ojemann and Ward, 1973). In the following discussion the only complications mentioned are those undesirable neurologic changes that have frequently followed apparently accurate placement of lesions in a particular target. Techniques of stereotaxis are not reviewed here (see Van Buren and Ratcheson, 1973).

The brevity and incomplete nature of many of the reports on stereotactic surgery in epilepsy add to the difficulties in evaluating this type of treatment. Within these limitations, reports of the effect of stereotactic operations on specific seizure types are reviewed by principal target for the stereotactic lesion.

Internal Capsule

Kalyanaraman and Ramamurthi (1970) placed lesions in the medial side of the posterior limb of the internal capsule which they believe destroy a premotor bundle related to the generalization of seizures. They have reported on seven adult patients with grand mal seizures. Three patients had unilateral capsulotomies. Two had their seizures abolished for follow-up periods of 2 years and 3 months, respectively (although one patient later underwent an amygdalotomy, the seizures were reportedly controlled by capsulotomy alone). The remaining patient improved considerably but continued to have seizures during a follow-up period of 4 years. Three other patients had simultaneous or spaced bilateral lesions with little improvement over 4 to 6 years, although one patient had "a considerable reduction in the frequency" of seizures. One patient died immediately postoperatively. Operations were done under general anesthesia. The anatomic target is 14 mm lateral to the midline on the line joining a point 1 mm above and 4 mm posterior to the anterior commissure, to a second point 5 mm above the midcommissural line. No motor responses were evoked with stimulation at this location although these were obtained in a position 4 mm more lateral. The right brain lesion is generally placed first. The second side is done during the same operation or at a later procedure if the first fails. The EEGs do not change following these lesions.

Jelsma, Bertrand, Martinez, and Molina-Negro (1973) reported on three cases with epilepsy partialis continua and right frontal electroencephalographic foci, in whom lesions were placed in the posterior limb of the ipsilateral internal capsule at the point of maximal motor response in the extremity affected by the seizures. In the first of these cases, an initial lesion abolished the seizures for 6 months, following which the seizures returned and a more posterior lesion was made. In the 8½ years following the second lesion this patient was free of epilepsy partialis continua but continued to have one to two focal and grand mal seizures monthly. The remaining two patients also were free of epilepsy partialis continua following lesions for 6 years and 17 months, respectively, although both continued to have focal seizures every 2 to 3 months. One case eventually came to cortical resection. These capsular lesions have been associated with permanent weakness only in the extremity where motor response had been evoked.

Mullan, Vailati, Karasick, and Mailis (1967) presented a series of cases with predominantly thalamic and subthalamic lesions, but several lesions also encroached on the internal capsule. In case 2, two lesions—one in the genu of the internal capsule, the other in inferior anterior thalamus—were followed by a very striking reduction in seizures for 3 years at the time of the report. Seizures originally were grand mal and absence attacks. Schaltenbrand, Spuler, Nadjimi, Hopf, and Wahren (1966) reported one case of combined capsular and globus pallidus lesions in a patient with partial motor seizures, following which the patient was seizure-free.

Pallidum

Spiegel and Wycis (Spiegel, Wycis, and Baird, 1958, 1962; Wycis, Baird, and Spiegel, 1966; Wycis, 1969) reported long-term follow-up on the effects of pallidal and combined pallidal-amygdala lesions in cases of generalized epilepsies, especially cases with clinical features of the "salaam" type: seizures with head nodding, extension of the arms, and flexion at the waist. Five cases of pallidotomy (four unilateral, one bilateral) and nine cases of pallidotomy combined with amygdalotomy (eight unilateral, one bilateral) were reported. Selection of pallidotomy or combined pallidotomy-amygdalotomy was based on the presence of spikes in depth recordings from these nuclei. Five of these 14 patients were not benefited by the operation, including one patient with only "salaam" seizures, one with partial seizures with secondary generalization, two with seizures of both grand mal and absence types, and one with partial seizures of the psychomotor type with secondary generalization. (This last patient was not helped with bilateral pallidotomy, a right amygdalotomy, and left fornicotomy.)

On the other hand, of the nine patients who had seizures of the salaam type, three have been seizure-free with follow-ups from 6 to 9½ years at last report. One other was seizure-free for 3 years after which the seizures returned. Three others have had a decrease in seizure frequency and in two there was no change. None was made worse. In 10 patients who had grand mal seizures, three have been seizure-free for follow-ups of 7 to 9½ years, seizures were diminished in five, and unchanged in two. Although the patients were seizure-free for such prolonged periods, the EEG generally remained abnormal. Absence seizures were present in two of these patients, and were diminished in one and not changed in the other. Grand mal seizures appeared postoperatively in one patient who had only salaam seizures preoperatively. It appears from the serial reports of these authors that the results in these types of seizures in general were better in the later follow-up periods than they were initially. The results of combined lesions of the pallidum and amygdala were more effective than those of the pallidum alone, especially for salaam seizures (Wycis et al., 1966). These results of operative treatment are also compared with the natural history of salaam seizures. About twice as many operated patients were seizure-free as would be expected from that natural history.

These reports present some of the more successful results of stereotactic lesions in seizure disorders with lengthy follow-up and seem to suggest a potentially useful role of pallidal lesions, perhaps combined with amygdala lesions in the generalized epilepsies, especially with features of the salaam type. Yet, despite these encouraging results, no later series of patients was reported by these authors.

Schaltenbrand et al. (1966), in reporting effects of a variety of lesions on several types of seizure disorders, included four patients with pallidal lesions. One patient with partial motor seizures had been seizure-free following a combined pallidal-internal capsule lesion. (This was the only seizure-free patient in the entire series.) One patient with psychomotor seizures was improved, with only minor seizures, following addition of a pallidal lesion to a previous fornix and anterior commissure lesion. In the two other patients—one with cerebral palsy and the other with posttraumatic epilepsy—pallidal lesions produced transient improvement. Orthner and Lohman (1966) also report on the effect of lesion of fornix and commissure, in addition to pallidum, in two patients with partial seizures. In one patient seizures decreased in a 3-year follow-up. In the other, with secondary generalization, no change in seizures occurred, and the patient showed memory impairment and micrographia.

Putamen

Dierssen (1966) briefly mentions placement of lesions of putamen in 11 patients with five seizure-free, three of these for more than 2 years. Hori, Terada, Kanazawa, and Miyamoto (1968) reported that 20% of 69 epileptics were seizure-free after bilateral putamen lesions, and another 44% improved. Best results occurred in "corticogenic" epilepsy.

Thalamus

Thalamic nuclei have been favorite targets for stereotactic intervention in seizure disorders, in part on theoretical grounds including the suspected relationship between thalamic nuclei and bilateral synchronous 3/sec spike-and-wave discharges. The efficacy of thalamic targets in dyskinesias has also made it an area with which stereotactic surgeons are well acquainted. Although the discussion of thalamic targets is subdivided by the particular nuclear area thought to be the center of the lesion, it should be recognized that many of these lesions extend into adjacent structures, particularly laterally and inferiorly, and it may be these extensions of the lesions which cannot be precisely delimited which are important to the therapeutic results.

Ventral Anterior Nucleus (VA)

Mullan et al. (1967) suggested that VA lesions should be particularly effective in the therapy of generalized epilepsy. In his patient group there were three cases in which lesions predominantly involved VA. Case 2 had generalized seizures of both the grand mal and falling varieties; two lesions were placed in this patient, one in inferior VA and a second laterally in the genu of the internal capsule. This patient was nearly seizure-free in the 3½-year follow-up. In case 3, two lesions were also placed, one in inferior VA, and a second posterio-laterally in the region of the lateralis posterior and a portion of the ventrolateral nucleus. This adult with seizures of the grand mal and salaam type had also been followed for 3½ years with a marked reduction in seizure frequency (he had one grand mal and four minor seizures of a sensory nature in that period). The third patient had partial seizures of a sensory nature with occasional secondary generalization. A right VA lesion in that patient was complicated by hemorrhage at the lesion site with hemiplegia, and only a slight reduction in seizure frequency in the 3-year follow-up period. Talairach (1952) placed bilateral VA lesions in five patients with mental illness, two of whom were also epileptics, apparently without benefit for the seizure disorder and without neurologic deficits. Sramka, Lojka, Nadvornik, and Ciganek (1972) recorded "epileptic spikes" in four patients from the anterior-lateral portion of "ventroanterior" thalamus—an area that lies at the boundary between caudate and thalamus. Coagulation in this area, the anterior thalamic reticulum, resulted in "significant improvement in the epileptic disease."

Pertuiset, Hirsch, Sachs, and Landau-Ferey (1969) placed lesions in VA and centromedian targets, identifying the VA target by the evoked recruiting response. Five of these 12 patients were significantly mentally retarded; in five of the 12 bilateral lesions were made. The patients' seizure disorders were of a grand mal nature. Two of the 12 patients were rendered seizure-free in 4- and 6-year follow-ups; two were considered failures. Bouchard and Umbach (1972) have added VA lesions to fornix and amygdala lesions in patients with primary generalized seizure disorders with bilaterally synchronous spike-and-wave complexes on EEG. In some cases bilateral lesions staged 4 to 6 months apart were placed. "No progression" in the seizure disorder was reported after short follow-up periods. The fornix and amygdala lesions alone were not of benefit in patients with this type of seizure disorder.

Following on the observations of Mullan et al. (1967), we studied the effects of VA lesions on the experimental model of partial epilepsy produced by injection of alumina cream into the monkey sensory motor cortex. A significant reduction in seizure frequency occurred in the month following placement of these VA lesions in animals continuously monitored for seizures, compared to the month before (Kusske et al., 1972). Based on this work, VA lesions were placed in three adult patients with medically intractable epilepsy. Results have not been encouraging. The first of these patients had generalized seizures, absence attacks associated with chewing movements, and occasional left facial twitching. The EEG demonstrated right temporal and generalized bilateral discharges. A lesion was placed in the lateral aspect of right VA extending into the genu of the internal capsule. This patient had two seizures in the immediate postoperative period, was then seizure-free for 7 weeks out of the hospital, after which his seizures returned at slightly less than their preoperative frequency for 6 months. Seizure frequency then increased to somewhat more than the preoperative level.

The second case had partial seizures of a psychomotor type with a right frontal-temporal electrographic focus. A lesion was placed in the medial half of VA at the very pole of the thalamus. Her seizure frequency was not altered in any way by this lesion. The third patient had partial seizures with a right superior frontal electrographic focus. A lesion was again placed in the medial side of VA. In the last two cases, recruiting responses were evoked by stimulation at the site of the lesion. In this third case only, interictal spikes associated with scalp EEG spikes could be recorded from the region of the VA nucleus. This patient, who had many seizures per day preoperatively, was free of seizures from the 4th to the 10th postoperative day, the seizures then recurring with a slightly increased frequency and intensity compared to the preoperative period. Extensive neuropsychologic testing of these three patients following their VA lesions showed only a minor decrease in motor agility of the left upper extremity following placement of these lesions, a finding which in the first two cases had cleared by the time of testing 6 months after the operation.

Ventral Lateral Nucleus (VL)

This thalamic nucleus, one of the preferred targets in dyskinesias, has also been utilized in some cases of intractable epilepsy. In the first case of Mullan et al. (1967), a strontium needle passed through this target as well as the internal capsule and centromedian nucleus. That case had a marked reduction in the partial seizures of temporal lobe origin over a 10-day period. Jelsma et al. (1973) reported a series of patients with partial seizures with secondary generalization, or primarily generalized seizures of both grand mal and absence variety. Simultaneous bilateral lesions centered on the inferior portion of VL diminished the secondarily generalized grand mal seizures in the three patients thus affected. Two of them had no grand mal seizures with follow-ups of 30 and 23 months. The focal seizures were also diminished in one patient. In two of these cases the cortical focus became evident in the postoperative EEGs when only the generalized component had been evident in the preoperative records. Only two of the seven cases with primarily generalized seizures appeared to benefit. One has had none and the other a very marked reduction in grand mal seizures, although both have had persisting absence attacks in follow-ups of 49 and 39 months (one patient had a unilateral, the other bilateral lesions). The effective lesions in these two cases appeared to be somewhat deeper and more medially placed than were the lesions in the other five patients of a similar seizure type who were followed for comparable periods without improvement. The effective lesions likely extend inferior-laterally from VL into adjacent structures.

Mullan et al. (1967) had two additional cases with unilateral VL lesions combined with other lesions. In his case 7 a VL lesion followed a subthalamic and centromedian lesion and was associated with no additional improvement in partial seizures of temporal lobe origin and secondary generalization. In case 8 the combination of VL and centromedian lesions was placed following a lesion in the field of Forel, again in a patient with partial seizures of temporal origin, in this case increasing the seizure frequency back to preoperative levels. Nesterov and Kulikov (1973) have made lesions in VL and centromedian nuclei in 55 patients with Kozhevnikov's epilepsy (partial continuous epilepsy with focus in the motor cortex). They report that 45 of these patients had "good or satisfactory" reduction in seizure frequency.

In general it would appear that VL lesions are somewhat less effective than the other thalamic lesions in altering seizure frequency. In many of the cases where lesions in the nucleus seem to have been of some benefit, they were either part of a combined lesion or had significant extension into the adjacent capsule or subthalamus.

Centromedian Nucleus (CM)

Centromedian lesions alone have been placed by Kalyanaraman and Ramamurthi (1970) in children with salaam seizures. In three patients, these seizures were abolished for follow-up periods of 4 months to 2½ years (one patient having serial bilateral, one only a unilateral, and one a unilateral CM lesion coupled with bilateral amygdalotomies); another patient had little improvement following simultaneous bilateral CM lesions. It was noted that the salaam seizures did not stop immediately postoperatively but did some time later. Other authors have combined CM lesions with ventral lateral thalamic lesions, either simultaneously or staged. The beneficial effects noted by Nesterov and Kulikov (1973) in Kozhevnikov's partial motor epilepsy have been mentioned. Similar are the cases of Mullan et al. (1967): in one an internal capsule lesion combined with CM lesion was of great benefit in a partial temporal lobe seizure disorder with a short followup; in the other two the combination of CM and ventral lateral thalamic lesions with previous subthalamic lesions did not seem to be of benefit in partial temporal lobe seizures. Combination of CM with ventral anterior thalamic lesions, effective in 2 of 12 patients with primary generalized seizure disorders, reported by Pertuiset et al. (1969) has also been mentioned. Koshino, Wakano, Miki, and Sakamoto (1973) reported that following CM and subthalamic lesions, "the epileptic fits showed signs of gradual improvement within several days," and the patients were then "well controlled on their continued medications 6 months to 3 years later." Seizure type was not specified.

Internal Medullary Lamina

Spiegel et al. (1962) reported a series of six patients with generalized seizures and absence attacks in whom lesions were centered in the internal medullary lamina. In three of the patients there was no change, in two the absence seizures were decreased for periods of 4 months and 1½ years, respectively, and in one the seizures stopped for a period of 3 months and then recurred at a very low frequency over a follow-up period of 11 years. Spiegel et al. (1962) also mentioned a report of Hassler and Riechert (1957) where in three cases of absence seizures only transient improvement followed coagulation in the internal medullary lamina. In case 4 of Mullan et al. (1967), the lesion extends into this area also, with a moderate reduction in partial psychomotor seizure frequency. Poblete, Palestini, Figueroa, Gallardo, Rojas, Covarrubias, and Doyharcabal (1970) placed lesions in the internal medullary lamina in the region of the mamillothalamic tract for aggressive psychopathy, sometimes associated with seizures. In "epileptic patients, seizures have become less frequent," including one case of apparently primary generalized seizures. Orthner and Lohman (1966) briefly mention four epileptics in whom unilateral medial thalamic lesions adjacent to the massa intermedia were placed without benefit.

The internal medullary lamina is an especially small target with considerable variability in its location, so it is quite likely that lesions directed at it extend into or are entirely in adjacent structures.

Fields of Forel

Jinnai (1966; and Nishimoto, 1963; and Mukawa, 1970) has presented a series of patients with various types of epilepsy treated by lesions in Forel's fields, immediately beneath the thalamus. Jinnai used a target 2 mm posterior to the midpoint of the intercommissural line, 4 mm inferior to the intercommissural line, and 8 mm lateral for these lesions in his patients. He placed the lesions bilaterally in the presence of bilateral clinical seizure patterns. He reports nine patients with "idiopathic" epilepsy with bilateral Forel lesions. Two of these patients had seizures of both the grand mal and absence types: neither had grand mal seizures postoperatively in follow-ups of 4½ years; in one there was a reduction and in the other no change in the absence attacks. Four patients had generalized epilepsy with grand mal and myoclonic seizure patterns. Two patients were seizure-free in follow-ups of 1 year and 3 years; the other two, although free of grand mal seizures, continued to have the myoclonic attacks with unchanged frequency. Three patients who had partial seizures of the psychomotor type with secondary generalization also had no further grand mal seizures following lesions in Forel's field: one was free of all seizures, and the other two continued to have psychomotor seizures with a reduced frequency. Jinnai relates improvement to the exactness of lesion placement within Forel's field.

The results of bilateral Forel lesions in nine patients with partial epilepsy are also reported. Secondary generalization was not present postoperatively in seven of the nine, with follow-up ranging from 2 to 5½ years. On the other hand, overall seizure frequency was reduced to zero in only one of the patients and by more than 50% in two others. Ten patients with unilateral Forel field lesions ipsilateral to the focus of their partial seizures were also reported, with follow-ups ranging from 6 months to 5 years. Only two of these 10 had secondary generalized seizures postoperatively. Six of the 10 were rendered seizure-free postoperatively with follow-ups ranging from 6 months to 1½ years. Again, lesions considered to be satisfactorily placed in the Forel field target appeared to be associated with relief of seizures. Jinnai concludes that Forel field lesions are indicated for grand mal and neocortical motor seizures but not for seizures arising in the limbic system or for myoclonic seizures.

Lesions in several of the cases of Mullan et al. (1967) center principally in Forel's field also. In their case 4, who had had a previous temporal lobectomy, the subcortical lesion extends from Forel's field anterio-superiorly toward the mammilothalamic tract and anterior nucleus. This patient with partial seizures of temporal lobe origin with secondary generalization had a significant reduction in seizure frequency as well as a change in the pattern to sensory seizures over a 3¼-year follow-up. Case 5 (with partial motor seizures and secondary generalization) also had a unilateral lesion centered in Forel's field and extending inferiorly, followed by a very substantial reduction in seizure frequency and, at last report (39 months postoperatively) was seizure-free. This represented one of the best results in Mullan's series. His case 6 had a lesion in a similar location although slightly more anteriorly, in front of the red nucleus extending anterior superiorly to the region of the mammilothalamic tract. This patient with unilateral partial seizures of a sensory motor type had only a moderate seizure reduction in a 3-year follow-up. Two other cases of Mullan's had Forel lesions as initial treatment. Both were cases of partial seizures with temporal lobe origin, one with secondary generalization. The Forel lesions in one case reduced seizure frequency for a 6-month period, with a subsequent increase to preoperative levels; the other had seizure frequency reduced to about 50% of preoperative level (this was not considered clinically adequate and the patient returned for further surgical treatment).

Chiorino, Donaso, Diaz, Aranda, Asenjo, and Garcia (1968) reported two patients with unilateral Forel field lesions with apparently generalized seizures with an EEG that showed "diffuse subcortical dysrhythmia." Grand mal seizures were reported to have been reduced postoperatively. One of these patients developed absence seizures postoperatively that had not been present preoperatively. Laitinen's (1967) subventral thalamotomies also seem to include principally part of Forel's fields. In seven patients with primary generalized seizures of grand mal and myoclonic type along with dyskinesias, these lesions decreased grand mal seizures in five (with 4- to 20-month follow-up) although myoclonia was little helped.

The fields of Forel seem to be a promising target in the treatment of seizures, particularly grand mal seizures, whether of the primary or secondary generalized type. Further clinical investigation with this target area in intractable epilepsy of these types would seem to be indicated.

Hypothalamus

Placement of posteromedial hypothalamic lesions to "calm down or correct . . . abnormal behavior" in 51 patients was reported by Sano, Mayanaji, Sekino, Ogashiwa, and Ishijima (1970). Twenty-two of these patients also had uncontrolled seizures, most grand mal seizures, a few absence or psychomotor attacks. Small lesions (3 to 4 mm) were placed bilaterally, staged 7 to 10 days apart, at the point in the posterio-medial hypothalamus where the most marked signs of sympathetic discharge could be evoked by stimulation. Average coordinates were 2 to 4 mm below the midpoint of the intercommissural line, and 2 mm lateral to the midline. At follow-up of 2 or more years, one of 16 patients with more than one seizure per month preoperatively had been seizure-free without medication since the operation. Six others had a decrease in seizure frequency to less than one per month, four of these on lower doses of anticonvulsant medication. Two patients died in status 5 and 7 years after operation. Patients were frequently more calm and placid after these lesions. EEGs were not changed. Stimulation at the lesion site on occasion evoked increased EEG spiking, especially in limbic structures.

Cingulum

Bilateral stereotactic cingulotomies were followed by a marked diminution or cessation of seizures in the three patients with generalized seizure disorders reported by Diemath, Heppner, Enge, and Lechner (1966).

Medial Temporal Lobe: Amygdala, Hippocampus, Fornix

Placement of stereotactic lesions in medial temporal lobe structures and/or in their major efferent pathways has developed in parallel with recognition of the importance of these structures in partial seizures of psychomotor type with temporal lobe foci. The effect of lesions in these structures on epilepsy has also been a "spin-off" of studies of the stereotactic amygdala lesions in aggressive behavior disorders, where some patients with pathologic aggressive behavior were also epileptic. The reports of Narabayashi, one of the early exponents of the placement of amygdala lesions in hyperkinetic behavioral disturbances, concern the latter group. Narabayashi and Mizutani (1970) recently reported the results of amygdala lesions in a series of epileptics. Three of those patients had partial seizures of psychomotor type. After unilateral amygdala lesions, both the seizures and epileptic discharges were largely absent for 6 months in two patients and a year in the other case, but they then recurred. On the other hand, in 25 patients (most of whom were children) with grand mal seizures, the seizures were abolished in nine (with six no longer on medication) and decreased in eight others. Narabayashi has not been able to determine appropriate indications for unilateral or bilateral amygdala lesions, although he suggests that the bilateral lesions are associated with better seizure control. He noted a distinct parallel between the degree of behavioral improvement and decrease in seizures. Epileptics in general showed more behavioral improvement after amygdala surgery than did the nonepileptic group. Narabayashi concludes that amygdalotomy has a role in preventing generalized seizures but the operation seems to be much less effective in partial psychomotor seizures. Schaltenbrand et al. (1966) also found only transient improvement in six patients with partial seizure disorders of either motor or psychomotor types following unilateral amygdala lesions.

On the other hand, Talairach and Szikla (1965) noted a cessation of seizures in nine patients (followed 7 to 14 months) and a diminished frequency in two others in a series of 14 patients with partial seizures with uni- or bitemporal foci, treated with amygdala and hippocampal lesions produced by stereotactically implanted yttrium 90 pellets. Beneficial effect on partial psychomotor seizures was also noted in the series of patients of Heimberger, Whitlock, and Kalsbeck (1966). Hostile, aggressive behavior abnormalities were the primary indication for amygdalotomy, but a number of these patients also had uncontrolled seizure disorders. After amygdalotomy, four of the 20 epileptic patients of various types were seizure-free and 12 improved. Partial psychomotor seizures were most often benefited and in at least one case ceased entirely. One case is reported with earlier left frontal and temporal lobectomies where subsequent right amygdalotomy diminished seizure frequency without behavioral, memory, or other neuropsychologic deficits. Similarly, the eight patients in this series with bilateral amygdala lesions showed no evidence of a Kluver-Bucy syndrome. As in most other reports, improvement did not correlate with changes in the scalp EEG.

Chitanondh and Laksanavicharn (1969) reported the use of amygdalotomy in 31 patients with partial psychomotor seizures. Twenty-five of these lesions were unilateral, six bilateral. Three of these patients were seizure-free with a 2-year or longer follow-up. Seven had a marked and eight a moderate decrease in their seizure frequency. As in the reports of Narabayashi and Mitzutani (1970) and Heimburger et al. (1966), few side effects were noted from placing the amygdala lesions, even staged bilateral lesions. Chitanondh (1966) separately reported three cases of partial seizures with olfactory aura and secondary generalization; each case was treated with a unilateral amygdalotomy on the side of maximal spiking as recorded in the scalp EEG and confirmed by spiking in the amygdala. These patients were reported to be transiently seizure-free, for 8 months in two cases. Chitanondh noted that the scalp EEG abnormalities disappeared following amygdalotomy.

Schwab, Sweet, Mark, Kjellberg, and Ervin (1965) reported the placement of amygdala lesions in 10 patients, nine with partial seizures of the psychomotor type, and one apparently a primary generalized seizure disorder. Three patients were seizure-free, with follow-ups ranging from 3 years in two to 3 months in the other; seizures were reduced in four and unchanged in three, including the patient with the generalized seizure disorder. These lesions were placed unilaterally in the posterior amygdala, behind the area of maximal spiking, the amygdala being approached from a parieto-occipital burr hole. Visual field defects were present in two of the 10 patients, a complication not otherwise reported from amygdala surgery. Vaernet (1972) performed amygdalotomies on 52 patients with partial psychomotor seizures, temporal lobe foci on scalp EEGs and spikes recorded from the amygdala. Forty-five of these patients have been followed over 1 year. In the 27 patients with unilateral foci on scalp EEG, five were seizure-free and 10 more had seizure frequency diminished at least 50% ("improved"). Ten patients with bilateral foci on scalp EEG had unilateral amygdala lesions placed: one of these was seizure-free and five improved. Eight patients with bilateral scalp EEG foci had bilateral amygdalotomies: two of these were seizure-free and two improved. No neuropsychologic deficits were noted in these patients.

Nashold, Flanigin, Wilson, and Steward (1973) reported on the effect of medial temporal stereotactic lesions in five patients with psychomotor seizures and bitemporal electrographic abnormalities. Lesions were placed unilaterally, in the amygdala only in two patients, and in the amygdala and hippocampus in the other three. The site of the lesions was determined from the location of maximal interictal spiking, spontaneous seizure activity, and the sites from which typical seizures could be evoked with stimulation, during a 4-week period of the study of chronic implanted electrodes in both amygdala, hippocampi, and sometimes globus pallidus and medial thalamus. After placement of the lesions, three patients had a decrease in the frequency and intensity of their seizures while on medication but were not seizure-free. One had a decrease in the intensity but not the frequency of the seizures, and one patient was felt to have had too short a follow-up for evaluation. One patient had a significant memory defect following a lesion in both amygdala and hippocampus in the dominant hemisphere.

Diemath (discussion in Vaernet, 1972) reported two patients with generalized grand mal seizures and generalized EEG abnormalities with amygdala lesions on one side and a staged dorsal medial thalamic lesion on the opposite side. After the second operation, these patients had been seizure-free, off drugs, for periods of 5 and 7 years, respectively. They were from a series of patients whose primary indication for operation was an aggressive behavioral disorder.

Adams and Rutkin (1969) reported on the effects of medial temporal stereotactic lesions in 25 epileptics—six with only partial seizures of the psychomotor type, 13 with primary generalized seizures initially who later developed a psychomotor seizure pattern, and six with both psychomotor and generalized seizures. Adams placed chronic depth electrodes in posterior and anterior hippocampus, dorsal medial nucleus of the thalamus, amygdala, and anterior commissure bilaterally, and placed his lesion at the site of an onset of spontaneous seizure discharge or where stimulation evokes a typical seizure. In 16 patients such a location could be identified and lesioned: in seven patients these lesions were exclusively in the amygdala; in four, in the amygdala and anterior commissure; in one, in the amygdala, anterior commissure, and globus pallidus; in one, in the amygdala, anterior commissure, and anterior hippocampus; in one, in the hippocampus and anterior commissure; and in two, in the hippocampus alone. Of this group of patients only one was seizure-free during a follow-up of 18 months; one had no further psychomotor seizures but continued to have other types of seizures; nine had a diminished severity of seizures; five had no change; and none became worse. Of those with a diminished severity, two patients were seizure-free for 23 and 10 months, respectively, before their seizures recurred. In discussion of this paper, Wycis mentions two cases of psychomotor seizures treated with amygdala lesions without benefit.

Ramamurthi (1970), in nine patients with psychomotor seizures and unilateral foci on scalp EEGs, placed depth electrodes in medial temporal structures and destroyed the area of maximal interictal discharge—in most cases apparently the amygdala and immediate adjacent structures. Five of these patients have been seizure-free without medication and two seizure-free on medication with follow-ups of from 6 months to 5 years.

A somewhat different approach has been that of Hassler and Riechert (1957) and of Umbach (1966). They placed lesions in the fornix at the posterior margin of the anterior commissure. Umbach reported 20 cases of partial seizures of the psychomotor type in which the lesions were placed unilaterally in the fornix at this level: in this group, five patients also had amygdala lesions, three also had lesions in the lamella medialis, and two also had hippocampal lesions. He reported on another group of five additional patients who had bilateral fornix lesions staged 6 to 8 months apart. In this group, one had an additional pallidal lesion and two also had amygdala and lamella medialis lesions. No neurologic disturbances of the Kluver-Bucy type or memory disturbances have been noted following the staged bilateral lesions. Placement of additional lesions outside of fornix was determined on the basis of depth electrode studies and the ability to evoke typical seizures from stimulation, particularly at low (4 to 8 Hz) frequencies. Umbach reports follow-up of 3 to 11 years for 18 cases, five of whom have been free of all attacks. In the 13 who had had grand mal seizures, 11 have been free of this type of seizure. He mentions one case in which a focus in the opposite temporal pole became apparent 3 years after fornicotomy, requiring subsequent temporal lobectomy without major neurologic (specifically, memory) deficits. A later report from this group (Bouchard and Umbach, 1972) includes 50 cases of epilepsy treated with fornix and anterior commissure lesions, more recently with a later ipsilateral basal-lateral amygdalotomy. Grand mal seizures have been diminished by 65%; smaller seizures by 62%. Associated psychic disturbances improved in 50%.

Schaltenbrand et al. (1966) reported effects of fornicotomies, mostly combined with anterior commissure lesions, in five patients with partial epilepsy of psychomotor or motor types. Three patients were improved, including two patients with partial motor seizures, and one other was transiently improved. The one patient with psychomotor seizures who was improved had both fornicotomy and pallidal lesions. Anterior commissurotomy alone seemed to be ineffective in one case. In this series, fornix lesions seem more effective than amygdala lesions.

Orthner and Lohman (1966) placed unilateral fornix lesions in two patients with partial seizures with temporal lobe signs, with a decrease in seizure frequency on a 9-year follow-up. Combined anterior commissure and fornix lesions in two other patients with similar seizures diminished but did not abolish their seizures. These lesions were combined with pallidal lesions in two others, with benefit in one and major neuropsychologic deficit in the other.

The decrease in seizure frequency following medial temporal stereotactic lesions generally is not as dramatic as that following standard temporal lobectomy in properly selected cases. On the other hand, the risks and complication of medial temporal stereotactic lesions in most reports are few. Thus these procedures deserve further evaluation for certain categories of patients.

(1) Patients with temporal lobe seizure disorders in whom there is ambiguity as to which temporal lobe is the site of the seizure discharges, and in whom this question is to be resolved by depth electrode studies. If a single temporal lobe can then be identified as the source of the seizure discharges, placement of the stereotactic lesion in the amygdala or one of the other medial temporal structures by way of the already implanted electrode would seem to then be a low-risk

procedure which, if therapeutically beneficial, avoids open craniotomy without precluding open temporal lobectomy at a later date if the stereotactic lesion fails to control seizures successfully.

(2) Patients who appear to have bilateral medial temporal discharges and who are generally not considered to be candidates for temporal lobectomy. In these cases, bilateral medial temporal lesions may well be therapeutically useful. If the lesions are confined to amygdala or fornix and staged, and perhaps even if not staged, the major neuropsychologic memory deficits associated with bilateral open medial temporal resections do not seem to occur (Heimburger et al., 1966; Umbach, 1966; Narabayashi, 1972; Vaernet, 1972). Bilateral hippocampal and hippocampal gyrus stereotactic lesions may not be quite so safe in terms of avoiding this complication (Narabayashi, 1972).

(3) Patients who have already undergone unilateral temporal lobe resection and who have recurrence of seizures with evidence for a contralateral temporal focus. In these cases, the stereotactic medial temporal lesions may well provide further seizure control with minimal risk of neuropsychologic disability—again with the suggestion that hippocampus-hippocampal gyrus lesions should be avoided. Indeed, it has been suggested (Umbach, 1966) that even in cases of psychomotor seizures which meet the usual criteria for a temporal lobectomy (i.e., a unilateral temporal lobe focus on scalp EEG), a stereotactic procedure should be undertaken initially because of its lower risk, with the temporal lobectomy reserved for those not achieving adequate seizure control by stereotaxy.

Summary of Effects of Subcortical Lesions on Various Forms of Epilepsy

Table 1 summarizes the reported results from stereotactic lesions at different subcortical sites on various types of seizure disorders. Success is indicated in terms of the criteria presented at the beginning of this chapter—i.e., on medication the patient reports either no seizures or less than one seizure per year with a minimum follow-up of 6 months. Lesser degrees of success are also indicated: abolition of a particular type of seizure (although more minor seizures may persist) and sometimes quite dramatic decreases in frequency of seizures (although not their cessation.)

Obviously the total experience with stereotactic lesions in seizure disorders has not been reported in the literature; this is particularly true of patients who fail to show any benefit from particular subcortical lesions. Thus the data in Table 1 are highly biased toward only favorable results, a fact which must be considered in evaluating the percentages of reported series achieving complete seizure control.

Stereoencephalography

A somewhat different approach to the stereotactic treatment of epilepsy is subsumed under the term "stereoencephalography." Here the effort is not to

TABLE 1. *Effect of stereotactic lesions in different subcortical sites on various types of seizure disorders*

Seizure type	Internal capsule (IC)	Globus pallidus (GP)	Putamen	Ventral anterior nucleus (VA)	Ventral lateral nucleus (VL)	Centro-median nucleus (CM)	Internal medullary lamina	Field of Forel (F)	Hypo-thalamus	Cingu-lum	Amygdala (Am)	Fornix (Fx)
					Thalamus							
Primary generalized												
grand mal	+33; +VA	+ +Am } 30		+1C, 33; +CM, 17	⊕14	+VA, 17	*	⊕100	+5	+	+37; +DM; +GP	+20; ⊕62
absence	+VA	*		+IC, 33	0		*	*				
salaam myoclonic		+ +Am } 33		⊕VL		+, 75		+0, 50			+GP	
Partial												
psychomotor with secondary generalization		*; Am-Fx		0	0CM + F; 0CM	0VL + F; 0VL	*	+33			+0, 88; +Hip, 85	
motor	+GP	+IC			+CM			+; ⊕60			0	⊕67
epilepsy partialis continua	⊕											
with secondary generalization					⊕, 66			⊕, 78–80				
other or unspecified		*Fx	+20	0			0					
Unspecified			+45	*		*F	0	*CM				

DM = Dorsomedial thalamic nucleus; Hip = hippocampus.
Symbols: +, A lesion in that site in patients with that type of seizure disorder has on at least one occasion been followed by either a complete cessation of seizures, or a reduction in seizure frequency to less than one seizure per year with at least 6 months follow-up. ⊕, That particular seizure type was controlled completely for 6 months or more by this type of lesion, but more minor seizures persisted. *, Improvement in a particular seizure type has been reported with lesions at that particular location but not to the criteria level outlined above. 0, No significant improvement followed lesions in this particular location. Numbers following the symbols indicate the percentages of patients in various series who achieve the criteria indicated by the symbols. Letters following the symbols identify multiple lesions, for example +VA under internal capsule represents the combination of an internal capsule and ventral anterior thalamic lesion. Although this table summarizes the data presented in this chapter, it is heavily biased toward successful results as cases which do not improve particular seizure patterns are frequently unreported.

relate destruction of a particular target site to improvement in a given class of epilepsy, but rather to identify the sites of origin and spread of seizure discharges in a particular patient. Then these apparent foci of origin or pathways of spread of the seizure discharges are ablated, either simultaneously or serially. The technique requires recording the seizure discharges simultaneously from many cortical and subcortical points in the brain. This is accomplished through the implantation of a number of multicontact electrodes using stereotactic techniques to place them in specific selected subcortical targets. The indications, interpretation, and hazards of these depth electrographic studies are discussed by Gloor in Chapter 5.

The name for this technique originated with and has been extensively popularized by Bancaud and Talairach (Talairach, Bancaud, Bonis, Szikla, and Tournoux, 1962; Bancaud and Talairach, 1965; Bancaud, Talairch, Geier, and Scaralin, 1973). They use both acute depth electrographic studies with many electrodes (as many as 300 contacts), conducted over 10 hr or so in the operating room, and preceding or later chronic implantation of a smaller number of electrodes followed over days. Simultaneous recording of spontaneous seizure activity for many sites, looking for earliest discharges, and the effects of electrical stimulation are the most useful signs for identifying a focus and preferred pathways of spread; interictal discharges are of little value. Choice of areas to be sampled in depth studies is "determined individually for each patient corresponding to the clinical, radiological and scalp electrocephalographic findings" (Talairach et al., 1962). In their report of results from surgical therapy based on these studies—either open resection of the focus or subcortical coagulation of focus or preferred pathways of spread with yttrium 90 beads—79% of the first 34 cases of all types of epilepsy, followed 1 to 3 years after operation, were either seizure-free or improved (Talairach et al., 1962). Use of chronic recording to determine location of lesions in patients with suspected temporal lobe foci has been described above (Adams and Rutkin, 1969; Nashold et al., 1973).

The use of subcortical EEG records from stereotactically placed electrodes, and the combination of discrete open resections and stereotactic lesions in patients with multifocal epilepsy, has been useful in a number of Russian clinics. Romodanov (1972) reports selecting a stereotactic procedure in the presence of generalized seizures without focal EEG signs, using the recording from subcortical areas to try to identify and destroy a focus or foci. He emphasizes the importance of obtaining new data if the first procedure proves ineffective, in an effort to identify a second focus which may only then be evident. Thus he has patients in whom multiple cortical foci were identified and resected, in whom multiple subcortial foci were destroyed stereotactically, and in whom combined cortical resection and stereotactic destruction were necessary to produce satisfactory seizure control. Similarly, Zemskaya (1972) used serial operative procedures in children with multiple foci, involving both cortical and subcortical sites. She recommends initial stereotactic procedure (thalamectomy) with subsequent cortical excision in these patients.

The selection of appropriate targets for sampling with depth electrodes and the temporal stability of patterns of seizure spread described in the finite sampling time available with even chronic recording are continuing problems with the stereoencephalographic techniques. Electrodes implanted in the brain obviously produce at least a small amount of local injury; this is probably greater with a chronic than an acute electrode. The degree of injury is usually not clinically significant with a single electrode but increases with larger numbers of brain penetrations. Whether these areas of injury may later serve as epileptic foci is unknown. The effectiveness of procedures which interrupt preferred pathways of spread, rather than destroying the focus, remains to be demonstrated. Continuing experimental investigation of this technique is most welcome (see Bancaud et al., 1973).

OTHER PROCEDURES FOR THE TREATMENT OF EPILEPSY

Stimulation

Possibilities for controlling seizures by electrical stimulation of different parts of the brain have recently provoked much interest. Based on animal studies relating cerebellar function and seizure control, described in Chapter 2, stimulation of cerebellum has been of most intense interest. Cooper (1973a, b; Cooper, Crighel, and Amin, 1973) has placed electrodes unilaterally on the cerebellar surface, contralateral to electrographic epileptic focus. In his first cases, an electrode was placed over the surface of the anterior cerebellum transtentorially. More recently, an additional electrode has been inserted posteriorly over the cerebellar hemisphere surface. Electrodes are platinum discs in multiples of four, on Dacron mesh, activated by transcutaneous inductive coupling similar to that used in implanted dorsal column stimulators. The initial seven cases reported by Cooper included patients with primary generalized grand mal and absence seizures, psychomotor seizures with secondary generalization, and partial motor seizures, recurrent after cortical resections. Five of these patients were improved by cerebellar stimulation at 8 to 13 month follow-up. Off medication, seizures were virtually absent in one patient with psychomotor seizures and secondary generalization. In patients with primary generalized seizures, grand mal attacks were absent and absence attacks reduced or absent when stimulation was functioning. In one case malfunction of the electrode was associated with a recurrence of seizures, control being reestablished after electrode repair. Initially, stimulation was applied when the patient noted an aura, aborting the expected subsequent spell. More recently, stimulation of 10-Hz, 1-msec pulse trains, 10 min on, 10 off, or alternating between anterior and posterior cerebellar electrodes every 10 min, 24 hr a day, has been found effective in reducing seizure frequency.[1] Stimula-

---

[1] The current levels of these effective stimulations are unknown due to use of transcutaneous inductive coupling. A dull headache has frequently accompanied stimulation, suggesting current spread to dura.

tion of anterior cerebellum at 200 Hz evoked a seizure in one patient. Scalp EEG recordings did not change even when seizures were controlled.

With the advent of implanted stimulators of considerable reliability, the possibilities of controlling seizures with electrical stimulation are certainly worth further evaluation. This experience with surface cerebellar stimulation seems encouraging, although more information from experimental animal models and from carefully controlled clinical trials is needed before the value of this technique will be known. Evaluation of stimulation at other brain sites in the control of seizures is also in order: cerebellar roof nuclei and caudate nucleus seem particularly promising. Stimulation of the caudate nucleus and adjacent white matter of anterior limb of the internal capsule in man produces an arrest of motor behavior (Van Buren, Li, and Ojemann, 1966), which, if triggered from an aura, might also inhibit the clinical seizure.

Cerebral Commissurotomy

The rationale behind using cerebral commissurotomy for medically intractable seizure problems is to diminish spread of the seizure discharge, and thus seizure intensity, by dividing the major commissural pathways between the cerebral hemispheres. Early experience with this procedure was that of Van Wagenen and Herren (1940) who sectioned portions of the corpus callosum through open craniotomy in some 27 cases. In most cases these were incomplete sections, and in only one was the entire corpus callosum and anterior commissure sectioned. Following these operations, 12 patients apparently had seizures restricted to only one side and did not lose consciousness in contrast to their preoperative seizures which were bilateral with loss of consciousness. The frequency of seizures was not reduced. Nor were absence attacks altered (Hursh, 1945). Some of the remaining patients continued to have status epilepticus (i.e., case 22, Akelaitis, 1942).

More recently Bogen, Sperry, and Vogel (1969) reported a series of 10 patients in whom the corpus callosum, anterior commissure, and probably hippocampal commissure were divided at a single open craniotomy; in three cases the massa intermedia was also divided. In a follow-up period of 2 or more years, they report that grand mal seizures have been absent in nine (longest follow-up free of grand mal seizures has been 7 years.) Most continued to have some focal seizures on medication, although these seizures were "improved." These patients have also been the subject of extensive neuropsychologic investigations (Gazzaniga, 1970). Although a group of very interesting neuropsychologic changes have been recorded, few of these have been of significance in the daily functioning of the patients.

Luessenhop, dela Cruz, and Fenichel (1970) reported the effects of open section of the corpus callosum, anterior commissure, and fornix at the level of foramen of Monro in children. Three of their patients had partial seizures, two with secondary generalization. Marked reduction in seizure frequency was noted in these patients in follow-ups of 1½ to 3 years. An infant with primarily generalized seizures showed no change following callosal section. A later communication from a relative of one of the patients considered to be a good result in this series illustrates some of the difficulties in the long-term evaluation of patients with complex seizure disorders (Byrne, 1970).

Stereotactic destruction of portions of the corpus callosum in conjunction with lesions of the fornix has been reported by Schaltenbrand et al. (1966) in three patients, with a diminished number of seizures in two cases (one had partial motor seizures) and a transient diminution of the third. Cerebral commissurotomy may prevent secondary generalization of partial seizure disorders with foci in one hemisphere. As with many of the procedures covered in this chapter, more detailed reports of long-term follow-ups of the patients would be of great value in determining the usefulness of this procedure.

Cooling

A number of studies suggest that reducing the temperature of the brain, either focally or with general body hypothermia, is associated with the cessation of ongoing seizure activity, and in some cases the seizures do not return with rewarming. Evidence for this effect in experimental animal models of epilepsy has been presented in Chapter 2.

Seizures reportedly ceased following ventricular irrigation with 5 to 10°C solutions in three children with generalized seizures and psychopathy (Tokuoka, Aoki, Higashi, and Tatebayashi, 1961). Primary generalized grand mal seizures in one patient ceased following subdural and ventricular profusion of 10 to 15°C for an hour; the seizures were absent with medication for a year, then returned off medication, but were absent following reinstallation of medication (Negrin, 1963). Cooling of one side of the brain lasting 45 min, and dropping brain temperature 1½ cm below the pial surface to 28 to 30°C, stopped seizures in seven patients in status from myoclonic and partial motor epilepsies, and was followed by a seizure-free interval for periods of at least weeks (Ommaya and Baldwin, 1963).

Ommaya and Baldwin (1963) felt that the ability of anticonvulsants to cross the blood-brain barrier was enhanced by hypothermia, and they proposed the combination of cooling and intravenous administration of large doses of anticonvulsants as a possible treatment for intractable seizure disorders. Sourek (1972; Sourek and Travnicek, 1970) has reported further on this technique, combining general body hypothermia with local extravascular brain cooling by irrigation of iced solutions through burr holes and catheters in the lateral ventricles and basal cisterns and i.v. injection of either 500 mg of thiopental or 20 to 30 mg of diazepam during the period of maximum hypothermia. Brain temperature was gradually lowered over 20 to 30 min to 18 to 27°C, in most cases below 24°C, for a 20- to 40-min period and then gradually rewarmed. Four of the initial 15 patients treated in this way and followed over 3 years were free of seizures off medication. All four had primary grand mal seizures and had been cooled to temperatures of 19 to 26°C. The type of drug injected at these hypothermic levels did not seem to have a bearing on the ultimate outcome. Five other patients (three with primary grand mal seizures and two with mixed seizure patterns) had no more than a single minor seizure in the 3-year or longer follow-up period, after cooling to 21 to 24°C with injection of various drugs. Two patients had a 50% reduction in seizures, and in four there was no change. In a total of 60 patients treated with this technique, transient neurologic deficit was noted in six and there was a single death from intracerebral hematomas early in the series. Cessation of intractable status epilepticus with total body hypothermia to 32 to 36°C was reported by Vastola, Homan, and Rosen (1969).

Surprisingly little functional change has been noted in patients following cooling, or even during cooling carried out under local anesthesia, including the failure to arrest speech when both the frontal and temporoparietal speech areas were locally cooled to 30°C, a depth of 1½ cm below the surface (Ommaya and Baldwin, 1963). Thus focal and general brain cooling may be useful in treatment of intractable partial epilepsies, and deserves more extensive clinical trials.

ACKNOWLEDGMENTS

The authors' research reported in this chapter is supported in part by U.S. Public Health Service grant NS 04053, from the National Institute of Neurological Diseases and Stroke. A portion of that research was conducted through the Clinical Research Center facility of the University of Washington, supported by NIH (RR-37).

REFERENCES

Adams, J., and Rutkin, B. (1969): Treatment of temporal lobe epilepsy by stereotactic surgery. *Confin. Neurol.*, 31:80-85.

Akelaitis, A. (1942): Studies on the corpus callosum. VI. Orientation (temporal-spatial gnosis) following section of the corpus callosum. *Arch. Neurol. Psych.*, 48:914–937.

Bancaud, J., and Talairach, J. (1965): *La Stereoencephalographic dans l'Epilepsia.* Masson et Cie, Paris.

Bancaud, J., Talairach, J., Geier, S., and Scaralin, J.-M. (1973): *Electroencephalographie et stereoelectroencephalographie dans les tumeurs cérébrales et l'epilepsie.* Edifor, Paris.

Bogen J., Sperry, R., and Vogel, P. (1969): Addendum: Commissural section and propagation of seizures. In: *Basic Mechanisms of the Epilepsies,* edited by H. Jasper, A. Ward, and A. Pope., Little, Brown, Boston.

Bouchard, G., and Umbach, W. (1972): Indications for the open and stereotactic brain surgery in epilepsy. In: *Present Limits of Neurosurgery,* edited by I. Fusek and Z. Kunc. Excerpta Medica, Amsterdam.

Byrne, T. (1970): Surgical disconnection of hemispheres for seizures [a letter]. *J. Am. Med. Assoc.,* 214:2339.

Chiorino, R., Donaso, P., Diaz, G., Aranda, L., Asenjo. A., and Garcia, C. (1968): Stereotaxic surgery in the treatment of epilepsy. Description of a new technique—Campotomy. *Neurocirugia,* 26: 143–147.

Chitanondh, H. (1966): Stereotaxic amygdalotomy in the treatment of olfactory seizures and psychiatric disorders with olfactory hallucination. *Confin. Neurol.,* 27:181–196.

Chitanondh, H., and Laksanavicharn, U. (1969): Stereotaxic amygdalotomy in the treatment of temporal automatism. *Excerpta Medica Int. Congress Series,* 193:9.

Cooper, I. S. (1973a): Effect of chronic stimulation of anterior cerebellum on neurologic disease. *Lancet,* 1:1321.

Cooper, I. S. (1973b): Chronic stimulation of cerebellar cortex in epilepsy and generalized myoclonus in man. Presentation to American Epilepsy Society Annual Meeting, New York, Dec. 6, 1973.

Cooper, I. S., Crighel, E., and Amin, I. (1973): Clinical and physiological effects of stimulation of the paleocerebellum in humans. *J. Am. Geriatrics Soc.,* 21:40–43.

Diemath, H. (1972): Discussion, in K. Vaernet, Stereotaxic amygdalotomy in temporal lobe epilepsy. *Confin. Neurol.,* 34:182.

Diemath, H., Heppner, F., Enge, S., and Lechner, H. (1966): Die stereotaktische vordere Cingulotomie bei therapieresistenter generalisierter Epilepsie. *Confin. Neurol.,* 27:144.

Dierssen, G. (1966): Discussion in H. Wycis, H. Baird, and E. Spiegel, Long range results following pallidotomy and pallidoamygdalotomy in certain types of convulsive disorders. *Confin. Neurol.,* 27:114–120.

Gazzaniga, M. (1970): *The Bisected Brain.* Appleton-Century-Crofts, New York.

Hassler, R., and Riechert, T. (1957): Uber einen Fall von doppelseitiger Fornicotomie bei sogenannter temporaler Epilepsie. *Acta Neurochir.,* 5:330–340.

Heimburger, R., Whitlock, C., and Kalsbeck, J. (1966): Stereotaxic amygdalotomy for epilepsy with aggressive behavior. *J. Am. Med. Assoc.,* 198: 165–169.

Hori, Y., Terada, C., Kanazawa, K., and Miyamoto, S. (1968): The effect of stereotaxic putamectomy for epileptic seizures. *Neurol. Med. Chir. (Tokyo),* 10:321–323.

Hursh, J. (1945): Origin of the spike and wave pattern of petit mal epilepsy. *Arch. Neurol. Psych.,* 53:274–282.

Jelsma, R., Bertrand, C., Martinez, S., Molina-Negro, P. (1973): Stereotaxic treatment of frontal-lobe and centrencephalic epilepsy. *J. Neurosurg.,* 39:42–51.

Jinnai, D. (1966): Clinical results and significance of Forel-H-tomy in the treatment of epilepsy. *Confin. Neurol.,* 27:129–136.

Jinnai, D., and Mukawa, J. (1970): Forel-H-tomy for the treatment of epilepsy. *Confin. Neurol.,* 32:307–315.

Jinnai, D., and Nishimoto, A. (1963): Stereotaxic destruction of Forel-H for treatment of epilepsy. *Neurochirurgia,* 6:164–176.

Kalyanaraman, S., and Ramamurthi, B. (1970): Stereotaxic surgery for generalized epilepsy. *Neurol. India,* 18 (Suppl. 1): 34–41.

Koshino, K., Wakano, M., Miki, M., and Sakamoto, Y. (1973): Stereotaxic operation for uncontrolled epilepsy and associated behavioral disorder. *Excerpta Medica Int. Congress Series,* 293:171.

Kusske, J., Ojemann, G., and Ward, A. (1972): Effects of lesions in ventral anterior thalamus on experimental focal epilepsy. *Exp. Neurol.,* 34:279–290.

Laitinen, L. V. (1967): Thalamotomy in progressive myoclonus epilepsy. *Acta Neurol. Scand.,* 43 (Suppl. 31):170–171.

Luessenhop, A., de la Cruz, T., and Fenichel, G. (1970): Surgical disconnection of the cerebral hemispheres for intractible seizures. *J. Am. Med. Assoc.,* 213:1630–1636.

Mullan, S., Vailati, G., Karasick, J., and Mailis, M. (1967): Thalamic lesions for the control of epilepsy. *Arch. Neurol.,* 16:277–285.

Narabayashi, H. (1972): Discussion of K. Vaernet, Stereotaxic amygdalotomy in temporal lobe epilepsy. *Confin. Neurol.,* 34:182.

Narabayashi, H., and Mizutani, T. (1970): Epileptic seizures and the stereotaxic amygdalotomy. *Confin. Neurol.,* 32:289–297.

Nashold, B., Flanigin, H., Wilson, W., and Steward, B. (1973): Stereotactic evaluation of bitemporal epilepsy with electrodes and lesions. *Confin. Neurol.,* 35:94–100.

Negrin, J. (1963): discussion in A. Ommaya and M. Baldwin, Extravascular local cooling of the brain in man. *J. Neurosurg.,* 20:19–20.

Nesterov, L., and Kulikov, A. (1973): Stereotactic operations on the subcortical structures of the brain in the treatment of Kozhevnikov's epilepsy. *Excerpta Medica Int. Congress Series,* 293:21.

Ojemann, G., and Ward, A. A., Jr. (1973): Abnormal movement disorders. In: *Neurological Surgery,* edited by J. Youmans. Saunders, Philadelphia.

Ommaya, A., and Baldwin, M. (1963): Extravascular local cooling of the brain in man. *J. Neurosurg.,* 20:8–19.

Orthner, H., and Lohman, R. (1966): (Experience with stereotaxic interventions in epilepsy). *Dtsch. Med. Wochenschr.,* 91:984–991.

Pertuiset, B., Hirsch, J., Sachs, M., and Landau-Ferey, J. (1969): Selective stereotaxic thalamotomy in "grand mal" epilepsy. *Excerpta Medica Int. Congress Series,* 193:72.

Poblete, M., Palestini, M., Figueroa, E., Gallardo, R., Rojas, J., Covarrubias, M., and Doyharcabal, Y. (1970): Stereotaxic thalamotomy (lamella medialis) in aggressive psychiatric patients. *Confin. Neurol.,* 32:326.

Ramamurthi, B. (1970): Stereotaxic surgery in temporal lobe epilepsy. *Neurol. India.,* 18 (Suppl. 1):42–45.

Romodanov, A. (1972): Combined surgical interventions on the brain for epilepsy. In: *Present Limits of Neurosurgery,* edited by I. Fusek and Z. Kunc. Excerpta Medica, Amsterdam.

Sano, K., Mayanaji, Y., Sekino, H., Ogashiwa, M., and Ishijima, B. (1970): Results of stimulation and destruction of the posterior hypothalamus in man. *J. Neurosurg.,* 33:689–707.

Schaltenbrand, G., Spuler, H., Nadjimi, M., Hopf, H., and Wahren, W. (1966): Die stereotaktische Behandlung der Epilepsien. *Confin. Neurol.,* 27:111–113.

Schwab, R., Sweet, W., Mark, V., Kjellberg, R., and Ervin, F. (1965): Treatment of intractible temporal lobe epilepsy by stereotactic amygdala lesions. *Tr. Am. Neurol. Assoc.,* 90:12–19.

Spiegel, E., Wycis, H., and Baird, H. (1958): Long-range effects of electropallidoansotomy in extrapyramidal and convulsive disorders. *Neurology,* 8:734–740.

Spiegel, E., Wycis, H., and Baird, H. (1962): Subcortical mechanisms in convulsive disorders. In: *Stereoencephalotomy,* part II, edited by E. Spiegel, and H. Wycis. Grune and Stratton, New York.

Sourek, K. (1972): General and local hypothermia of the brain in the treatment of intractible epilepsy. In *Present Limits of Neurosurgery,* edited by I. Fusek and Z. Kunc. Excerpta Medica, Amsterdam.

Sourek, K., and Travnicek, V. (1970): General and local hypothermia of the brain in the treatment of intractible epilepsy. *J. Neurosurg.,* 33:253–259.

Sramka, M., Lojka, J., Nadvornik, P., and Ciganek, L. (1972): Relation of the anterior thalamic reticulum to epilepsy. In: *Present Limits of Neurosurgery,* edited by I. Fusek and Z. Kunc. Excerpta Medica, Amsterdam.

Talairach, J. (1952): Destruction du noyau ventral anterieur thalamique dans le traitement des maladies mentales. *Rev. Neurol.,* 87:352–357.

Talairach, J., Bancaud, J., Bonis, A., Szikla, G., and Tournoux. P. (1962): Functional stereotaxic exploration of epilepsy. *Confin. Neurol.,* 22:328–330.

Talairach, J., and Szikla, G. (1965): Destruction partielle amygdalohippocampique par l'yttrium 90 dans le traitement de certaines epilepsies a expression rhinencephalique. *Neuro-Chirurgie,* 11: 233–240.

Tokuoka, S., Aoki, H., Higashi, K., and Tatebayashi, K. (1961): Cooling irrigation of the cerebral ventricular system. *Excerpta Medica Int. Congress Series,* 36:E148–E149.

Umbach, W. (1966): Long-term results of fornicotomy for temporal epilepsy. *Confin. Neurol.,* 27: 121–123.

Vaernet, K. (1972): Stereotaxic amygdalotomy in temporal lobe epilepsy. *Confin. Neurol.,* 34:176–180.

Van Buren, J., and Borke, R. (1972): *Variations and Connections of the Human Thalamus.* Springer-Verlag, New York.

Van Buren, J., Li, C.-L., and Ojemann, G. (1966): The fronto-striatal arrest response in man. *Electroencephalogr. Clin. Neurophysiol.,* 21:114–130.

Van Buren, J., and Ratcheson, R. (1973): Principles of stereotaxic surgery. In: *Neurological Surgery,* edited by J. Youmans. Saunders, Philadelphia.

Van Wagenen, W., and Herren, R. (1940): Surgical division of commissural pathways in the corpus callosum. *Arch. Neurol. Psych.,* 44:740–759.

Vastola, E., Homan, R., and Rosen, A. (1969): Inhibition of focal seizures by moderate hypothermia. *Arch. Neurol.,* 20:430–439.

Wycis, H. (1969): Discussion in J. Adams and B. Rutkin, Treatment of temporal lobe epilepsy by stereotaxic surgery. *Confin. Neurol.,* 31:80–85.

Wycis, H., Baird, H., and Spiegel, E. (1966): Long range results following pallidotomy and pallido-amygdalotomy in certain types of convulsive disorders. *Confin. Neurol.,* 27:114–120.

Zemskaya, A. (1972): Focal epilepsy (uni and multifocal) in children and some aspects of its surgical treatment. In: *Present Limits of Neurosurgery,* edited by I. Fusek and Z. Kunc. Excerpta Medica, Amsterdam.

Advances in Neurology, Vol. 8, edited by D. P.
Purpura, J. K. Penry, and R. D. Walter. Raven
Press, New York © 1975.

13
Postoperative Management and Criteria for Evaluation

Paul H. Crandall

INTRODUCTION

In the earliest reports on surgery for focal or partial epilepsies, effectiveness of treatment was judged primarily by the yardstick of relief from seizures (Penfield and Steelman, 1947; Falconer, Hall, Meyer, Mitchell, and Pond, 1955; Penfield and Paine, 1955; Picaza and Gumá, 1956; Bloom, Jasper, and Rasmussen, 1960; Falconer and Serafetinides, 1963. The following subdivision has been widely used in applying this criterion:

Group A (success group)—either completely free of seizures after the first year or almost so, i.e., having not more than two or three seizures in any one year;

Group B (worthwhile improvement)—improved by at least 50% in frequency of attacks;

Group C (unimproved group)—frequency of seizures is the same or worse.

While the main objective of treatment is to render the patient seizure-free, this is only one part of the total handicap of this disability. Psychological, social, educational, and vocational limitations are also imposed on those with epilepsy. The epileptic patient should be viewed as an individual with a complex disability. The related problems of retardation, psychological abnormalities, and troublesome social situations often create a larger and more difficult therapeutic challenge.

The time has come to establish common criteria by which to evaluate medical and surgical treatment of epilepsy, associated social services, and employment standards. For example, the efficacy of drug treatment is frequently assessed on the basis of a reduction in seizure frequency and/or severity without toxic side effects. However, the value of the treatment can hardly be determined without repeated psychological evaluations of possible cognitive problems or observations concerning postdrug social relationships. The latter impairments cannot be dismissed as "natural or inevitable" in epileptics. Similarly, a high success of surgical treatment must be based on abolition or reduction in frequency of seizures without cognitive or neurologic deficits and without aggravation of psychiatric status or lowered social status. The important aspects of employment evaluations of epileptics have been the severity and frequency of seizures, type of neurologic or psychological defect, and careful placement. The general personality trait of social competence is a major element in successful employment of persons with epilepsy.

In a recent opinion, an ad hoc "Consensus Committee" of the Epilepsy Foundation of America defined which epileptics are "substantially handicapped" to aid in determining services and benefits due epileptics: ". . . persons substantially handicapped by the epilepsies include . . . those whose seizures are of such severity as to interfere with their educability, employability, or social adjustment. 'Substantial handicap to employment' means that a physical or mental disability (in the light of attendant medical, psychological, vocational, educational, cultural, social, or environmental factors) impedes an individual's occupation performance, by preventing his obtaining, retaining, or preparing for a gainful occupation consistent with his capacities and abilities." While this definition lists many qualifications and entails complexities in interpretation, it indicates the kind of information which will be requested by those concerned with the care and welfare of epileptic persons.

A reasonably comprehensive assessment of the changing status of the patient can be gained by repeated documentation of seizure types and frequency, psychological status, psychiatric condition, and social adaptation. The ictal, mental, psychological, and social status can be related to the factors in any mode of treatment. As Taylor and Falconer (1968) pointed out, "outcome is measured by the reduction of incapacity." A continuous appreciation of these four features in each epileptic patient allows an examination of the nature of the incapacity, its relationship to the epilepsy, and the determinants of change. It avoids the problems of vague "clinical impressions" since these four factors can be formulated into rating scales which have been worked out and appear to be valid when used by different examiners (Taylor and Falconer, 1968; Horowitz, Cohen, Skolnikoff, and Saunders, 1970).

In contrast to many neurosurgical disorders, which usually require acute care, it is essential in the care of patients with a chronic disability such as epilepsy to have a team of therapists prepared to offer continuous care from the preoperative phase through several years of postsurgical management. The surgical treatment of epilepsy also requires the development of special facilities. For these reasons it is likely that epilepsy will be treated surgically only in a few regional centers. Yet, despite the excellence of the central facilities, little will be accomplished unless there is strong support for the patient from a family member or close associate, preferably one living with the patient. Much information about the patient is second-hand, since he is often unaware of his seizures or amnesic, and observations about the seizures are generally made by untrained persons. Behavioral states are possibly better described by such informants, but patients have been known to manipulate close associates into emphasizing or de-emphasizing their accounts of the seizure state, and even parents may alter their descriptions according to whether their perception is for more or less treatment of their child. Despite these occasional misleading circumstances, we have found that many epileptic patients do have a strong, reliable individual interested in their welfare. The continuity of this support is a major factor in the outcome.

I can best express the principles of postoperative management by relating the results of our treatment of 53 patients with temporal lobe epilepsy over the past 14 years. The original UCLA team consisted of a neurologist-*cum*-electroencephalographer (R. D. Walter), a neurosurgeon (P. H. Crandall), and a clinical psychologist (Loring Chapman). Psychiatric evaluation was infrequent and acquired by referral to one of our psychiatric staff. Then, in 1966, a mass survey of patients was carried out by a team that included a psychiatrist (Mardi J. Horowitz, University of California, San Francisco), social worker, and a research psychologist. Living situations, work, family situation, social activity, interpersonal relations, and self-image of the patients were evaluated (Horowitz and Cohen, 1968) in addition to determinations of seizures, neurologic and psychological status, and electroencephalographic findings. This revealed to us the deficiencies in our psychosocial analysis, but the survey did not fill the needs of psychotherapy. Since 1971 the UCLA group has consisted of two neurologists (Walter and G. O. Walsh), two neurosurgeons (Crandall and S. M. Weingarten), a psychiatrist (E. A. Serafetinides), and two psychologists. The group would be further strengthened by adding a social worker to improve liaison with social welfare and rehabilitation agencies.

CHARACTERISTICS OF OUR PATIENT GROUP

General Characteristics

All patients in our series shared two characteristics: one of their clinical patterns of seizure was diagnosed as an automatism, and there was some evidence of a temporal EEG focus (three exceptions), although it was frequently intermingled with other electrographic abnormalities and bilateral independent discharges. Their seizures were refractory to medications.

Patients with a mixture of several seizure patterns, with marked frequency, or with a history of long duration were not excluded, although these are generally regarded as prognostically unfavorable indices. Most patients had preoperative and postoperative batteries of IQ tests, other tests of cognitive function, a psychiatric diagnosis, and an assessment of socioeconomic adjustment such as interfamily and outside personal relations, working ability, and sexual adjustment. Patients with an IQ below 70 were excluded.[1] There was no evidence of space-occupying lesions or arteriovenous malformations by radiographic procedures. Following these examinations, 53 patients underwent approximately 3 to 5 weeks of depth electrode studies using stereotactically implanted electrodes in bilateral amygdala and hippocampal formations, and calvarial electrodes distributed in the international 10–20 EEG pattern (except for occipital leads) to record from neocortical sites (Crandall, Walter, and Rand, 1963). Thirty-nine patients were

---

[1] In this series, additional diagnostic verification was obtained by depth electrode analysis, a procedure considered unsafe in patients with too diminished an intellectual capacity. Also, this finding may be associated with severe, bilateral hippocampal sclerosis, a contraindication to lobectomy.

diagnosed as having a unilateral seizure focus in one temporal lobe. Many were based on ictal recordings. The EEG characteristics of the seizure foci were:

(1) Autonomous, high amplitude interictal epileptiform potentials occurred nearly constantly, day and night, in the epileptogenic focus, which was most commonly in a limbic site. Often these abnormalities were not reflected in the convexity temporal electrodes.

(2) There were periodic paroxysms of sustained electrical seizure activity in these local sites, but not necessarily associated with a clinical concomitant.

(3) Ictal activity was associated with a local onset of rhythmical discharges progressively spreading to adjacent sites followed by abrupt involvement of all contralateral limbic sites, which was then associated with the patient's clinical seizure pattern.

(4) Three or more similar ictal EEG patterns were recorded from most patients during periods of continuous monitoring by radiotelemetry—available since 1969.

(5) The ictal behavior of the patients was observed by special nurses.

The surgical procedure used in 38 patients diagnosed in this fashion consisted of a modified anterior temporal lobectomy including removal of the temporal tip, the amygdala, and the hippocampal formation to a distance of 3 to 4 cm from its tip and the inferotemporal cortex. An attempt was made to spare the superior and middle temporal gyri behind the Sylvian point. The ablation was more or less standardized at 5.5 cm on the speech-dominant lobe as measured on the middle temporal gyrus behind the pole and 6.0 to 6.5 cm on the nondominant side. The procedure was modified in this fashion to remove limbic structures while sparing temporal neocortex in much of the superior and middle temporal gyri. Depth electrode studies had shown the maximal epileptogenic activity to be in limbic structures with only two patients who had primarily a temporal convexity seizure focus.

Ictal States

Our 53 patients have been followed for at least 3 years, not more than 11 years. Personal follow-up examinations were possible in 50 patients; in three, reports were available from other physicians. Near-relatives or personal friends accompanying the patients were interviewed. In regular periodic follow-up care it seemed that the point of eventual outcome in postlobectomy patients for both seizures and neuropsychological status was reached between the end of the first and second postoperative year. In 1966, 1971, and 1973 mass follow-up examinations were conducted to again check neurologic, psychiatric, and EEG status.

There were 33 males and 20 females. At the time of surgical treatment, most were between 15 and 25 or 25 and 45 years old (Table 1). Thirty patients had onset of seizures at a prepubertal age, 14 in early childhood before the age of five (Table 2). Most of the patients had seizures for more than 10 years prior to operation.

TABLE 1. *Age at operation of 53 patients*

Age at operation (yr)	No. of patients
<15	3
15–24	24
25–44	24
45–49	2

TABLE 2. *Age at onset and duration of epilepsy in 53 patients*

Years	Age at onset	Duration
	(No. of patients)	
<5	14	6
5–9	16	14
10–14	8	15
15–19	3	11
20–24	9	6
25–29	1	0
30–34	2	1

Auras

Somewhat more than half the patients had pre-ictal auras prior to automatism (Table 3). In fact, the depth electrode recordings showed that these auras were associated with localized, early discharges in various limbic structures. The auras

TABLE 3. *Clinical patterns of attacks*

Pre-ictal auras	No. of patients	Percent
Visceral	15	28
Special sensory		
visual	3 ⎱	
auditory	2	
olfactory	2 ⎰	15
gustatory	1	
vertigo	0	
Sensory phenomena		
central	7 ⎱	17
peripheral	2 ⎰	
Psychic illusions	9	
Déjà vu	6	
Emotional states		
fear or panic	5	60
rage	5	
depression	3	
pleasure	1	
Amnesia or no aura	24	45

were an integral part of the seizure, a phenomenon Penfield surmised many years ago. Forty-five percent of the patients reported no aura or did not remember. The latter is probably the case in some patients who uttered exclamations and displayed typical appearances of fear prior to automatism, although they denied having any aura later. Most automatisms were accompanied by bilateral epileptic activity in the hippocampal formations, which possibly accounts for their amnesia.

The characteristic auras reflect functional activities of the limbic system. Twenty-eight percent had visceral symptoms of midline axial location such as epigastric aura, sensations mounting in the chest and throat, and pressure in the head. Other sensory phenomena were about equally divided between truncal or peripheral tactile sensations and special sensory effects involving the domain of the cranial nerves. The largest group of auras or behavioral reactions reported to the observers were psychic hallucinatory and affective responses (60%).

Ictal Clinical Actions

The behavioral manifestations during the ictus were quite varied (Table 4). In four patients external stimuli such as noises or startle could either precipitate or abort attacks. Violent behavior during the ictus occurred in five patients. These actions were brief in duration, nonspecific in nature, and not goal-directed. Twitching facial movements or head turning during the attack occurred in 10 patients but they were not of lateralizing value. There were 10 patients with unilateral neurologic deficits including tremor, hemiparesis, apraxia or aphasia, or malformation of a limb. All these deficits were mild in degree.

There were 20 patients whose sole seizure manifestations throughout their life

TABLE 4. Clinical patterns of attacks: Ictal activities[a]

Ictal activity	No. of patients	Percent
Automatisms		
arrest, stare, defensive	15	28
fumbling	12	22
masticatory	11	22
disrobing actions	4	8
destructive actions	5	9
wandering or circling	4	
urinary loss	3	6
speech		
iterative or mumbling	8	17
aphasia	1	
Attacks precipitated by		
external stimuli	2	8
Attacks inhibited by		
external stimuli	2	

[a] Observed by trained personnel during patients' hospitalization for depth electrode studies.

TABLE 5. *Clinical patterns of attacks: Combinations*

Combination	No. of patients	Percent
Automatisms alone	20	38
Automatisms and generalized	33	62
Mixed seizures (3+)	14	26
adversive	10	
absences	4	

had been automatisms (Table 5). However, 33 patients also had generalized seizures at some time in the course of their history. For the most part these generalized seizures occurred only rarely, were often the initial type of seizure, and were frequently well controlled on medication. Patients were classified as experiencing mixed seizures if they had automatisms, generalized convulsions, and a third pattern, e.g., adversive or unilateral motor phenomena or absences (absence: consciousness lost, staring expression, posture unchanged, continues with activities as soon as seizure is over at precisely the point at which he/she had been interrupted as a result of seizure, and no sleep after seizure).

With respect to frequency of temporal lobe attacks or automatisms, 45% of the group had attacks in excess of 30 per month, 14% more than 20 per month, 32% more than 10 per month, and 9% more than one per month.

EEG Findings

EEGs were interpreted and classified by Walter and Walsh (Table 6). The classification of unilateral temporal abnormalities refers to those readings with strictly unilateral or predominantly one-sided temporal discharges. Thirty-six percent of the group had bitemporal independent discharges in which there was no indication for lateralization based on interpretation of scalp recordings. Twenty-six percent of the patients had highly complex, widespread abnormalities

TABLE 6. *EEG classifications (scalp recordings)[a]*

Classification	Right	Left	No. of patients	Percent
Unilateral temporal	Right	Left	17	30
spike focus	2	2		
spike and slow wave	7	2		
slow wave	4			
Bitemporal independent			19	36
Generalized abnormalities with intermingled focal temporal discharges			14	26
Ill-defined or no change			3	6

[a] Three or more recordings in all patients; recordings made in interictal periods during sleep.

TABLE 7. *Temporal lobe seizure foci defined by depth electrode studies of interictal and ictal discharges*[a]

Focus	No. of patients	Percent
Unilateral right	28	73
Unilateral left	11	
Bilateral ictal foci	2	4
Generalized abnormalities	12	23

[a] The most certain evidence for or against a seizure focus was derived from recordings of three or more ictal episodes by means of indwelling depth electrodes.

in the EEG with occasional unilateral interictal, focal temporal discharges. A last group (6%) had definite clinical signs and symptoms of temporal lobe epilepsy, but despite sleep recordings, sphenoidal recordings, activation procedures, and repeated EEGs, had never shown clear-cut epileptiform discharges in the EEG.

Depth electrode studies were indispensable to subsequent surgical treatment in the second group of patients—those with bitemporal discharges—and in the last group, those without clear-cut scalp EEG discharges. In the group with widespread EEG abnormalities these diagnostic recordings were valuable in distinguishing those patients whose automatisms represented temporal lobe epilepsy from those whose automatisms were manifestations of generalized epilepsy. In the unilateral temporal group there were four patients in whom depth electrode studies showed an opposite lateralization to the scalp EEG findings. Also, two patients had independent, bilateral, multifocal seizure foci in the temporal lobes. In summary, depth electrode studies with recordings made during the ictus were successful in verifying a single seizure focus in approximately three-fourths of our patients (Table 7).

Results Concerning Seizures

Thirty-eight patients of the total group (53) have had anterior temporal lobectomy (one patient had a localized focus but refused lobectomy). More than twice as many had right-sided resections as left. This does not represent a selection on our part but may represent a selectivity from referral sources.

The overall results with regard to relief from seizures were gratifying in that 27 patients (71%) are in Group A and seven patients (18%) are in Group B (Table 8). Long duration of epilepsy, age at operation, or type of preliminary scalp EEG abnormality apparently were not unfavorable factors in the net result. However, all of our recurrences were in patients with mixed seizures. It is well known that patients with mixed as well as frequent seizures are in the difficult-to-manage category under any regimen of treatment, including drug treatment (Rodin, 1968).

The success of the operation in terms of seizure control was largely evident

TABLE 8. *Results of surgery: Relief from seizures*

Seizure data	Group A: free or almost free of seizures	Group B: worthwhile reduction	Group C: remaining patients	Totals
Laterality				
right	19	3	4	26
left	8	4	0	12
Age at onset (yr)				
<10	15	2	2	19
10–14	5	2	0	7
15–24	7	3	1	11
25–44	0	0	1	1
over 45	0	0	0	0
Seizure patterns				
Automatisms alone	11	3	0	14
Automatisms and generalized	13	4	0	17
Mixed seizures	3	0	4	7
Totals	27 (71%)	7 (18%)	4 (11%)	38

by the end of the first year. Only two patients had recurrence of automatisms among those who remained seizure-free for 1 year or more. However, there have been several instances of recurrence of isolated, generalized convulsions. For this reason, it has been our practice in patients with a history of generalized convulsions to continue diphenylhydantoin indefinitely in postsurgical therapy. The recurrence of even a single seizure carries such a social penalty that we believe this is justified.

Most postlobectomy complications were temporary disabilities (Table 9). Severe neurologic handicaps of a permanent nature occurred in six patients, often combined with cognitive defects. Three patients have a permanent hemiparesis, mainly affecting the upper extremity. Some of these patients with postsurgical complications have cognitive and psychiatric defects, described below.

TABLE 9. *Complications of anterior temporal lobectomy*

Complication	No. of patients
Hemiparesis	
transient	2
permanent	3
Dysphasia (slight)	3
Epidural hematoma	1
Transient third nerve palsy	3
Memory disorder	2
Meningitis and occult hydrocephalus	1
Tremor of upper limb	1

Psychological and Mental States

Preoperative Cognitive States

Many cognitive and intellectual deficiencies in our patients existed prior to surgical intervention for epilepsy. A brief summary of preoperative intelligence tests as provided by our psychologists is indicated in Table 10. This spectrum corresponds generally with other reports of epileptic subjects (Tarter, 1972). Most of our patients were functioning within the low normal to borderline mental retardation range as defined in the rating scale of the International Classification of Disease. Thirty percent were within normal range and three had superior

TABLE 10. *Preoperative psychological and psychiatric status of temporal lobe epileptic patients*

Mental status	No. of patients	Percent
By psychometrics		
Superior	3	6
Normal range	16	30
Subnormal	17	32
Retarded	6	11
Not tested	11	21
Psychiatric aspects		
Normal	12	23
Inadequate personality	6	11
Aggressive	5	9
Depressive	10	19
Schizoid (simple)	4	8
Paranoia	2	4
Florid psychiatric disorder		
Hysteria	2	4
Schizophrenia	5	9
Anxiety neurosis	0	0
Severe depression	0	0
Psychiatric diagnosis not available	8	15

intellectual capacity. Despite these relatively favorable IQ scores, all but five patients had been excluded from school or employment, for both seizures and failure in intellectual performance. Patients' relatives and friends implied that there had been a gradual deterioration in abilities and frequent episodes of confused behavior. Problems were encountered in clarifying patients' cognitive state by testing since there was much test–retest variability, probably due to such factors as high levels of medication, frequent seizures, and emotional turmoil.

Preoperative Psychopathology

Psychopathology as diagnosed by the psychiatrists was frequently present, only 23% being without any personality disorder (Table 10). Certain florid psychiatric abnormalities were separated as a group because of their prognostic significance.

Patients with inadequate personality were attended by irritability, suspiciousness, tension, "adhesiveness" in social relationships, and predisposition to circumstantial and irrelevant speech, all of which had been obstacles to their social development. Aggressive tendencies in patients were aggravated during periods of frequent seizures, and were present in four young men with mild retardation and one intelligent adult female. Depression was prevalent in adult female patients.

Florid psychosis and/or hysteria were encountered in seven patients. It was noted that epileptic psychoses seem to have better preserved social, affective responses and insight compared with nonepileptic psychoses. Clinically, epilepsy has been related to increased suicidal tendencies. Although several patients had histories of attempted suicide, none was suicidal pre- or postoperatively in this series.

Postoperative Cognitive Function

It was found that relief of epilepsy was almost essential to improved cognitive function and improved psychopathology.

Anterior temporal lobectomy by the method used here results in the removal of areas TG, TF, HA, HB, the basolateral amygdala, and the anterior 3 to 4 cm of the pes hippocampi (cytoarchitectural areas according to Bailey and von Bonin, 1951).

Briefly, cognitive dysfunction after ablation on the nondominant lobe results in subtle deficits in pattern recognition, visual memory for new faces, impaired discrimination of tone quality, timbre, and tonal patterns. In our patients, we did not find any handicap affecting the functional capacity of everyday life attributable to these particular cognitive deficits.

Speech and memory assessments in patients with lobectomy on the dominant side showed important changes. It is well known that recent memory impairment occurs with bilateral hippocampal loss, and it has recently been noted that laterality on the dominant lobe may also be a factor (Serafetinides, 1968).

Further confirmatory evidence was found in the examination of 30 patients after anterior temporal lobectomy (Cherlow and Serafetinides, *in preparation*). This group of 30 did not include two patients with the complication of slight dysphasia. The assessment of patients' speech was made by the Boston Diagnostic Aphasia Examination (Goodglass and Kaplan, 1972).

There were no significant differences between any of the groups of subjects for either of two speech tests. The patients were assessed for recent and long-term memory on a specially devised verbal auditory learning test and questionnaire on past general and personal information. Patients with left or dominant temporal lobectomies showed significant differences in amount recalled/amount learned, number of pieces learned, amount learned/number of repetitions. They took longer to learn comparable material, learned less of it, and remembered less of what they did learn than those with lobectomies on the right side. Since the left lobectomy patients showed no language deficit, a laterality effect was demonstrated for recent memory in these patients independent of language function. This is not to infer that the deficit approached in any degree that of an amnesic syndrome.

Within Group A were 23 patients who experienced remarkably good rehabilitation with distinctly improved cognitive function. In addition, when preoperative characteristics existed such as belligerence, verbal expansiveness, negativism, nervousness, and hyperactivity, there was significant postoperative improvement. Of the seven patients in Group B, two had memory disorders. In Group C, patients whose seizures continued, there were cognitive impairments of the organic brain syndrome, intermittent confusional states, perseveration, confabulation, and errors in sequencing.

Cognitive deficits can result from temporal lobe ablations, tumors, and congenital abnormalities, all due to tissue loss. However, they occur more commonly from epileptic disruption of function. The definite improvement in certain cognitive functions, especially in young patients in the series, followed relief from seizures, and was observed in follow-ups by different observers in 1966 (Horowitz and Cohen, 1968) and later in 1971 and 1973.

Postoperative Psychopathology

In the younger age group in this series (15 to 25 years), with the exception of one patient with florid schizophrenia, relief from seizures was associated with improvement in all psychiatric states. In the older age group (25 to 45 years), with long duration of psychomotor epilepsy, there were more frequent psychiatric problems encountered in rehabilitation. It should be mentioned that in patients with no preoperative psychopathology rehabilitation was relatively easily accomplished. With the others the original observation of James (1960) held, that while new postoperative complications are relatively uncommon, transient depressions and confusional states are not unusual for a 2-year period following complete control of seizures. Therefore, professional psychiatric attention is a necessity in postsurgical management of temporal lobe epileptics with evidence of preoperative psychopathology.

Three patients who were diagnosed as having intermittent psychotic states preoperatively had anterior temporal lobectomy with subsequent relief from seizures, but their psychotic states have intensified. Two patients with preoperative psychosis in Group B have continuing psychosis. In our limited experience there is no indication that amelioration of seizures will also aid schizophrenia.

Social Status

The preoperative and postoperative social status of the 38 patients receiving anterior temporal lobectomy is shown in Fig. 1. Patients with seizure activity not

SOCIOECONOMIC STATUS

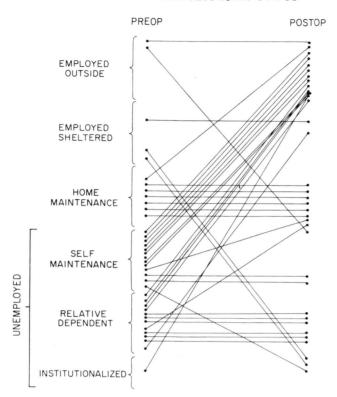

FIG. 1. Socioeconomic status and progression of patients after anterior temporal lobectomy for psychomotor epilepsy.

localized by depth electrode studies have continued with medical management and are unchanged from their preoperative intractable epilepsy.

Preoperatively, five patients were able to maintain employment in the face of their severe epilepsy and seven patients could manage family matters and the work involved in maintaining a home. Twenty-six patients were dependents, including one who was institutionalized.

Postoperatively, 16 patients are now employed and fully independent in functional capacity. Nine persons maintain a home. A total of 23 patients (60%) in our series have been relieved of functional incapacity due to seizures and psychological and psychiatric impairments. Twenty-five patients (66%) had an excellent overall result.

Of the seven patients in Group B—those with worthwhile reduction of seizures—two have psychosis (mentioned above) and one has hemiparesis. The remaining four patients take care of themselves but are unable to secure employment. The four patients in Group C have unrelieved seizures and dependent social status.

Psychosocial rehabilitation is very worthwhile after surgical treatment of epilepsy (except that it is ineffectual in psychosis). Some of the most striking examples occurred in adolescent patients. In this group, after onset of seizures, the person's ability to do school work and their relationships with peers and parents usually declined sharply. Nevertheless, seizure relief in adolescents or young adults makes it possible for them to reestablish identity and resume maturation in social relationships. Patients with seizures in early childhood and adolescence have an additional problem in that adequate personality development has not taken place during the various phases of maturation. If these patients have strong family support as well as relief from seizures, the overall results may be very good. When an adult has been disabled by seizures for most of his life, and when he is suddenly freed, social rehabilitation does not occur automatically; there are likely to be many difficult relationships within his family because of excessive expectations or withdrawal of support. His peers may require excessive revision of the patient's role or may adopt an overprotective role which does not allow the patient to reestablish identity along a developmental route.

CONCLUSION

The management of the epileptic patient in the immediate postoperative period differs little from that of other neurosurgical patients. However, for most epileptic patients, the road to successful rehabilitation will be peopled by the neurosurgeon, neurologist, psychologist, psychiatrist, and nurse in the medical center. Outpatient therapy requires support by family members, teachers, vocational or rehabilitation counselor, and possibly volunteers providing a variety of services. I have emphasized this therapeutic team approach as being essential to the management of more complex forms of temporal lobe epilepsy.

The beginning of rehabilitation requires that a preoperative, well-delineated clinical, EEG, and psychosocial profile of the total patient be available. Even if seizures are relieved by surgery it must be recalled that one starts with an individual who has lived a life of uncertainty and anxiety in the face of unpredictable seizures. The patient has a continued feeling of being different and has experienced a certain amount of rejection in the past. Epilepsy engenders a particular form of dependency. The objective of postoperative rehabilitation is to attain for him or her a meaningful, independent life.

The patient will develop a certain psychosocial relationship to each member of the therapeutic team. There are serial phases of rehabilitation. The neurosurgeon and neurologist, by their continued interest and commitment to continuing care, can offer authoritative reassurance and encouragement. Performance of serial EEG, psychological, and psychiatric studies also serve as evidence of commitment. Continued medical therapy may prove to be effective after surgical therapy in difficult cases. With relatively little effort family members can usually be educated to set realistic goals for the patient and to encourage favorable attitudes and behavior. In this way the anxiety and depression so often associated with epilepsy can be alleviated. Regular follow-up examinations appear to be essential during the first 2 postoperative years even in seizure-free patients. Serial studies of the total profile of the patient are of more than academic interest.

ACKNOWLEDGMENTS

This research was supported by U.S. Public Health Service grant NS 02808. Acknowledgment to the numerous individuals during the 12 years of this program is impossible. However, I wish to thank the directors of the Brain Research Institute, Reed Neurological Research Center, and UCLA Neuropsychiatric Institute, as well as the department chairmen of Neurology, Surgery, and Psychiatry, the program investigators, staff physicians, nurses, technicians, and others who have contributed to this study.

REFERENCES

Bailey, P., and von Bonin, G. (1951): *The Isocortex of Man.* University of Illinois Press, Urbana.
Bloom, D., Jasper, H., and Rasmussen, T. (1960): Surgical therapy in patients with temporal lobe seizures and bilateral EEG abnormality. *Epilepsia,* 1:351–365.
Crandall, P. H., Walter, R. D., and Rand, R. W. (1963): Clinical applications of studies on stereotactically implanted electrodes in temporal lobe epilepsy. *J. Neurosurg.,* 21:827–840.
Falconer, M. A., Hill, D., Meyer, A., Mitchell, W., and Pond, D. A. (1955): Treatment of temporal-lobe epilepsy by temporal lobectomy. *Lancet,* 1:827–835.
Falconer, M. A., and Serafetinides, E. A. (1963): A follow-up study of surgery in temporal lobe epilepsy. *J. Neurol. Neurosurg. Psychiat.,* 26:154–165.
Goodglass, H., and Kaplan, E. (1972): The assessment of aphasia and related disorders. Lea and Febiger, Philadelphia.
Horowitz, M. J., and Cohen, F. M. (1968): Temporal lobe epilepsy: Effect of lobectomy on psychosocial functioning. *Epilepsia,* 9:23–41.
Horowitz, M. J., Cohen, M. J., Skolnikoff, A. Z., and Saunders, F. A. (1970): Psychomotor epilepsy: Rehabilitation after surgical treatment. *J. Nerv. Ment. Dis.,* 150:273–290.
James, I. P. (1960): Temporal lobectomy for psychomotor epilepsy. *J. Ment. Sci.,* 106:543–558.
Overall, J. E., and Gorham, D. R. (1962): The brief psychiatric rating scale. *Psychol. Rep.,* 10:799–812.
Penfield, W., and Steelman, H. (1947): The treatment of focal epilepsy by cortical excision. *Ann. Surg.,* 126:740–761.
Penfield, W., and Paine, K. (1955): Results of surgical therapy for focal epileptic seizures. *Can. Med. Assoc. J.,* 73:515–531.
Picaza, J. A., and Gumá, J. (1956): Experience with the surgical treatment of psychomotor epilepsy. *Arch. Neurol. Psychiat.,* 75:57–61.
Rodin, E. A. (1968): *The Prognosis of Patients with Epilepsy.* Charles C Thomas, Springfield, Ill.
Serafetinides, Ε. A. (1968): Brain laterality: New functional aspects. In: *Main Droite et Main Gauche,* edited by R. Kourilsky and P. Grapin. Presses Universitaires de France, Paris pp. 167–181.
Tarter, R. E. (1972): Intellectual and adaptive functioning in epilepsy: A review of 50 years of research. *Dis. Nerv. Syst.,* 33:763–770.
Taylor, D. C., and Falconer, M. A. (1968): Clinical, socio-economic, and psychological changes after temporal lobectomy for epilepsy. *Brit. J. Psychiat.,* 114:1247–1261.

Advances in Neurology, Vol. 8, edited by D. P. Purpura, J. K. Penry, and R. D. Walter. Raven Press, New York © 1975.

14
Factors Contributing to the Success or Failure of Surgical Intervention for Epilepsy

William Feindel

INTRODUCTION

Repeated reviews from a number of neurosurgical centers now provide adequate evidence that surgical treatment of epilepsy can result in significant reduction or arrest of seizures in about 70% of patients (Penfield and Erickson, 1941; Penfield and Steelman, 1947; Walker, 1949; Penfield and Flanigin, 1950; Penfield and Paine, 1955; Bailey, 1961; Rasmussen and Branch, 1962; Falconer and Serafetinides, 1963; Green, 1967; Feindel, 1974).

Success or failure of surgical intervention can evidently be documented only by persistently following the progress of each patient after operation and by comparing this record with an adequate preoperative history of seizure frequency and other disabilities.

When a progressive pathologic lesion can be eliminated as the cause of the seizures, the benefits of operation must also be judged against the preoperative results of thorough trials of anticonvulsant medication. In such patients, surgery is recommended only when the seizures are intractable to medical treatment. For reasons not understood at present, there may be variation in the frequency, pattern, and severity of clinical seizures in many patients who are eventually considered for surgery. Thus, a period of at least 2 to 5 years after operation is needed to assess properly the value of surgery. Moreover, in about one quarter of the patients in the series from the Montreal Neurological Institute, postoperative seizures have occurred occasionally during the first 1 or 2 years and have then become less frequent or absent. If the follow-up had not been continued in this group of patients, the long-term results of surgery might well have been considered unsatisfactory.

Systematic supervision of the patient does not, of course, stop with surgical treatment. These patients still require rehabilitation to derive maximum benefit from surgical therapy. All patients in our series have been maintained on standard dosages of diphenylhydantoin (Dilantin®) and phenobarbital for up to 2 years after operation. In about half the patients who have received surgical treatment, medication is reduced or stopped at the end of 2 years, depending on the degree of seizure control and the electroencephalographic findings. Another 20% of patients have effective control of their seizures on medication, where before operation this had not been possible. One third of the large series have received

Montreal Neurological Institute Reprint No. 1168.

only moderate or no reduction of seizure control after surgery. Obviously they require expert management from the medical point of view. But the importance of follow-up is emphasized here as well, since these patients may not be identified in the total series until a period of a year or 2 has elapsed since operation.

Just over 2,000 patients have now been operated on for the treatment of epilepsy at the Montreal Neurological Institute. A review of results (Table 1) in patients in whom no evidence of progressive lesions such as tumor was discovered, supports the statements made above. Follow-up was inadequate in 6.5% of patients. Note also that there were 15 deaths occurring in the postoperative period, a mortality rate of 1.1%. No operative deaths occurred in a series of 501 consecutive patients operated on for temporal lobe seizures between 1950 and 1967.

Follow-up review of the patients in this surgical series is also needed to assess the role of the EEG in the selection and prediction of surgical success or failure, to document residual neurologic deficits (many of these are transient over a period of a few weeks after operation), and to evaluate the psychological and social performance of the patient where satisfactory control of seizures has been obtained. Certain psychological defects are sufficiently subtle so that specific testing techniques are needed to identify them. It is evident that patients who harbor pathologic lesions associated with focal or regional epilepsy require follow-up examination to mark any change in the progress of these lesions which in itself could indicate modification of treatment.

Thus, to define the factors which contribute to the success or failure of surgical intervention for focal epilepsy, a systematic method for selection of the patients must be established and a long-term follow-up program maintained. The experi-

TABLE 1.

Results of Cortical Excision for Focal Epilepsy

Patients with non-tumoral lesions operated upon 1928 through 1970

Seizure free since discharge	234 pts. (21%)	430 pts. (39%)	747 pts. (67%)	1112 pts. with follow-up data of 2-41 yrs.
Became seizure free after some early attacks	196 pts. (18%)			
Free 3 or more years then rare or occasional attacks	105 pts. (9%)	317 pts. (28%)		
Marked reduction of seizure tendency	212 pts. (19%)			
Moderate to no reduction of seizure tendency	365 pts. (33%)			median 11 yrs.
Inadequate follow-up data	81 pts.			
Deaths in first 2 years	22 pts.			
Postoperative deaths	15 pts.			
Total	**1230 pts.**			

ence, judgment, and technical skill of the surgeon play a primary role in the treatment of these patients, but the overall results also depend on the expertise of a team which includes the neurologist, radiologist, anesthetist, neuroscientist, and a specially trained neurologic nursing staff. The members of this team must be prepared to tackle the complex and difficult problem of intractable epilepsy as it affects the individual patient (Walker, 1949; Penfield and Jasper, 1954; Rasmussen and Jasper, 1958; Falconer, 1966).

GENERAL COMMENT

While the ultimate purpose of surgical treatment in this series of patients is to afford relief from seizures, there are substantial secondary benefits. These include the early detection, differential diagnosis, and removal of a progressive pathologic lesion other than atrophy or cicatrix. It is clearly advantageous to be able to excise small, low-grade tumors or benign lesions whose presence is heralded by the onset of focal attacks.

A further contribution to success following surgery is the psychological readjustment and improvement of the patient. This is related to reduction of anticonvulsant medication, reduction or arrest of seizures, and a return to a life style which was impossible while the patient was subject to attacks.

Finally there is the important retrieval of psychosocial and economic status following control of seizures. This return of the patient to a more normal life clearly represents the eventual aim of any well-directed program of surgical treatment.

SPECIAL PROBLEMS IN THE ANALYSIS OF SURGICAL RESULTS

Certain factors make it difficult to give a precise analysis of the results of surgical treatment for focal epilepsy. Because of these, a survey of the results is necessarily pragmatic and must be based mainly on longterm follow-up results and the presence or absence of neurologic and psychological complications. These factors may be noted under several categories.

Incomplete Knowledge

(1) Despite extensive and active research, our knowledge of the basic mechanism of epilepsy still remains incomplete (Penfield and Jasper, 1954; Gloor and Feindel, 1963; Jasper, Ward, and Pope, 1969). It is evident that surgery is not the final answer, but must be reserved for those patients where medical treatment does not at present provide an adequate solution.

(2) This lack of precise knowledge is reflected in the continuing controversy over classification and various hypotheses explaining different types of generalized and focal epilepsy. For example, the epileptogenic lesion of the mesial part of the temporal lobe has been interpreted as being caused in many cases by birth

injury ("incisural sclerosis" of the Montreal school), or as being associated mainly with febrile illness and infantile seizures ("mesial sclerosis" as proposed by Falconer and his group). The practical importance of excising the amygdala and uncus and a portion of the hippocampus, however, is now recognized by protagonists of both points of view (Feindel, Penfield, and Jasper, 1952; Penfield and Baldwin, 1952; Feindel and Penfield, 1954; Morris, 1956; Feindel, 1961; Falconer and Serafetinides, 1963).

(3) Certain seizures appear to be related to epileptic discharge involving the supplementary motor cortex of the frontal lobe. The reason for this particular localization and pattern is uncertain. Increasing evidence is being obtained that the involvement in this region of cortex of the so-called "watershed" between the territorial supply of the middle and anterior cerebral artery may be an important feature.

(4) Some patients with well-defined occipital damage in the distribution of the posterior cerebral artery have clinical attacks which are related to temporal lobe discharge. One interpretation of this situation is that the ischemic cortex is eventually supplied by collateral flow from the more anterior branches of the posterior cerebral artery as well as the middle cerebral and anterior choroidal arteries, so that their supply to their primary arterial territory may be partly reduced (Remillard, Ethier, and Andermann, 1974).

(5) The effect of the healing process following surgery requires more precise study. At present the technique of subpial resection or resection to a sulcus or pial bank appears to be the most rational approach.

(6) The long latency between the time of brain injury, which may occur at birth or infancy, and the appearance of persistent seizures is at present poorly understood. This "ripening" of the epileptogenic lesion appears in part to be a progressive change in the gliovascular component of the epileptogenic zone.

(7) The contrasting process—a gradual disappearance of epileptic attacks, particularly those sustained after brain injury in adult life—also remains to be clarified. A similar condition, as mentioned above, involves some patients who show a reduced frequency of attacks after operation and then a cessation of attacks at the end of the first year or 2 following surgery.

The Variability of Related Factors

(1) The etiology of epilepsy is heterogeneous. Since seizures represent a symptom rather than a disease, a great variety of lesions are evidently capable of producing this common setting which results in seizures.

(2) The process of selection of patients for surgery varies somewhat from one medical center to another. The surgical results will be affected by the number of patients in the series who have associated psychiatric disorders, who are mainly examples of posttraumatic epilepsy, or who have seizures related on one hand to birth injury or on the other hand to the presence of brain tumors. Some of these lesions may be discovered only at the time of surgery and the pathologic nature of the lesion clearly will influence the long-term results.

Anatomic Factors

(1) The degree of localization of the epileptogenic lesion, insofar as it can be determined before operation and identified at the time of operation, will strongly influence the results of surgical treatment. The presence of a focal seizure pattern, as observed clinically, may be associated at times with a cerebral lesion which can be regional or diffuse. Conversely, certain focal lesions which respond satisfactorily to fairly limited excision may be judged at operation as being more diffuse in character.

(2) Inadequate excision of the epileptogenic lesion may result either because of improper identification or because of recognized physiologic and anatomic limitations. An example is the epileptogenic region which involves or is adjacent to the sensory or motor cortex or the cortex subserving speech function. A difficult decision must be made by the surgeon in these cases to balance the benefit of adequate excision of epileptogenic tissue against residual permanent neurologic deficit. It is reasonable in such a circumstance to defer additional excision to a second operation, with a careful interim evaluation of the results. This is important, since persistent electrographic abnormality at the time of operation and even a persistent but reduced seizure tendency in the early postoperative period do not always indicate a surgical failure.

DETAILED ANALYSIS OF CASE EXAMPLES

The reports of three patients, each with a follow-up record of more than 10 years, will illustrate the evaluation of factors concerned in surgical success or failure.

Case Report 1. Patient P. J., age 20. At the age of 13, he struck his right temple while sledding and sustained a depressed fracture of the right frontal bone. At 16 he had attacks with head-turning to the left and twitching of the left side of the face. During the 4 years before admission, the frequency of attacks had increased to about once a week.

A depressed fracture, with cranial erosion, was shown on X-ray, just anterior to the pterion. The EEG showed bilateral spike-and-wave abnormality, sometimes maximal on the left, but with unclear lateralization in most recordings. This was interpreted as a secondary bilateral synchronous discharge coming possibly from the orbital surface of the frontal lobe.

First operation: October 8, 1953. Operation showed a bony spicule in a dural defect 3.0 cm wide with scarring of the frontal cortex beneath this. The cicatrix with the neighboring opercular and orbital cortex was excised under corticographic control (Figs. 1 and 2). Postexcision record (Fig. 2) showed no further high-voltage spikes.

On the first postoperative day the patient had eight attacks with turning of head and eyes to the *right*. The EEG still showed bilateral synchronous sharp waves at 2/sec, greater on the side opposite to the operation. Reoperation was proposed and carried out 1 month later. The mesial frontal cortex gave slow waves at 2½

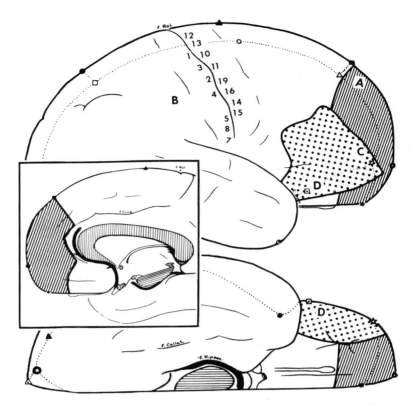

FIG. 1. Brain map and excision in patient P.J. The hatched area indicates the excision at the second operation. Inset: mesial aspect of the frontal lobe.

cycles/sec. Further excision (Fig. 1) included the frontal polar cortex, but spike-and-slow-wave activity were still recorded from the mesial surface of the opposite frontal lobe. Both the electroencephalographer and the surgeon concluded that the excision had not satisfactorily eradicated the epileptogenic lesion, but it was considered that removal of the large area of scar tissue might favor medical control of the attacks.

After operation he had five generalized attacks, some of which began with head and eye turning to the right. His attacks then stopped. Three years later the EEG, even after hyperventilation, showed no epileptiform changes. Six years later, in 1959, his anticonvulsant medication was stopped. At the most recent follow-up report, 18 years after operation, he has remained free of attacks.

Comments. This patient had a classical focal posttraumatic lesion, but the EEG gave a diffuse bilateral spike-and-wave pattern, suggesting subcortical abnormality. Failure to eradicate this, even after the second operation, appeared to strengthen this conclusion. The electrographic abnormality and the clinical pattern of some of his attacks suggested an origin in the opposite frontal region. The

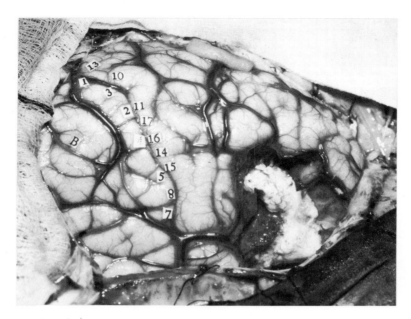

FIG. 2. Photograph of the operative field, patient P.J. The motor and sensory cortices are indicated by stimulation tickets and the extent of the first excision of the cerebral cicatrix is shown.

EEG remained abnormal, even after the second operation, but returned to normal 3 years later.

The attacks occurred during the third week after the first operation and then stopped, at which time the seizure discharges appeared to involve mainly the left frontal lobe. It is impossible to answer the question of whether the more extensive excision was necessary and whether the seizure tendency might have declined in time without the second procedure. This patient is certainly rated as a surgical success, but we must recognize our failure to understand properly the scientific basis for that result.

Case Report 2. J. D., age 11. This patient began to have attacks at the age of 5. There was no obvious antecedent cause, but the boy's paternal uncle was known to have seizures. The seizure pattern involved turning of the head and eyes to the right, preceded by blurring of vision and followed by right-sided movements, mastication, and unconsciousness. He sometimes had as many as 30 attacks a day despite heavy medication. The EEG showed 2 to 4/sec sharp waves and spikes of high amplitude, mainly left frontal but occasionally temporal and bilateral occipital.

Operation: In July 1960, operation showed a thickened area of pia-arachnoid just in front of the motor cortex. From here, marked spike-and-wave abnormality was recorded, with no abnormality noted from the temporal or mesial frontal cortex. Toughened and partly buried fingers of cortex were noted in this region

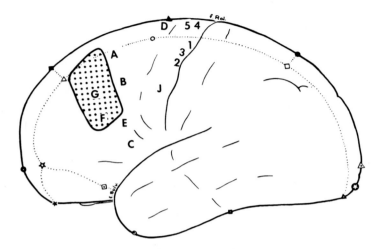

FIG. 3. Brain map, patient J.D. Numbers indicate the motor cortex, letters indicate sites of maximal electrographic abnormality. Area of the final excision is shown.

during excision, which measured 4.0×3.0 cm (Fig. 3). The recording then improved, with only some minor sharp-wave activity remaining. He had no seizures in the 13 years after operation and has had no medication for the past 10 years.

Comments. We note that the etiology here was unknown and that there was some family history of seizures. The relatively local excision of an atrophic lesion was successful, although the EEG before operation had indicated some temporal and bilateral occipital abnormality. As in the previous case, medication was completely withdrawn and the patient has led a very active life, becoming at one stage a champion long-distance cyclist.

Case Report 3. D. R., age 39. This patient had numerous convulsive seizures during the first 2 weeks of life, and then again beginning at the age of 17. He had a left homonymous hemianopsia and an external squint of the left eye. There was extensive atrophy in the posterior part of the right hemisphere, but no occlusion of the posterior cerebral artery. The EEG showed maximum abnormality in the right posterior temporal and occipital regions. At operation in October 1962, as the thinned-out occipital cortex was excised, a large cavity was seen to extend into the greatly dilated temporal horn, with much of the inferior part of the temporal lobe being absent. Further excision was made anteriorly to include most of the amygdala, until the corticographic abnormality was reduced (Fig. 4). He has had no attacks since operation. His medication has been withdrawn and he has held a steady job.

Comments. The visual field deficit was long-standing and made it possible to carry out a large excision of the damaged occipital cortex without further disability. The epileptogenic lesion here was clearly related to the territory of supply of the posterior cerebral artery.

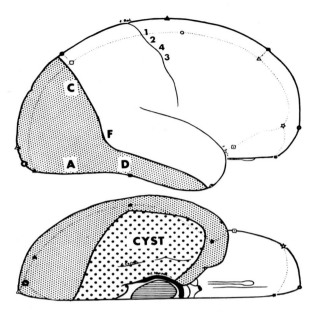

FIG. 4. Diagram of operative findings, patient D.R. Letters indicate the sites of electrographic abnormality; shaded area indicates the extent of excision.

This case is an early example of an ischemic lesion in the occipital region being associated with focal cerebral seizures, involving also the temporal lobe. It is suggested that the collateral flow toward the ischemic zone may have the effect of reducing circulation in the neighboring distribution of the middle cerebral artery (Remillard et al., 1974). Recognition of this temporal lobe involvement is important to successful surgical excision.

LOCAL AND REGIONAL EXCISION

In these cases, the clinical features and electrographic findings indicated a focal or restricted epileptogenic area. Excision carried out under corticographic guidance was followed by arrest of attacks. Limited cortical excision appears to be most successful in the frontal, parietal, or occipital region. When the epileptogenic process involves the mesial frontal or temporal lobe, the spread of the initial epileptic discharge may be more complex and the approach to the surgical removal somewhat different.

In our experience, successful surgery in temporal lobe epilepsy has depended on the recognition that the mesial temporal region and particularly the amygdala and anterior hippocampus are crucially involved in the seizure discharge. This factor, which was recognized by Hughlings Jackson (1888), was supported by evidence obtained from using stimulation to produce temporal lobe automatism from the peri-amygdaloid region (Feindel et al., 1952; Feindel and Penfield, 1954), and by the demonstration that these mesial structures were particularly vulnerable to compressive ischemia at birth (Earle, Baldwin, and Penfield, 1959) and susceptible also to damage during febrile illnesses in early life (Meyer and Beck, 1955). Before this knowledge was available, earlier patients in this series whose EEGs pointed to an anterior sylvian abnormality were subjected to excision of the lateral or polar cortex of the temporal lobe. Almost uniformly, the results in this small series of early cases were unsatisfactory. Some were converted into successes by a second operation with excision of the amygdala and anterior part of the hippocampus (see Penfield and Jasper, 1954, for case examples).

The important distinction concerning the extent of the mesial excision needed to obtain satisfactory relief of seizures requires more detailed study. In two series of patients treated by temporal lobectomy, 50% of the patients with the most satisfactory postoperative results had complete hippocampus removal. By contrast, of those with less satisfactory control, only 10% had complete hippocampal removal and a much larger number, 57%, had only partial removal of the hippocampus (Bengzon, Rasmussen, Gloor, Dussault, and Stephens, 1968).

The separation of the roles of the hippocampus and amygdala in relation to surgical success is also of considerable importance, since removal of the amygdala and uncus has not been shown so far to be related to any significant memory deficit. In the dominant temporal lobe, removal of the hippocampus, even in the absence of contralateral temporal lobe pathology, may produce some impairment in the learning of specific new verbal material. On the nondominant side, subtle reduction in certain test patterns may be identified. Stimulation of the hippocampus rarely produces automatism at operation, although active epileptic discharge can frequently be recorded directly from the hippocampus. On the other hand, automatism can consistently be produced by stimulation within the amygdala. More exact comparison of these two types of removal should be made where the extent of the surgical excision has been precisely documented.

In addition to the extent of the hippocampal removal, Bengzon et al. (1968) have indicated that certain other factors tend to favor a better surgical prognosis in temporal lobe epileptic patients. Younger age at the time of operation, the presence mainly of focal rather than generalized clinical attacks, confirmation of localization by psychological testing and EEG localization, and right-sided rather than left-sided abnormality are all favorable features. A normal postexcision corticogram and postoperative EEG and the absence in the early postoperative period of seizures are also found in patients with the most successful results. It should be noted, however, that these features show considerable overlap among cases with satisfactory and unsatisfactory results.

In the presence of a gross lesion, the excision should include not only the pathologic tissue, but also adjacent cortical areas which give electrographic evidence of epileptogenic abnormality. When the lesion is in the temporal lobe, even though it is limited in extent, it has been our practice to do an anterior temporal lobectomy with removal of the amygdala, uncus, and anterior hippocampus.

TABLE 2.

Etiology in M.N.I. Surgical Studies 1928-1967

	All Excisions		Temporal Excisions	
	No. Patients	%	No. Patients	%
Tumors	257	19	93	13.5
Vascular lesions	17	1.5	5	<1
Non-tumor Lesions				
Birth trauma, anoxia or compression	345	25	213	30.5
Postnatal trauma	265	20	93	13.5
Postinflammatory brain scarring	166	12	99	14
Miscellaneous	74	5.5	29	4
Unknown	231	17	164	23.5
Total	**1355 pts.**	**100%**	**696 pts.**	**100%**

Curiously, many lesions occurring in the brain, especially in the temporal lobe, may not be associated with seizures (Haymaker, Pentschew, Margoles, and Bingham, 1958). The variety of pathologic lesions related to epilepsy is well illustrated in the analysis of cases operated on between 1928 and 1967 (Table 2). The four major groups identified include tumors, perinatal injury, postnatal trauma, and postinflammatory brain scarring. In the excisions related to the temporal lobe region, tumors were somewhat fewer and the incidence of birth injury somewhat higher than in the total series. Different etiologic agents may, of course, involve different regional systems or areas of the brain and indicate regions of various extent for surgical excision. Severely damaged hemispheres may call for radical hemispherectomy.

PREOPERATIVE FACTORS

A detailed analysis of surgical procedures and techniques can be found in previous papers (Penfield and Baldwin, 1952; Penfield, 1958; see especially Penfield and Jasper, 1954, Chapter 18). But it is useful to review some points briefly and to mention certain new factors.

(1) The focal nature of the seizures must be established by accurate clinical observation of the pattern and by repeated preoperative EEG examination. The initial feature of the seizure is of great significance and certain postictal deficits such as aphasia or mild paresis are helpful in indicating localization.

(2) The nature of the lesion responsible for the seizures should be searched out to determine whether it is atrophic, neoplastic, or vascular.

(3) Radiologic contrast studies including pneumoencephalography and angiography, radioisotopic brain scanning and, more recently, computer encephalography (Ambrose, 1973), will provide the surgeon with information on which he can make a judgment and which can be of value during operation.

(4) Detailed psychometric studies with properly designed tests give increasing

support in the selection and postoperative assessment of the epileptic patient (Milner, 1959; Kimura, 1961).

(5) Lateralization of speech function and assessment of memory function must be carried out in patients in whom there is a question of cerebral dominance or bitemporal abnormality. This is done by the carotid Amytal test.

(6) A thorough medical trial of anticonvulsants is indicated if there is a diagnostic clearance of the presence of a focal progressive lesion.

(7) Certain general features of the patient's attitude and disability should be assessed. Motivation, prospects for rehabilitation, degree of neurologic deficit, and extent of behavioral defect should all be evaluated.

(8) In patients with bitemporal electrographic abnormality, repeated recording with sphenoidal electrodes or with fine indwelling depth electrodes to record spontaneous seizure activity may provide evidence for lateralization. Special EEG activation procedures are indicated in problem cases.

(9) Computer EEG telemetry is invaluable in cases where it is difficult to obtain a recording of spontaneous seizures during the usual standard examination.

FACTORS DURING SURGERY

General Features

(1) Surgery is carried out insofar as possible under local anesthesia. This is supplemented by analgesic drugs, by injection of local anesthetic agents to reduce pain from the sensitive meningeal arteries, and occasionally by injection into the trigeminal ganglia or into the dura of the tentorium and falx.

(2) With the patient awake and cooperative, essential cortical areas such as the motor, sensory, and speech regions can be defined exactly.

(3) Reproductions of subjective features of the patient's aura by surface or depth stimulation can be helpful in supporting other evidence of localization of the seizure discharge.

(4) Monitoring of the patient's functions such as speech and motor ability during various stages of the excision guides the surgeon in avoiding neurologic deficit (Penfield and Jasper, 1954; Feindel, 1964).

(5) Electrocorticography is not masked by anesthetic drugs so that more adequate localization of epileptic discharge can be determined. Certain drugs may also be used, as well as hyperventilation, to activate the epileptogenic discharge.

(6) Caution must be taken during stimulation to proceed in precisely graded levels of stimulation strength in order to avoid overt seizures.

Technical Aids

(1) Cortical excision is carried out whenever possible to the sulcus so that the pia-arachnoid is left intact on the adjacent convolutional bank. In small excisions

near the motor, sensory, or speech areas, removal of the cortex is made by careful subpial suctioning through a small opening in the pia-arachnoid. These maneuvers preserve the arteries and veins which supply the cortex adjacent or distal to the point of excision. This is especially critical when removal is made in the posterior sylvian region or in the lower central region. The larger veins should be spared whenever possible, depending on the variations in epicerebral venous patterns. Our experimental work has shown that occlusion of some of the larger bridging veins entering the midline sinus causes reduced cerebral flow and subpial hemorrhages.

(2) Electrocorticography provides direct confirmation of the focal or regional epileptogenic zones, and permits both comparison of the recording from surface and depth electrodes and monitoring of afterdischarge during cortical stimulation and depth stimulation. Frequently, additional tissue is excised because of persistent electrical abnormality until a clear record is obtained. The identity of any residual abnormality which cannot be dealt with surgically is carefully noted.

(3) Detailed documentation of the operative procedure is essential to a proper analysis of the role of surgical treatment in epilepsy. Each patient has a photographic record of the exposed area of the brain with stimulation responses identified by small tickets and corticographic abnormalities marked in a similar way. The surgeon draws the main features on a brain map. The size of the lesion and of the cortical excision are measured. The findings, dictated in the operating room, are supplemented by the electroencephalographer's report.

(4) The surface of the brain is protected during surgery by a moistened transparent plastic membrane and frequent irrigation with artificial cerebrospinal fluid. Accepted details of neurosurgical technique must be rigorously followed, including meticulous hemostasis and gentle handling of tissue. In patients undergoing temporal lobe excision, great care must be taken to avoid manipulation of the middle cerebral artery and its branches by stretching or by too vigorous retraction. Failure to do so may cause a degree of permanent hemiparesis (Penfield, Lende, and Rasmussen, 1961). Insular cortex need not be removed as a rule, since, even when small spikes appear there, they have no relation to persistence of seizures (Silfvenius, Gloor, and Rasmussen, 1964).

To control infection, ultraviolet lights are used in the operating room and the wound is irrigated during closure with microcrystals of sulfanilamide and with bacitracin solution. The postoperative infection rate in this surgical series has been less than 1% over the past 15 years.

During the final stages of the operation, corticosteroids and anticonvulsants are added to the intravenous infusion. Fluid is restricted to about 1,500 ml in 24 hr for adult patients for the first 5 days after operation.

RECENT IMPROVEMENTS

Some techniques which have become available to the neurosurgeon only in recent years can be predicted to have a beneficial future effect on the results of surgery for focal epilepsy. First among these is the use of microsurgical methods. The operating microscope with its elegant enlargement of detail in the operative field and excellent lighting, combined with the use of microinstruments, miniature suction, and precise bipolar cautery, all allow the surgeon to carry out more exact excision with minimal disturbance of the surrounding areas and essential blood vessels.

Display of the microcirculation patterns in and around the epileptogenic lesion by fluorescein angiography, and measurement of focal cerebral blood flow are now providing more detailed information on the vascular factors related to certain focal epileptic lesions (Feindel, Yamamoto, and Hodge, 1967). Areas of impaired microcirculation in the cortex are shown which could not be otherwise recognized. These surgical findings can now be correlated with anatomic evidence derived from X-ray microangiography (Saunders, Feindel, and Carvalho, 1965; Saunders and Bell, 1971). The important role of the circulation in relation to epilepsy, which has long been recognized, demands further investigation with these newer techniques (Penfield, 1937, 1971; Penfield, von Santha, and Cipriani, 1939; Feindel and Perot, 1965). The role of norepinephrine, serotonin, and prostaglandins in the control of blood flow in brain tissue is under active study (Peerless, 1969; Peerless and Yasargil, 1971; Yamamoto, Feindel, Wolfe, and Hodge, 1973).

Early detection of small tumors, cystic lesions, and infarcts, with exact disposition in the brain, can now be made by computer encephalography (EMI scan). Focal lesions which in their early stages may give only equivocal findings with conventional diagnostic methods are well defined in three dimensions, in relation both to grey and water matter in the ventricles and to the area of surrounding edema. The examination is rapid, taking only 30 min, and the patient is subjected to no discomfort or risk. The technique marks one of the most significant ad-

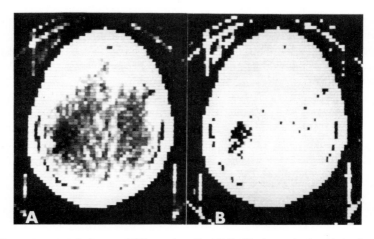

FIG. 5. Computer encephalogram (EMI scan), patient D.K. (A) shows the low X-ray density area in the left parietal region which, on (B), is brought out by a contrast window setting.

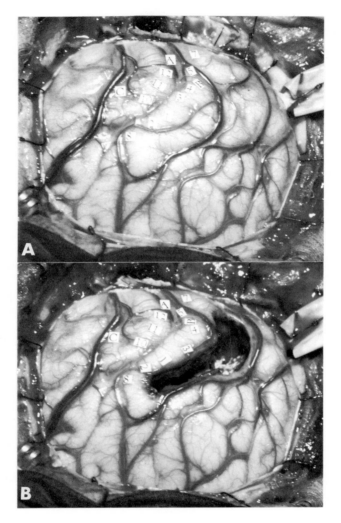

FIG. 6. Operative findings, patient D.K. (A): minimal enlargement of the postcentral gyrus; (B): area of excision of a grade I glioma, corresponding exactly to the scan localization.

vances in neurologic diagnosis and is of particular interest for the early detection and definition of the etiologic factors in patients with focal and regional epilepsy. A single example will make this evident.

Case Report 4. D. K., aged 43. The patient had focal seizures for 5 years which began with tingling of the right side of the mouth and the right hand, followed by clonic movements of the right hand and trouble in speaking. Pneumoencephalography and angiography shortly after the onset of his attacks were normal. Repeat angiography recently suggested the presence of an avascular lesion in the left parietal region, but with poor definition. The EEG showed mild abnormality on the opposite side and radioisotope scan was normal. Computer encephalography revealed a region of low X-ray absorption density, well-demarcated in the left parietal region (Fig. 5). At operation this proved to be a grade I glioma which was infiltrating the convolution just posterior to the sensory cortex (Fig. 6). Of particular value to the surgeon in this new method is the detailed information on the location, size, and shape of the abnormality.

SUMMARY

(1) Surgical treatment of epilepsy can provide benefit in about 70% of patients.

(2) Selection of patients for surgery, the surgical procedure itself, and evaluation of postoperative results demand a team which can provide expertise on the various aspects of the epileptic patients' complex problems.

(3) The importance of long-term follow-up is emphasized in the light of our incomplete knowledge of the basic mechanism of epilepsy.

(4) The difficulties of evaluating the factors leading to success or failure in the surgical treatment are illustrated by several case reports.

(5) The extent of local or regional excision must be based on preoperative information and on the surgical findings correlated with the anatomic and physiologic knowledge of different cerebral regions.

(6) Factors which appear to be significant in the various phases of surgical management are catalogued.

(7) New approaches which include microsurgical techniques, fluorescein angiography, measurement of focal cerebral blood flow, and computer encephalography can be expected to bring increasing benefit and provide further insight into the problem of the surgical treatment of epilepsy.

REFERENCES

Ambrose, J. (1973): Computerized transverse axial scanning (tomography). Part 2: Clinical application. *Brit. J. Radiol.,* 46:1023–1047.

Bailey, P. (1961): Surgical treatment of psychomotor epilepsy. Five-year follow-up. *South. Med. J.,* 54:299–301.

Bengzon, A. R. A., Rasmussen, T., Gloor, P., Dussault, J., and Stephens, M. (1968): Prognostic factors in the surgical treatment of temporal lobe epileptics. *Neurology,* 18:717–731.

Earle, K. M., Baldwin, M., and Penfield, W. (1959): Incisural sclerosis and temporal lobe seizures produced by hippocampal herniation at birth. *Arch. Neurol. Psychiatry,* 69:27–42.

Falconer, M. A. (1966): Problems in neurosurgery: Temporal lobe epilepsy; the assessment of patients for surgical treatment. *Trans. Med. Soc. Lond.,* 82:111–126.

Falconer, M. A., and Serafetinides, E. A. (1963): A follow-up study of surgery and temporal lobe epilepsy. *J. Neurol. Neurosurg. Psychiatry,* 26:154–165.

Feindel, W. (1961): Response patterns elicited from the amygdala and deep temporal insula cortex. In: *Electrical Stimulation of the Brain,* edited by D. E. Sheer. Texas University Press, Austin.

Feindel, W. (1964): Memory and speech function in the temporal lobe in man. In: *Brain Function, Vol. 2, R.N.A. and Brain Function: Memory and Learning,* edited by M. A. Brazier. University of California Press, Los Angeles.

Feindel, W. (1974): Temporal lobe seizures. In: *The Epilepsies. Vol. 15, Handbook of Clinical Neurology,* edited by P. J. Vinken and G. W. Bruyn. North Holland, Amsterdam.

Feindel, W., and Penfield, W. (1954): Localization of discharge in temporal lobe automatism. *Arch. Neurol. Psychiatry,* 72:605–630.

Feindel, W., Penfield, W., and Jasper, H. H. (1952): Localization of epileptic discharge in temporal lobe automatism. *Trans. Amer. Neurol. Soc.,* 77:14–17.

Feindel, W., and Perot, P. (1965): Red cerebral veins: A report on arteriovenous shunts in tumours and cerebral scars. *J. Neurosurg.,* 22:315–325.

Feindel, W., Yamamoto, Y. L., and Hodge, C. P. (1967): Intracarotid fluorescein angiography: A new method for examination of the epicerebral circulation in man. *Can. Med. Assoc. J.,* 96:1–7.

Gloor, P., and Feindel, W. (1963): The Temporal Lobe and Affective Behavior. In: *Physiologie des Vegetativen Nerven Systems, Vol. 2.* Hippokrates Verlag, Stuttgart.

Green, J. R. (1967): Temporal lobectomy. With special reference to selection of epileptic patients. *J. Neurosurg.,* 26:584–593.

Haymaker, W., Pentschew, A., Margoles, C., and Bingham, W. G. (1958): Occurrence of lesions in the temporal lobe in the absence of convulsive seizures. In: *Temporal Lobe Epilepsy,* edited by M. Baldwin and P. Bailey. Charles C Thomas, Springfield, Ill.

Jackson, J. H. (1888): On a particular variety of epilepsy ("Intellectual Aura"): One case with symptoms of organic brain disease. *Brain,* 11:179–207.

Jasper, H. H., Ward, A. A., and Pope, A. (1969): *Basic Mechanisms of the Epilepsies.* Little, Brown, Boston.

Kimura, D. (1961): Some effects of temporal lobe damage on auditory perception. *Can. J. Psychol.,* 15:156–165.

Meyer, A., and Beck, E. (1955): The hippocampal formation in temporal lobe epilepsy. *Proc. Roy. Soc. Med.,* 48:457–462.

Milner, B. (1959): The memory defect in bilateral hippocampal lesions. *Psychiat. Res. Rep.,* 11:43–52.

Morris, A. A. (1956): Temporal lobectomy with removal of uncus, hippocampus, and amygdala. *Arch. Neurol. Psychiatry,* 76:479–496.

Peerless, S. J. (1969): The cerebral vaculature. In: *Microsurgery Applied to Neurosurgery,* edited by M. G. Yasargil. Georg Thieme Verlag, Stuttgart.

Peerless, S. J., and Yasargil, M. G. (1971): Adrenergic innervation of the cerebral blood vessels in the rabbit. *J. Neurosurg.,* 35:148–154.

Penfield, W. (1937): The circulation of the epileptic brain. *Res. Publ. Assoc. Nerv. Ment. Dis.,* 18:605–637.

Penfield, W. (1958): Pitfalls and success in surgical treatment of focal epilepsy. *Brit. Med. J.,* 1:660–672.

Penfield, W. (1971): Remarks on incomplete hypotheses for the control of cerebral circulation. *J. Neurosurg.,* 35:124–127.

Penfield, W., and Baldwin, M. (1952): Temporal lobe seizures and the technique of cerebral sub-total temporal lobectomy. *Ann. Surg.,* 136:625–634.

Penfield, W., and Erickson, T. (1941): *Epilepsy and Cerebral Localization.* Charles C Thomas, Springfield, Ill.

Penfield, W., and Flanigin, H. (1950): Surgical therapy of temporal lobe seizures. *Arch. Neurol. Psychiatry,* 64:491–500.

Penfield, W., and Jasper, H. H. (1954): *Epilepsy and the Functional Anatomy of the Human Brain.* Little, Brown, Boston.

Penfield, W., Lende, R. A., and Rasmussen, T. (1961): Manipulation hemiplegia. An untoward complication in the surgery of focal epilepsy. *J. Neurosurg.,* 18:760–776.

Penfield, W., and Paine, K. W. E. (1955): Results of surgical therapy for focal epileptic seizures. *Canad. Med. Assoc. J.,* 73:515–531.

Penfield, W., and Steelman, H. (1947): The treatment of focal epilepsy by cortical excision. *Ann. Surg.,* 126:740–762.

Penfield, W., von Santha, K., and Cipriani, A. (1939): Cerebral blood flow during induced epileptiform seizures in animals and man. *J. Neurophysiol.,* 2:257–267.

Rasmussen, T., and Branch, C. (1962): Temporal lobe epilepsy: Indications for and results of surgical therapy. *Postgrad Med.,* 31:9–14.

Rasmussen, T., and Jasper, H. H. (1958): Temporal lobe epilepsy: Indications for operation and surgical techniques. In: *Temporal Lobe Epilepsy,* edited by M. Baldwin and P. Bailey. Charles C Thomas, Springfield, Ill.

Remillard, G. M., Ethier, R., and Andermann, F. (1974): Temporal lobe epilepsy and perinatal occlusion of the posterior cerebral artery. *Neurology (in press).*

Saunders, R. L. de C. H., and Bell, M. A. (1971): X-ray microscopy and histochemistry of the human cerebral blood vessels. *J. Neurosurg.*, 35:128–140.

Saunders, R. L. de C. H., Feindel, W. H., and Carvalho, V. R. (1965): X-ray microscopy of the blood vessels of the human brain. *Med. Biol. Illus.*, 15:108–122, 234–246.

Silfvenius, H., Gloor, P., and Rasmussen, T. (1964): Evaluation of insular ablation in surgical treatment of temporal lobe epilepsy. *Epilepsia*, 5:307–320.

Walker, A. E. (1949): *Post-traumatic Epilepsy.* Charles C Thomas, Springfield, Ill.

Yamamoto, Y. L., Feindel, W. H., Wolfe, L. S., and Hodge, C. P. (1973): Inhibition and reversal of cerebral vasospasm induced by prostaglandins. *Stroke*, 4:356–357.

Advances in Neurology, Vol. 8, edited by D. P.
Purpura, J. K. Penry, and R. D. Walter. Raven
Press, New York © 1975.

15
Psychological Aspects of Focal Epilepsy and Its Neurosurgical Management

Brenda Milner

BACKGROUND

Since 1950, most patients at the Montreal Neurological Institute undergoing a cortical excision for the relief of epilepsy have been subjected beforehand to extensive psychological testing on a variety of tasks. They have been retested from 2 to 3 weeks postoperatively and, whenever possible, a follow-up study has been carried out a year or more later. In a small but growing number of cases we have been able to reexamine the patient from 5 to 20 years after removal of the epileptogenic area. These late observations, in patients who have remained seizure-free, serve to delineate the residual effects of a known brain lesion.

The Patient Sample

The total group now comprises 955 cases of unilateral brain operation carried out to control seizures arising from long-standing atrophic lesions. This excludes cases where the seizures were secondary to brain tumor or other progressive brain disease and cases of large arteriovenous malformation.

When the 955 patients are subdivided according to the locus of cortical excision, we find 649 cases of anterior temporal lobectomy (352 in the left hemisphere, 297 in the right), constituting two-thirds of the total sample. For the frontal lobes, the numbers are much smaller (barely 8% of the total), but are still substantial: there are 73 cases in which the resection was limited to parts of the frontal cortex (37 left frontal lesions and 36 right). In contrast, pure cases of occipital lobectomy (6) or of parietal lobe excisions sparing the postcentral gyrus (9) are too few for separate statistical treatment.

Nearly all the remaining patients had lesions invading more than one lobe of the brain. Because of our special interest in cortical sensory function (Corkin, Milner, and Rasmussen, 1970), we have classified them in different groups, depending on whether the excision encroached upon the central region. The central, or Rolandic, group comprises 117 patients, including 12 with focal lesions of the precentral or postcentral gyrus, or both, as well as cases of more massive brain injury. The noncentral group contains 101 patients, most of whom had circumscribed removals of parieto-temporal, temporo-occipital, or fronto-temporal cortex.

Montreal Neurological Institute Reprint No. 1167.

Salient Findings and Their Diagnostic Implications

Few patients have shown any lasting postoperative impairment of general intelligence as measured by standard tests, and many have shown slight but significant long-term gains if their seizures have been brought under control. In this sense, then, there is some support for the view that an actively discharging lesion can interfere with the functions of other areas, so that when the damaged cortex is excised there is a measurable improvement in overall intellectual efficiency (Hebb and Penfield, 1940).

At the same time, the continuing study of patients with well-lateralized focal lesions has uncovered specific changes related to damage to particular cortical areas. Thus, by appropriate techniques one can show that chronic epileptogenic lesions tend to be accompanied by specific psychological deficits that vary according to the locus of the lesion (temporal, frontal, or central) and according to whether or not it is in the dominant hemisphere for speech (Milner, 1958, 1963, 1967). The deficits, described below, are evident in cases of birth injury (Milner, 1958) as well as in postnatal trauma (Milner, 1969), and have been found not only in adults but also in children with focal seizures (Fedio and Mirsky, 1969). Such specific changes are accentuated, not diminished, by removal of the malfunctioning cortical tissue, with residual deficits demonstrable in postoperative follow-up study many years later (Milner, 1962, 1963, 1967).

These deficits tend to be mild and to interfere little if at all with the patient's daily life. Yet they have lateralizing and localizing significance, and the fact that they are often detectable preoperatively explains why the psychological examination has come to play an increasing role in the assessment of patients who are candidates for seizure surgery. In such cases, the preoperative test profile may provide clues to areas of damage, not necessarily epileptogenic, that would not have been picked up by other means. One must, of course, be cautious in interpreting the performance of patients with active epileptogenic lesions. If the psychological findings suggest more widespread cortical abnormality than is indicated in the EEG, this could in principle be due to the interfering effect of the focal lesion on other areas, an effect potentially reversible by excision of the epileptogenic area. Such reversible deficits have occasionally been seen (Milner, 1958). An alternative interpretation would be that the site and extent of damaged cortex had not been adequately revealed by the EEG studies. On this view, one would expect persistence of the deficits after operation and possibly a continuing seizure tendency. In support of this interpretation is the finding of Bengzon, Rasmussen, Gloor, Dussault, and Stephens (1968) that whether or not the psychological examination points to extratemporal damage has a significant bearing on how well the patient's seizures are controlled by a subsequent temporal lobectomy.

A further purpose of the preoperative psychological tests is to draw attention to possible instances of right-hemisphere speech representation that would otherwise have been missed, because the patients were right-handed. Since the introduction of the technique of intracarotid injection of sodium amobarbital (Amytal®) to determine the lateralization of speech (Wada, 1949; Wada and Rasmussen, 1960), all our left-handed and ambidextrous patients who were surgical candidates have been routinely tested in this way (Branch, Milner, and Rasmussen, 1964). It has not, however, been thought necessary to subject right-handers to these procedures, unless there was reason to suspect an anomaly of speech representation. Here the patients at risk are those few right-handers who are right-hemisphere dominant for speech and yet have a right-hemisphere lesion. In such cases (and we have several), the surgeon may be alerted by a psychological test profile suggestive of a dominant-hemisphere lesion, and preoperative Amytal tests can then be carried out. Additional safeguards come from the use of special auditory tasks (Broadbent, 1954) that have been shown to be more dependable than handedness as indicators of speech lateralization (Kimura, 1961). Although these are valuable screening tasks, they are occasionally misleading and therefore cannot take the place of the direct demonstration of speech interference that the Amytal technique provides.

Risk to Memory

In rare cases, the operation of unilateral temporal lobectomy (including the hippocampus) has produced a global and persistent amnesic syndrome that is a more serious handicap than the epilepsy itself (Milner and Penfield, 1955; Baldwin, 1956; Walker, 1957; Dimsdale, Logue, and Piercy, 1964). To account for this unexpected result in two cases of left temporal lobectomy, Penfield and Milner (1958) supposed that in each case there had been an additional and possibly more extensive lesion in the hippocampal region of the opposite hemisphere. If so, when the surgeon removed the epileptogenic but still partially functioning hippocampus on the left, he effectively deprived the patient of hippocampal function bilaterally. This notion is consistent with the fact that bilateral surgical destruction of the hippocampus and hippocampal gyrus causes severe and lasting memory loss (Scoville, 1954; Scoville and Milner, 1957).

The hypothesis of a bilateral hippocampal lesion has since been confirmed for one of Penfield and Milner's patients (P. B.) who died in 1965 of a pulmonary embolism. On section of the brain, the right hippocampus was found to be shrunken and pale, and subsequent histologic studies revealed dense gliosis in the pyramidal cell layer and to a lesser extent in the dentate gyrus. The amygdala was intact, as was the parahippocampal gyrus and the temporal cortex. On the left side (the side of operation), approximately 22 mm of the posterior hippocampus remained (Penfield and Mathieson, 1974).

These cases of memory loss have led us to look carefully for possible signs of bilateral temporal lobe abnormality in all patients being considered for an unilateral temporal lobectomy. This has meant taking into account not only EEG findings but also the psychological test pattern and any radiologic evidence of bilateral damage. As a result, we have had no further cases of persistent amnesia despite the long series of temporal lobectomies.

At first this safety was achieved only by refusing operation to any patient showing evidence of bilateral temporal lobe abnormality, even though most of the clinical attacks might seem to originate from one side. Since 1960, however, we have been testing memory in all such patients after intracarotid injection of sodium Amytal, and thus have been able to screen out the few individuals likely to incur serious memory loss if the hippocampus on one side were excised (Milner, Branch, and Rasmussen, 1962; Milner, 1972).

The main features of the psychological examination currently used at the Montreal Neurological Institute to assess seizure patients are described below, followed by a discussion of some of the specific deficits associated with particular cortical lesions. The final section reviews results obtained with the intracarotid Amytal technique and indicates how this procedure is used to protect patients from undue risk to speech or memory in the neurosurgical treatment of epilepsy.

THE PSYCHOLOGICAL EXAMINATION OF SEIZURE PATIENTS

Our present basic examination for adult patients includes the complete Wechsler-Bellevue Intelligence Scale, the Wechsler Memory Scale, the Rey-Osterrieth Visual Reproduction Test, the McGill Picture Anomaly Series, and the Chapman-Cook Speed of Reading Test. The Chicago Word Fluency Test and the Wisconsin Card Sorting Test are also given regularly, as is a paced test of object naming (Oldfield and Wingfield, 1964) designed to uncover slight word-finding difficulties in patients not otherwise dysphasic. Matched versions are available for all these tasks except the last three, so that Form I can be used preoperatively and in 1-year follow-up, Form II in the early postoperative period. This is a prerequisite for tests of learning and memory and is desirable on most speeded tasks, in order to reduce practice effects.

Some of the tasks listed above will be described more fully (with appropriate references) in the context of the specific lesions, temporal or frontal, to which they are especially sensitive. A further aim of the psychological examination is to provide more refined and if possible more quantitative measures of sensory and motor function than are offered by the standard neurologic examination, as well as to explore with specially designed auditory tasks the question of cerebral dominance for speech. These issues are discussed in greater detail below.

Tests of Sensory and Motor Function

Sensory discrimination on the hand is assessed by quantitative techniques that have been standardized on a normal control group (Semmes, Weinstein, Ghent, and Teuber, 1960; Corkin et al., 1970). The measures include two-point discrimination, point localization, pressure sensitivity, and finger position sense (Taylor,

1969), as well as a test of tactual object recognition. Similar techniques (where applicable) are now being used by Taylor to assess sensory discrimination on the face and feet in normal subjects and in patients whose epileptogenic lesions are suspected of encroaching on the face or foot area of the postcentral gyrus.

Two further somesthetic tests (one limited to the fingers of both hands, the other involving the face, forearm, and shin) make use of the technique of double simultaneous stimulation of corresponding or differing points on the two sides of the body (Loeb, 1884; Oppenheim, 1885). In all cases the tactile stimulation is well above the patient's absolute threshold for a single touch. The purpose is to look for possible "extinction," or erroneous localization, of stimuli to one side of the body in the presence of competing input to the other (Bender, 1945). Such effects can have lateralizing value in patients whose sensory status is otherwise intact.

Hand dynamometer:[1] The force of the patient's handgrip is measured by having him pull on an easily manipulable wooden handle connected to a Dillon Tensile-Type Force Gauge graduated in pounds (Stevens and Mack, 1959). This instrument is more sensitive than the standard commercial dynamometers and enables us to test young children and also to measure residual strength in most hemiparetic patients. Three readings are taken for each hand, in a balanced order, beginning with the preferred hand.

Handedness Questionnaire (Adapted from Crovitz and Zener, 1962)

Hand preference is estimated on a scale from 18 to 90 by asking the patient to indicate on a 5-point scale (right always, right mostly, both equally, left mostly, left always) which hand he would normally use to perform each of 18 common actions. For bimanual activities, half the questions refer to the action of the nonpreferred hand (e.g., "Which hand would you use to hold the nail when hammering?"). This is to control for response bias by making the subject reflect on the action before answering. If there is uncertainty about any particular item, the patient is asked to make the appropriate gesture. A score over 30 suggests that the subject is not completely right-handed and a score of over 55 indicates strong left-handed tendencies.

The patient is also questioned as to the handedness of other members of his family and as to any changes in hand use brought about by schooling or by injury. The aim throughout is to determine his basic propensities.

Auditory Tasks—A Possible Indicator of Speech Lateralization

A pure-tone audiogram is obtained on all patients as a screening procedure for performance on more complex auditory tasks. If there is no hearing loss in either ear for the frequencies of ordinary speech, then the results of dichotic

---

[1] This apparatus was built for us in the M.I.T. laboratories, by courtesy of Professor H-L. Teuber.

listening tasks (Broadbent, 1954) can provide clues to the side of speech representation (Kimura, 1961). In the traditional verbal form of this task, different strings of digits are presented simultaneously to both ears, by means of a dual-channel tape recorder and stereophonic earphones. For example, two digits, 4 and 7, might be presented together, 4 to the left ear and 7 to the right, followed half a second later by another pair and then by a third pair; after this the subject reports all the numbers that he has heard, in any order. With this competing verbal input, Kimura showed that most normal right-handed subjects, and most patients with focal epilepsy, report more digits correctly for the right ear than for the left. In contrast, most patients proven by the Wada technique of intracarotid Amytal injection (Wada 1949; Wada and Rasmussen, 1960) to be right-hemisphere dominant for speech show a left-ear superiority on the same task.

On dichotic tasks using a musical input (melodies), the direction of ear asymmetry is the reverse of that for speech (Kimura, 1964), but this is a more fragile effect and can be disrupted by the presence of a right temporal lobe lesion (Shankweiler, 1966). Both tasks are used in the preoperative examination of seizure patients, dichotic digits routinely and dichotic melodies only when some anomaly is suspected.

Testing Children with Focal Epilepsy

For normal children below the age of 11 years and for older children who are obviously retarded, the Wechsler Intelligence Scale for Children must be used instead of the adult scales and stories more appropriate to a child's interests and vocabulary must be substituted for the prose passages of the Memory Scales. Laughlin Taylor has devised two pairs of stories, matched for difficulty, which we use together with the Wechsler Associate Learning tests to assess verbal memory before and after operation in those few children whose seizure problem is severe enough to warrant surgical treatment at an early age. In such cases the Rey-Osterrieth figure can still be used to test memory for visual patterns. We have also found that alert 7-year-old children can perform the Wisconsin Card Sorting Test quite well.

Among the more specialized procedures, dichotic listening tests suitably modified for younger subjects can be used with patients of 4 years of age and upwards (Kimura, 1963b), but the sensory tests are apparently more exacting and should be omitted altogether with children below the age of 6. Between the ages of 6 and 10, sensory testing should probably be limited to measures of pressure sensitivity and two-point discrimination on the hands.

General Testing Strategy

The complete adult examination as outlined above requires a minimum of three testing sessions of approximately 2 hr each and may take longer if the patient works slowly or has many seizures. We try to carry out the preoperative tests as soon as possible after the patient has been admitted to the hospital and medication withdrawn. Because a postpneumogram headache can invalidate the test results as well as being stressful for the patient, it is advisable to delay the pneumogram until after the psychological examination, or to allow a few days for the patient to recover from it before testing begins.

Since one of the main purposes of the psychological examination is to assess memory capacities, we measure *delayed recall,* and not merely immediate recall, for both verbal and nonverbal material. For this reason we try to give the tests always in the same order, maintaining constant the amount of interfering intellectual activity that occupies the interval between immediate and delayed recall. Thus, the Logical Memory, Associate Learning, and Visual Reproduction subtests of the Wechsler Memory Scale are followed by the complete Wechsler Intelligence Scale, with delayed-recall tests given without warning at the end. Similarly, in the next session, the delayed recall of the Rey figure is obtained after a 40-min interval taken up with various verbal tasks.

GENERAL INTELLIGENCE

Preoperative and Postoperative IQ Levels in Focal Epilepsy

In patients whose focal seizures are attributable to an early static brain lesion, the preoperative IQ reflects in part the severity of the original injury. Hence, when there is gross destruction of most of one cerebral hemisphere, the IQ tends on the average to be considerably lower than in the normal population (Basser, 1962; Milner, 1969), whereas this is not true when the cortical lesion is more circumscribed (Meyer and Jones, 1957; Milner, 1958, 1965; Meier and French, 1966).

Patients retested about 2 weeks after a focal cortical resection typically show some lowering of the IQ, owing to the postoperative edema that affects areas bordering the excision; with the introduction of cortisone therapy these transient postoperative changes have become less pronounced (Rasmussen and Gulati, 1962). In any case, the 1-year follow-up study typically shows a return to the preoperative level, except for patients over 40 years old with removals near the posterior temporal speech zone of the left hemisphere.

Long-term beneficial effects of the surgery can be seen in the IQ changes of patients examined at least 5 years after operation and who are no longer having seizures. Figure 1 shows the results for 51 such subjects tested from 5 to 20 years postoperatively and classed according to the side and site of their cortical excision. Their mean age at the time of follow-up was 35 years, with a range from 18 to 59 years, and the average follow-up interval was 10 years. All patients were left-hemisphere dominant for speech.

The mean preoperative IQ for each of the groups depicted in Fig. 1 is well within the normal range and any apparent group differences are due to the small size of the sample. As expected, the IQ declines in the early postoperative period

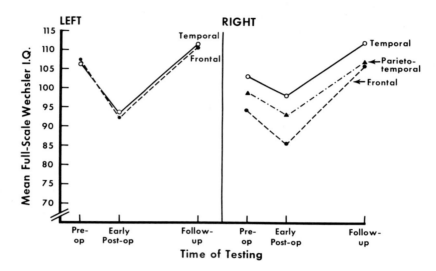

Fig. 1. Mean preoperative, early postoperative, and long-term follow-up Wechsler IQ ratings for 51 patients (38 male, 13 female), classed according to side and site of the cortical excision carried out to relieve epilepsy. (Number of cases: left temporal, 19; left frontal, 6; right temporal, 13; right frontal, 6; right parieto-temporal, 7).

for all groups but in every case the mean level attained in follow-up is significantly higher than before removal of the epileptogenic area. It is most unlikely that such consistent improvement could be an artifact of repeated testing, because in most cases no intelligence tests had been given since the first postoperative year and in some patients this was the first follow-up examination of any kind. These gains therefore suggest quite strongly that the mere presence of epileptogenic tissue disturbs the functioning of other cortical regions, although how this interictal effect is related to such factors as frequency of seizures or severity of lesion is still unknown (Blakemore, Ettlinger, and Falconer, 1966).

Stability of the IQ in Patients with Static Lesions

The preoperative test findings in our patient population indicate that whatever interfering effect the focal lesion may have must be quite stable. In those patients who have had repeated IQ testing several years apart, only minor and insignificant changes have been seen from one examination to another, even though different forms of the tests have been used. This is consistent with the fact that in the much larger number of patients who have been tested only once, the pattern of subtest scores on the Wechsler Scale rarely suggests deterioration. When one does see such a pattern, in which scores on tests requiring sustained attention and rapid problem-solving are consistently inferior to scores on tests of acquired knowledge, then one should probably suspect a chronic encephalitis (Aguilar and Rasmussen, 1960) or other progressive brain disease.

Hints to Lateralization

Up to now we have been considering only the full-scale IQ, but clues to lateralization of a focal lesion can be sought preoperatively in the difference between the Verbal IQ (based on verbal and numerical tasks) and the Performance IQ (based on spatial and other perceptual tasks). In native English-speaking subjects with temporal-lobe seizures, a difference of more than seven IQ points in favor of the Performance Scale suggests a dominant-hemisphere lesion (Meyer and Jones, 1957; Milner and Rovit, 1961), with larger differences in this direction indicating more extensive involvement of the speaking hemisphere.

The converse picture, with the Verbal IQ higher than the Performance IQ, can be seen in patients with various cortical lesions and has been a conspicuous finding in our cases of cortico-reticular epilepsy. In patients with temporal lobe seizures, a difference of more than 12 IQ points in favor of the Verbal Scale is more typical of a minor- than of a dominant-hemisphere lesion (Milner, 1958; Milner and Rovit, 1961; Meier and French, 1966).

Nonetheless, these are weak and variable effects (Meier and French, 1966). In the preoperative assessment of patients with cerebral seizures, the main value of the Wechsler Intelligence Scale is to provide a frame of reference within which to interpret performance on more specialized tasks, some of which will be discussed below.

SPECIFIC EFFECTS OF FOCAL CORTICAL LESIONS

Temporal Lobes

A comparison of the effects of left and right anterior temporal lobectomy in epileptic patients has revealed certain partial memory deficits that vary with the side of the lesion. Unlike the global amnesia that follows bilateral damage in the hippocampal zone, these milder effects of unilateral lesions are limited to a particular kind of stimulus material, though not to a particular sense modality. Thus, a dominant left temporal lobectomy impairs the learning and retention of verbal information (Meyer and Yates, 1955; Milner, 1958), whether the words are spoken or written (Blakemore and Falconer, 1967; Milner, 1967), but does not affect memory for perceptual material such as melodies, faces, or nonsense patterns. Conversely, removal of the right, nondominant temporal lobe leaves verbal memory intact but impairs the recall and recognition of visual and auditory patterns that cannot easily be coded in words (Milner, 1962, 1967, 1968; Kimura, 1963*a;* Shankweiler, 1966; Warrington and James, 1967; Taylor, 1969). Right temporal lobectomy (including the hippocampus) also retards the learning of stylus mazes, whether visually or proprioceptively guided (Corkin, 1965; Milner, 1965), whereas left temporal lobectomy does not. These findings argue for a complementary specialization of the two temporal lobes with respect to memory processes.

   The memory deficit for complex visual patterns shown by patients with right
temporal lobe lesions is often accompanied by milder perceptual deficits for the
same kind of material. These effects are subtle, and can only be demonstrated
in conditions where the normal perceptual cues are reduced. This can be achieved
by a brief exposure, as in a tachistoscope (Kimura, 1963*a*), or by eliminating some
of the contour lines (Milner, 1958; Meier and French, 1965; Lansdell, 1968).

Verbal Memory Function of the Left Temporal Lobe

   The verbal memory defect of patients with left temporal lobe seizures can
usually be detected preoperatively, and indeed such impairment can be among
the earliest signs of a left temporal lobe tumor (Meyer and Falconer, 1960).
Because the Wechsler Memory Scale is heavily loaded with verbal tests, the
Memory Quotient in these cases tends to be about 12 points lower than the IQ,
whereas no such difference is seen with a corresponding lesion of the right
hemisphere (Milner, 1958). The Memory Quotient is, however, an impure measure, being affected also by nonspecific disorders of attention, so that we prefer
to assess verbal memory by itself, using a combined measure based on the *delayed-
recall* scores for the Logical Memory and Associative Learning subtests. The
composite score is the sum of the mean number of items correctly recalled from
the two prose passages plus the number of correct word associations.
   In Fig. 2, the mean delayed-verbal-recall scores have been plotted for the
various patient groups represented in Fig. 1. It can be seen that the left temporal
lobe group is impaired relative to other groups at each testing period, and that
in long-term follow-up their performance is worse than preoperatively. These

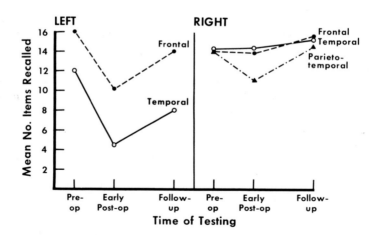

FIG. 2. Mean preoperative, early postoperative, and long-term follow-up scores for delayed
recall of verbal material (prose passages and word pairs) for 48 of the patients represented in
Fig. 1. (Number of cases: left temporal, 18; left frontal, 5; right temporal, 13; right frontal, 5; right
parieto-temporal, 7).

findings illustrate the residual selective deficits apparent years after a focal corti-cal excision, despite the fact that the IQ is now higher than before (Fig. 1) and that the seizures have been controlled. Such lasting postoperative changes run counter to the observations of Blakemore and Falconer (1967), who found sponta-neous recovery of verbal learning ability in patients tested 3 or more years after a left temporal lobectomy. It is possible, however, that this disagreement merely reflects differences in testing techniques.

Because the verbal memory impairment can be quite troublesome, it is desira-ble to give the patient some mnemonic technique by which he can compensate partially for his disability. Jones (1974) has shown that after left temporal lobec-tomy patients can learn to use visual imagery as a prop to facilitate the recall of verbal material, although they cannot be brought to the level of other patient groups by this device.

Perceptual and Memory Functions of the Right Temporal Lobe

Attention was first drawn to the perceptual difficulties of patients with right temporal lesions by their poor performance on the McGill Picture Anomalies and the Wechsler Picture Arrangement tests, both of which require the rapid comprehension of sketchy, cartoon-like drawings (Milner, 1958, 1969; Meier and French, 1966). The Picture Anomalies task is still included in our basic examina-tion of seizure patients, although the published norms (Hebb and Morton, 1943) have long since ceased to be applicable (Milner, 1958, 1969). It is retained because in our patient population a poor score on the test almost invariably denotes right temporal lobe abnormality; few patients, however, obtain low scores.

We find no evidence of verbal-memory defect in patients with well-lateralized lesions of the nondominant temporal lobe. Instead, one looks for impairment in the recall of visual patterns. Although such impairment is sometimes found in

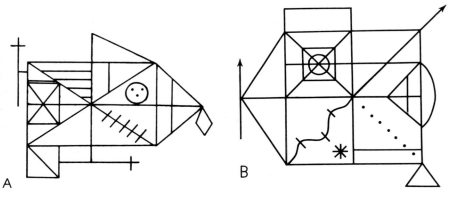

FIG. 3. (A) Rey-Osterrieth complex figure (Rey, 1942; Osterrieth, 1944). The patient copies the figure; then, 40 min later, he tries to reproduce it from memory. (B) Taylor's version of the Rey figure used in early postoperative testing (Taylor, 1969).

the delayed recall of the geometric designs in the Wechsler Memory Scale, this task is too simple for intelligent patients because the drawings can be easily verbalized. In such cases, Rey's complex figure (Rey, 1942; Osterrieth, 1944) is more apt to uncover the poor memory for visual patterns typical of patients with right temporal lobe damage. Figure 3A shows the original Rey figure, Fig. 3B the matched form designed by Taylor (1969) for use in the early postoperative examination.

As a group, patients with epileptogenic lesions of the right temporal lobe show a defective memory of the Rey figure and patients with left temporal lobe lesions do not, but the difference is less clear-cut than for verbal memory. Postoperatively the two groups diverge, with the right temporal group showing further impairment, which is still demonstrable in long-term follow-up (Taylor, 1969).

Role of the Hippocampus

Because severe amnesia results from bilateral destruction of the hippocampus, the question naturally arises as to whether the severity of the specific memory disorders seen after unilateral temporal lobectomy may not also depend on the extent of hippocampal removal. By using formally similar verbal and nonverbal tasks, Corsi (1972) has shown that these specific changes are in fact directly related to how much of the hippocampus on one side was excised in the temporal lobectomy (Milner, 1971, 1974). These results taken alone would suggest that the hippocampus should be spared unless it is clearly epileptogenic, but this must be weighed against the fact that the outcome with respect to seizures is usually better if the hippocampus is removed (Bengzon et al., 1968).

Frontal Lobes

Conventional intelligence and memory tests are notoriously insensitive as indicators of frontal lobe dysfunction, perhaps because these tests tend to be made up of unrelated items. Patients with frontal lobe lesions seem to experience their greatest difficulty on continuous, self-paced, trial-and-error tasks, in which they have to use feedback from their own previous response to guide their next choice (Luria, 1966; Milner, 1964). Maze tasks are of this kind (Porteus, 1959), and striking impairments are seen after frontal lobectomy in the learning of stylus mazes, whether proprioceptively or visually guided (Corkin, 1965; Milner, 1965). The fact that the deficits are greater after right frontal lobectomy than after left appears to reflect the spatial component in the tasks and not merely the greater size of the right frontal lesions.

Impairment of Card-Sorting after Dorsolateral Frontal-Lobe Excision

The first task on which we found impairment in patients undergoing frontal lobectomy for epilepsy was the Wisconsin Card Sorting Test (Berg, 1948; Grant

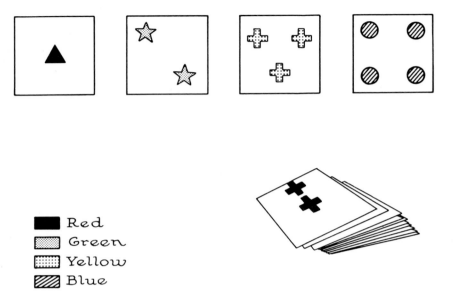

■ Red
▦ Green
▥ Yellow
▨ Blue

FIG. 4. Wisconsin Card Sorting Test, showing the material as presented to the subject. Above, the four stimulus cards; below, the pack of 128 response cards (Berg, 1948; Grant and Berg, 1948; Milner, 1963).

and Berg, 1948), and this continues to be our main diagnostic tool for evaluating frontal lobe function preoperatively. The procedure is described below in some detail, because slight changes in method can determine whether or not a deficit is seen.

Figure 4 shows the test material as it appears to the patient. He is faced with four stimulus cards, bearing designs that differ in color, form, and number, and is given a pack of response cards that vary along these same dimensions. Thus, in Fig. 4, the two red crosses on the response card correspond in color to the first stimulus card, in number to the second, and in form to the third. The patient is told that he should place each response card in front of one or other of the stimulus cards, wherever he thinks it should go, and that the examiner will then inform him whether he is "right" or "wrong." His task is to use this information to get as many cards "right" as possible. No other cues are given and a noncorrection procedure is used throughout.

The subject is arbitrarily required to sort first to color, all other responses being called wrong; once he has achieved 10 consecutive correct responses, the principle shifts from color to form, *without warning,* so that color responses are now called wrong. After 10 consecutive correct responses to form, the principle shifts to number, and then back to color once more. Testing continues until the subject has successfully completed six sorting categories (color, form, number, color, form, number) or until all 128 cards have been placed.

On this task, patients with an excision invading the dorsolateral frontal cortex tend to be abnormally perseverative, continuing to sort to a particular category, say color, long after this has ceased to be appropriate. They therefore complete fewer sorting categories than patients with lesions in other cortical areas. No impairment is found if the unilateral lesion is restricted to the orbital or inferior frontal cortex (Milner, 1963, 1964).

Not all patients with frontal lobe seizures show preoperative deficits on this task, presumably because not enough of the critical area is involved. In the early postoperative period, impairment is seen after either left or right frontal lobectomy, but in follow-up there is some recovery of function in the right-sided cases but rarely in the left. This finding is consistent with the observations of McFie and Piercy (1952) for a more traditional sorting task, and it is particularly convincing because the removals on the left are usually smaller than those on the right. It is of interest to note, however, that the functions tapped by this test are dissociable from the language functions of the left hemisphere; the same deficit is found after left frontal lobectomy in cases where an early left-hemisphere lesion has caused speech to develop on the right.

Word Fluency and the Left Frontal Lobe

A frontal lobectomy in the dominant hemisphere, sparing Broca's area, is not followed by any lasting dysphasia, and scores on most verbal tests rapidly return to the preoperative level. However, such patients show remarkably little spontaneous speech and this apparent reduction in fluency can be demonstrated objectively, both orally (Benton, 1968) and in writing (Milner, 1964, 1967). For this purpose, we include the Chicago Word Fluency task (Thurstone and Thurstone, 1943) in our routine examination. This test, in which the subject is allowed 5 min in which to write down as many words as possible beginning with the letter S and, after this, another 4 min for the harder task of writing down four-letter words beginning with C, is more discriminating than fluency tasks in which the subject has to name as many objects as possible belonging to a given category.

Central Area

Quantitative tests of sensory discrimination on the hand have uncovered lasting postoperative deficits only in patients with cortical excisions invading the postcentral gyrus and severe deficits only with a lesion of the contralateral hand area (Corkin et al., 1970). These orderly results mean that slight sensory impairment (defined always in terms of a normal control group) can provide reliable lateralizing and localizing clues to a damaged area. This is particularly useful because, with central-area lesions, EEG studies are less likely to pick up small areas of abnormality than in the case of a temporal lobe or frontal lobe lesion. The sensory deficit cannot of course define the epileptogenic area.

Corkin, Milner, and Taylor (1973) analyzed the patterns of sensory defect on the hand for point localization, position sense, and two-point discrimination in

139 patients with unilateral cortical excisions. They confirmed the high incidence of bilateral defects in point localization from unilateral lesions (Semmes et al., 1960), but found no evidence that such bilateral defects were more common after left-hemisphere lesions than after right.

CONSEQUENCES OF SEVERE EARLY INJURY TO THE LEFT HEMISPHERE

In patients who have incurred severe injury to the speech areas of the left cerebral hemisphere in infancy, language processes can be mediated by the right side of the brain but the price paid for this flexibility is a general lowering of the IQ (Hebb, 1942; Basser, 1962; Lansdell, 1969; Milner, 1974). In such cases, a radical excision of the damaged area, typically involving the anterior or posterior two-thirds of the hemisphere (Rasmussen, Chapter 10, *this volume*), rarely causes even a temporary intellectual setback and there is the expected gain on long-term follow-up if the patient's seizures have been controlled.

Figure 5 illustrates these results for a group of nine patients retested from 4 to 11 years after an extensive cortical removal from the nondominant left hemisphere. It should be noted also that the preoperative verbal-recall scores of these patients are higher than would be predicted from their low IQ ratings. This confirms the notion that some verbal processes tend to become established at the expense of nonverbal aspects of intelligence when, through early injury, one hemisphere has to take over the functions of the other side (Sperry, 1974; Teuber, 1974).

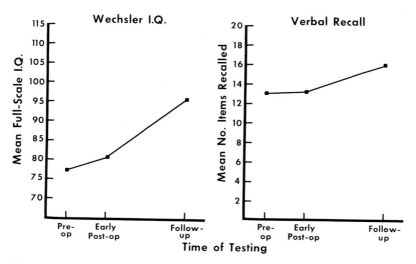

FIG. 5. Preoperative, early postoperative, and long-term follow-up mean IQ ratings and verbal recall scores for nine patients with early left-hemisphere lesions and speech lateralized to the right hemisphere. (Mean follow-up time: 7.5 yr; range: 4 to 11 yr).

PREOPERATIVE INTRACAROTID AMYTAL STUDIES OF SPEECH AND MEMORY

Indications for Tests

The Wada (1949) technique of intracarotid injection of sodium Amytal has proven a safe and valid method of determining how speech is represented in left-handed and ambidextrous patients who are being considered for brain surgery. We have by now tested over 400 patients without encountering any serious clinical complication. Yet the test must carry the slight but definite risks that accompany any puncture of the carotid artery and therefore should be used only when the knowledge it affords will have a direct bearing on the patient's clinical problem.

It is clearly worthwhile to determine in advance the lateralization of speech processes in any doubtful case, because this knowledge will enable the surgeon to decide how much epileptogenic tissue can safely be excised (Rasmussen and Milner, *in press*). Such questions arise in the case of all non–right-handed patients and in those of strongly left-handed stock, as well as in all cases of severe early trauma to the left cerebral hemisphere. Attention must also be drawn to those instances where the psychological test profile runs exactly counter to the EEG lateralization and where results of dichotic listening tasks point to right-hemisphere dominance for speech. These various signs, individually or together, constitute sufficient indication for intracarotid Amytal testing to be carried out.

Amytal tests are also performed routinely in patients who show evidence of bilateral temporal lobe damage but in whom the bulk of the seizures appear to arise from one side only. Here the clinical problem is to determine whether the major epileptogenic focus, which may involve the hippocampus, can be removed in a temporal lobectomy without risk to global memory loss.

To answer such questions properly, it is always necessary to test both hemispheres, using a standard procedure, in order that the relative contributions of the two sides to various aspects of speech and memory can be assessed. In this comparison, the right and left carotid arteries are injected on different days to ensure that no lingering generalized effect of the injection of Amytal into one hemisphere can invalidate the results obtained from the other side. All patients are tested for both speech and memory, so that each clinical group can serve as a control for the other.

General Procedure and Speech Tests

In more than 300 patients the injections have been made into the common carotid artery, using a standard dose of 200 mg of 10% sodium Amytal injected within 3 sec (Branch et al., 1964). In our current procedure, 175 mg of 10% Amytal are injected through a catheter placed well up in the internal carotid artery of one side. The speech and memory tests are then followed by a 2-cc arteriogram, permitting us to visualize the distribution of the drug and to assess the symmetry of the arterial supply to the two cerebral hemispheres. This procedure has the further advantage of providing a safer and more comfortable testing situation than the needle injection, should the patient have a seizure.

Speech is tested by asking the patient to name a number of common objects presented in quick succession and to count and recite the days of the week forward and backward, as well as by simple reading and spelling. In the typical right-handed subject with speech represented in the left hemisphere, these functions are disturbed together and recover together, but in about half the patients whom we have classed as having bilateral speech representation one finds a dissociation between disorders of naming and disorders of series repetition (Milner et al., 1964, 1966; Rasmussen and Milner, *in press*). This shows why it is important to use both kinds of task and to test each hemisphere in turn.

In analyzing the relationship between handedness and cerebral dominance for speech, we took into account the fact that many neurologic patients are mandatory left-handers as a result of severe left-hemisphere injury. In such cases, one would expect speech to be represented on the right more often than in the normal population. We therefore subdivided our 371 patients into those with evidence of early damage to the left hemisphere (109 cases) and those without such evidence (262 cases). Table 1 gives the results for the latter group.

The findings listed in Table 1 alert us again to the possibility of right-hemisphere speech representation in a right-handed patient. They also suggest that in the normal population at least two-thirds of left-handed and ambidextrous people will be left-hemisphere dominant for speech.

Table 2 shows the corresponding results for the group of patients with clinical evidence of early left-hemisphere injury. One notes again a high incidence of bilateral speech representation in the left-handed and ambidextrous group. Perhaps more striking is the fact that in 30% of the left-handers and 81 per cent of the right-handers the damaged left hemisphere is still dominant for speech. As far as we can tell, these are all patients in whom the early left-hemisphere injury spared the primary speech zones (Milner, 1974).

TABLE 1. *Speech lateralization as related to handedness in 262 patients with no clinical evidence of early damage to the left cerebral hemisphere*

Handedness	No. of cases	Speech representation		
		left	bilateral	right
Right	140	134	0	6
		96%	0%	4%
Left or mixed	122	86	18	18
		70%	15%	15%

TABLE 2. *Speech lateralization as related to handedness in 109 patients with clinical evidence of an early left-hemisphere lesion*

Handedness	No. of cases	Speech representation		
		left	bilateral	right
Right	31	25 81%	2 6%	4 13%
Left or Mixed	78	23 30%	15 19%	40 51%

Memory Testing

In interpreting the results of memory testing after carotid Amytal injection, we assume that inactivation of one temporal lobe is not sufficient to produce generalized amnesia, and therefore that no such memory loss would follow the injection unless there were a preexisting lesion in the medial temporal region of the opposite hemisphere. If there were such a lesion, then the action of the drug should produce transiently the generalized memory disorder characteristic of patients with bilateral hippocampal damage (Milner et al., 1962; Milner, 1966, 1972).

Because the effects of the drug wear off within a few minutes, only very simple memory tests can be used. Figure 6 shows the actual test items, different material being used on the two days. The pictures are taken from the Stanford-Binet Vocabulary Test and could be named easily by a young child. The sentences are equally simple, those used after the injection being taken from nursery rhymes and therefore not requiring new verbal learning.

The procedure is as follows. Before the injection is made, the patient is shown two pictures (e.g., the cup and the hand) and told to name and remember them. He is then distracted briefly by digit repetition and mental arithmetic before being asked to recall the names. Recall of the preinjection sentence is obtained similarly after an interpolated distraction.

Once this baseline has been established, the injection is made and memory testing resumed after some preliminary speech testing but before the hemiparesis has cleared. Here the critical test is for anterograde amnesia. To assess this, we show the patient two new pictures (the umbrella and the basket), asking him to name them and remember them, and give him the line from the nursery rhyme to repeat and remember. If, after distraction, he is unable to recall some of this material (as is often the case), we proceed to recognition testing, using a multiple choice procedure. Retention of the sentence is tested first by minor prompting and finally also by multiple choice.

Table 3 summarizes our findings for the first 123 patients, all of whom were tested with injection into the common carotid artery. Excluding tests carried out when all neurologic deficit had cleared and also those in which the injection had precipitated a seizure, we are left with 226 memory tests, 105 after injection into

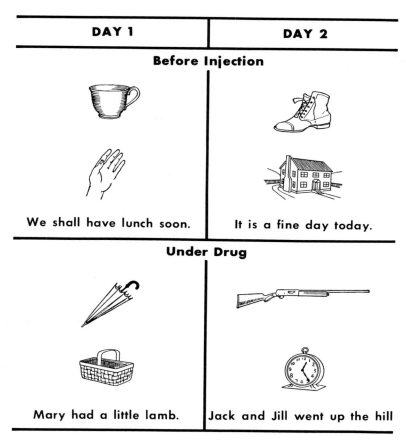

DAY 1	DAY 2
Before Injection	
We shall have lunch soon.	It is a fine day today.
Under Drug	
Mary had a little lamb.	Jack and Jill went up the hill

FIG. 6. Material used to test memory after intracarotid injection of sodium Amytal (from Milner, 1972).

TABLE 3. *Incidence of anterograde amnesia after intracarotid injection of sodium Amytal, as related to side and site of preexisting lesion*

	Locus of lesion	
Side of injection	temporal	nontemporal
Ipsilateral to lesion	0/87 (0%)	0/29 (0%)
Contralateral to lesion	18/82 (22%)	0/28 (0%)

the dominant hemisphere for speech, 111 after injection into the nondominant. If we take two recognition errors as the criterion of memory impairment, then anterograde amnesia occurred 18 times, always after injection contralateral to a known temporal lobe lesion.

Such systematic findings argue for the validity of the method, which has now been adopted, with slight modifications, by other workers (Kløve, Trites, and Grabow, 1969; Fedio and Weinberg, 1971; Blume, Grabow, Darley, and Aronson, 1973). Subsequent experience with over 50 patients tested with catheterization of the internal carotid artery has yielded only a slightly higher incidence of memory defect and has demonstrated that filling of the posterior cerebral artery is not a prerequisite for obtaining memory loss.

ACKNOWLEDGMENTS

This work has been supported mainly by the Medical Research Council of Canada through research grant MT2624 and through a Medical Research Associateship to the author. Support for the early studies came partly from U.S. Public Health Service research grant NB 02831 from the National Institute of Neurological Diseases and Blindness to the author and from Canadian Federal-Provincial health grant 604–5–89 to Dr. T. Rasmussen.

REFERENCES

Aguilar, M-J., and Rasmussen, T. (1960): The role of encephalitis in epilepsy. *Arch. Neurol.*, 22: 663–676.

Baldwin, M. (1956): Modifications psychiques survenant après lobectomie temporale subtotale. *Neurochirurgie*, 2:152–167.

Basser, L. S. (1962): Hemiplegia of early onset and the faculty of speech with special reference to the effects of hemispherectomy. *Brain*, 85:427–460.

Bender, M. B. (1945): Extinction and precipitation of cutaneous sensations. *Arch. Neurol. Psychiatry*, 55:1–9.

Bengzon, A. R. A., Rasmussen, T., Gloor, P., Dussault, J., and Stephens, M. (1968): Prognostic factors in the surgical treatment of temporal lobe epileptics. *Neurology*, 18:717–731.

Benton, A. L. (1968): Differential behavioral effects in frontal lobe disease. *Neuropsychologia*, 6:53–60.

Berg, E. A. (1948): A simple objective technique for measuring flexibility in thinking. *J. Gen. Psychol.*, 39:15–22.

Blakemore, C. B., Ettlinger, G., and Falconer, M. A. (1966): Cognitive abilities in relation to frequency of seizures and neuropathology of the temporal lobes in man. *J. Neurol. Neurosurg. Psychiatry*, 29:268–272.

Blakemore, C. B., and Falconer, M. A. (1967): Long-term effects of anterior temporal lobectomy on certain cognitive functions. *J. Neurol. Neurosurg. Psychiatry*, 30:364–367.

Blume, W. T., Grabow, J. D., Darley, F. L., and Aronson, A. E. (1973): Intracarotid amobarbital test of language and memory before temporal lobectomy for seizure control. *Neurology*, 23:812–819.

Branch, C., Milner, B., and Rasmussen, T. (1964): Intracarotid sodium Amytal for the lateralization of cerebral speech dominance: Observations in 123 patients. *J. Neurosurg.*, 21:399–405.

Broadbent, D. E. (1954): The role of auditory localization in attention and memory. *J. Exp. Psychol.*, 47:191–196.

Corkin, S. (1965): Tactually-guided maze learning in man: Effects of unilateral cortical excisions and bilateral hippocampal lesions. *Neuropsychologia*, 3:339–351.

Corkin, S., Milner, B., and Rasmussen, T. (1970): Somatosensory thresholds. Contrasting effects of postcentral gyrus and posterior parietal-lobe excisions. *Arch. Neurol.*, 22:41–58.

Corkin, S., Milner, B., and Taylor, L. (1973): Bilateral sensory loss after unilateral cerebral lesion in man. *Trans. Am. Neurol. Assoc.*, 98:118–122.

Corsi, P. M. (1972): *Human Memory and the Medial Temporal Region of the Brain*. Unpublished Ph.D. thesis, McGill University.

Crovitz, H. F., and Zener, K. (1962): A group test for assessing hand- and eye-dominance. *Am. J. Psychol.*, 75:271–276.

Dimsdale, H., Logue, V., and Piercy, M. (1964): A case of persisting impairment of recent memory following right temporal lobectomy. *Neuropsychologia*, 1:287–298.

Fedio, P., and Mirsky, A. F. (1969): Selective intellectual deficits in children with temporal-lobe or centrencephalic epilepsy. *Neuropsychologia*, 7:267–300.

Fedio, P., and Weinberg, L. K. (1971): Dysnomia and impairment of verbal memory following intracarotid injection of sodium Amytal. *Brain Res.*, 31:159–168.

Grant, D. A., and Berg, G. A. (1948): A behavioral analysis of degree of reinforcement and ease of shifting to new responses in a Weigl-type card-sorting problem. *J. Exp. Psychol.*, 38:404–411.

Hebb, D. O. (1942): The effect of early and late brain injury upon test scores, and the nature of normal adult intelligence. *Proc. Am. Phil. Soc.*, 85:275–292.

Hebb, D. O., and Morton, N. W. (1943): The McGill Adult Comprehension Examination: Verbal Situation and Picture Anomaly Series. *J. Educ. Psychol.*, 34:16–25.

Hebb, D. O., and Penfield, W. (1940): Human behavior after extensive bilateral removal from the frontal lobes. *Arch. Neurol. Psychiatry*, 44:421–438.

Jones, M. K. (1974): Imagery as a mnemonic aid after left temporal lobectomy: Contrast between material-specific and generalized memory disorders. *Neuropsychologia*, 12:20–30.

Kimura, D. (1961): Cerebral dominance and the perception of verbal stimuli. *Can. J. Psychol.*, 15:156–165.

Kimura, D. (1963*a*): Right temporal-lobe damage. *Arch. Neurol.*, 8:264–271.

Kimura, D. (1963*b*): Speech lateralization in young children as determined by an auditory test. *J. Comp. Physiol. Psychol.*, 56:899–902.

Kimura, D. (1964): Left-right differences in the perception of melodies. *Q. J. Exp. Psychol.*, 16:355–358.

Kløve, H., Trites, R. L., and Grabow, J. D. (1969): Evaluation of memory functions with intracarotid Sodium Amytal. *Trans. Am. Neurol. Assoc.*, 94:76–80.

Lansdell, H. C. (1968): Effect of extent of temporal lobe ablations on two lateralized deficits. *Physiol. Behav.*, 3:271–273.

Lansdell, H. C. (1969): Verbal and nonverbal factors in right-hemisphere speech. *J. Comp. Physiol. Psychol.*, 69:734–738.

Loeb, J. (1884): Die Sehstörungen nach Verletzung der Grosshirnrinde. *Pflügers Arch. Ges. Physiol.*, 34:67–172.

Luria, A. R. (1966): *Higher Cortical Functions in Man.* (Translated by B. Haigh.) Tavistock, London.

McFie, J., and Piercy, M. F. (1952): The relation of laterality of lesion to performance on Weigl's sorting test. *J. Ment. Sci.*, 98:299–308.

Meier, M. J., and French, L. A. (1965): Lateralized deficits in complex visual discrimination and bilateral transfer or reminiscence following unilateral temporal lobectomy. *Neuropsychologia*, 3:261–272.

Meier, M. J., and French, L. A. (1966): Longitudinal assessment of intellectual functioning following unilateral temporal lobectomy. *J. Clin. Psychol.*, 22:22–27.

Meyer, V., and Falconer, M. A. (1960): Defects of learning ability with massive lesions of the temporal lobe. *J. Ment. Sci.*, 106:472–477.

Meyer, V., and Jones, H. G. (1957): Patterns of cognitive test performance as functions of the lateral localization of cerebral abnormalities in the temporal lobe. *J. Ment. Sci.*, 103:758–772.

Meyer, V., and Yates, A. J. (1955): Intellectual changes following temporal lobectomy for psychomotor epilepsy; Preliminary communication. *J. Neurol. Neurosurg. Psychiatry*, 18:44–52.

Milner, B. (1958): Psychological defects produced by temporal-lobe excision. *Res. Publ. Assoc. Nerv. Ment. Dis.*, 36:244–257.

Milner, B. (1962): Laterality effects in audition. In: *Interhemispheric Relations and Cerebral Dominance,* edited by V. B. Mountcastle. Johns Hopkins Press, Baltimore.

Milner, B. (1963): Effects of different brain lesions on card sorting. *Arch. Neurol.*, 9:90–100.

Milner, B. (1964): Some effects of frontal lobectomy in man. In: *The Frontal Granular Cortex and Behavior,* edited by J. M. Warren and K. Akert. McGraw-Hill, New York.

Milner, B. (1965): Visually-guided maze learning in man: Effects of bilateral hippocampal, bilateral frontal, and unilateral cerebral lesions. *Neuropsychologia*, 3:317–338.

Milner, B. (1966): Amnesia following operation on the temporal lobes. In: *Amnesia,* edited by C. W. M. Whitty and O. L. Zangwill. Butterworth, London.

Milner, B. (1967): Brain mechanisms suggested by studies of the temporal lobes. In: *Brain Mechanisms Underlying Speech and Language,* edited by F. L. Darley. Grune and Stratton, New York.

Milner, B. (1968): Visual recognition and recall after right temporal-lobe excision in man. *Neuropsychologia,* 6:191–209.

Milner, B. (1969): Residual intellectual and memory deficits after head injury. In: *The Late Effects of Head Injury,* edited by A. E. Walker, W. F. Caveness, and M. Critchley. Charles C Thomas, Springfield, Ill.

Milner, B. (1971): Interhemispheric differences in the localization of psychological processes in man. *Brit. Med. Bull.,* 27:272–277.

Milner, B. (1972): Disorders of learning and memory after temporal-lobe lesions in man. *Clin. Neurosurg.,* 19:421–446.

Milner, B. (1974): Hemispheric specialization: Scope and limits. In: *The Neurosciences: Third Study Program,* edited by F. O. Schmitt and F. G. Worden. M.I.T. Press, Boston.

Milner, B., Branch, C., and Rasmussen, T. (1962): Study of short-term memory after intracarotid injection of sodium Amytal. *Trans. Am. Neurol. Assoc.,* 87:224–226.

Milner, B., Branch, C., and Rasmussen, T. (1964): Observations on cerebral dominance. In: *Disorders of Language (Ciba Foundation Symposium),* edited by A. V. S. De Reuck and M. O'Connor. Churchill, London.

Milner, B., Branch, C., and Rasmussen, T. (1966): Evidence for bilateral speech representation in some non–right-handers. *Trans. Am. Neurol. Assoc.,* 91:306–308.

Milner, B., and Penfield, W. (1955): The effect of hippocampal lesions on recent memory. *Trans. Am. Neurol. Assoc.,* 80:42–48.

Milner, B., and Rovit, R. L. (1961): The relationship between psychological test patterns and electroencephalographic findings in patients with temporal-lobe seizures. Paper read at 13th Annual Meeting, American Academy of Neurology, Detroit, Mich., Apr. 24–29.

Oldfield, R. C., and Wingfield, A. (1964): The time it takes to name an object. *Nature,* 202:1031–1032.

Oppenheim, H. (1885): Ueber eine durch eine klinisch bisher nicht verwertete Untersuchungsmethode ermittelte Form der Sensibilitätsstörung bei einseitigen Erkrankungen des Grosshirns. *Neurol. Centralbl.,* 4:529–532.

Osterrieth, P. (1944): Le test de copie d'une figure complexe. *Arch. Psychol.,* 30:206–356.

Penfield, W., and Mathieson, G. (1974): An autopsy and a discussion of the role of the hippocampus in experiential recall. *Arch. Neurol.,* 31:145–154.

Penfield, W., and Milner, B. (1958): Memory deficit produced by bilateral lesions in the hippocampal zone. *Arch. Neurol. Psychiatry,* 79:475–497.

Porteus, S. D. (1959): *The Maze Test and Clinical Psychology.* Pacific Books, Palo Alto.

Rasmussen, T., and Gulati, D. R. (1962): Cortisone in the treatment of postoperative cerebral edema. *J. Neurosurg.,* 19:535–544.

Rasmussen, T., and Milner, B.: Clinical and surgical studies of the cerebral speech areas in man. In: *Otfrid Foerster Symposium on Cerebral Localization,* edited by K. J. Zülch, O. Creutzfeldt, and G. Galbraith. Springer, Heidelberg *(in press).*

Rey, A. (1942): L'examen psychologique dans les cas d'encéphalopathie traumatique. *Arch. Psychol.,* 28:No. 112.

Scoville, W. B. (1954): The limbic lobe in man. *J. Neurosurg.,* 11:64–66.

Scoville, W. B., and Milner, B. (1957): Loss of recent memory after bilateral hippocampal lesions. *J. Neurol. Neurosurg. Psychiatry,* 20:11–21.

Semmes, J., Weinstein, S., Ghent, L., and Teuber, H-L. (1960): *Somatosensory Changes After Penetrating Brain Wounds in Man.* Harvard University Press, Cambridge, Mass.

Shankweiler, D. (1966): Effects of temporal-lobe damage on perception of dichotically presented melodies. *J. Comp. Physiol. Psychol.,* 62:115–119.

Sperry, R. W. (1974): Lateral specialization in the surgically separated hemispheres. In: *The Neurosciences: Third Study Program,* edited by F. O. Schmitt and F. G. Worden. M.I.T. Press, Boston.

Stevens, J. C., and Mack, J. D. (1959): Scales of apparent force. *J. Exp. Psychol.,* 58:405–413.

Taylor, L. B. (1969): Localisation of cerebral lesions by psychological testing. *Clin. Neurosurg.,* 16:269–287.

Teuber, H-L. (1974): Why two brains? In: *The Neurosciences: Third Study Program,* edited by F. O. Schmitt and F. G. Worden. M.I.T. Press, Boston.

Thurstone, L. L., and Thurstone, T. G. (1943): *The Chicago Tests of Primary Mental Abilities.* Science Research Associates, Chicago, Ill.

Wada, J. (1949): [A new method for the determination of the side of cerebral speech dominance. A preliminary report on the intra-carotid injection of sodium Amytal in man]. *Igaku to Seibutsugaki* [*Medicine and Biology*], 14:221–22 (In Japanese).

Wada, J., and Rasmussen, T. (1960): Intracarotid injection of sodium Amytal for the lateralization of cerebral speech dominance: Experimental and clinical observations. *J. Neurosurg.*, 17:266–282.

Walker, A. E. (1957): Recent memory impairment in unilateral temporal lesions. *Arch. Neurol. Psychiatry,* 78:543–552.

Warrington, E. K., and James, M. (1967): An experimental investigation of facial recognition in patients with unilateral cerebral lesions. *Cortex,* 3:317–326.

Advances in Neurology, Vol. 8, edited by D. P. Purpura, J. K. Penry, and R. D. Walter. Raven Press, New York © 1975.

16
Psychosocial Aspects of Neurosurgical Management of Epilepsy

E. A. Serafetinides

The purpose of this article is not to discuss the psychiatric aspects of temporal lobe or psychomotor epilepsy. This has been done recently in a number of reviews (Mignone, Donnelly, and Sadowsky, 1970; Flor-Henry, 1972; Taylor, 1972), from which two points seem to emerge: first, the difficulty at present of drawing firm and relevant conclusions regarding the relationship between epilepsy and behavior, and second, the desirability for better defined evidence in the matter. Nor is it my purpose to focus on the social aspects and prognosis of epilepsy, for which the reader is referred to Rodin's monograph (1968) and a recent special issue of *Epilepsia* (1972, Vol. 13, No. 1). Rather, as the title states, the scope of this chapter is limited to the psychosocial aspects of the neurosurgical management of epilepsy, based on two psychiatric studies of psychomotor epileptics selected and studied according to strict clinical and neurophysiologic criteria. Details of these criteria have been reported elsewhere (Falconer and Serafetinides, 1963) and in this volume (Walter, Chapter 4, and Crandall, Chapter 13), but they can be briefly summarized for present purposes in terms of long-standing seizures, mainly psychomotor, uncontrollable by anticonvulsant medication and hence investigated for possible neurosurgical treatment, i.e., temporal lobectomy. The tests employed were psychiatric interviews and—for the second study only—the Brief Psychiatric Rating Scale (BPRS) (Overall and Gorham, 1962), the Iowa Hostility Inventory (IHI) (Buss, Durkee, and Baer, 1956), and the Self-Rating Depression Scale (SDS) (Zung, 1965). The first of the two studies was conducted at the Maudsley Hospital, London, and the second at the UCLA Hospital, Los Angeles.

FIRST STUDY (MAUDSLEY HOSPITAL, LONDON)

The psychiatric features of patients who had had temporal lobectomy, as tabulated in the original report (Table 1) of the first 100 cases (Falconer and Serafetinides, 1963), reveal that "personality disorder" is the most frequent diagnosis and that of such disorders, "aggressive personality disorder" is the most common. Depression is next, followed by the diagnoses of inadequate personality and psychosis. Hysterical and anxiety symptoms complete the list. Paranoid personality disorder was found in only seven cases, but paranoid symptoms of various degrees are common, especially in patients with aggressive disorders. Many patients had more than one type of psychiatric symptom. Only four were psychiatrically normal, but it should be remembered that the sources of referral

TABLE 1. Correlation of changes in psychiatric disorders with postoperative improvement in epilepsy[a]

Psychiatric status	Group A: free or almost free of seizures (53 cases)				Group B: worthwhile improvement (30 cases)				Group C: remaining patients (17 cases)			
		Postop. rating[b]				Postop. rating[b]				Postop. rating[b]		
	Preop.	X	Y	Z	Preop.	X	Y	Z	Preop.	X	Y	Z
Normal	3	3	0	0	1	1	0	0	0	0	0	0
Personality disorder												
aggressive	19	16	2	1	7	2	5	0	10	1	6	3
inadequate	10	6	4	1	3	1	2	0	2	0	2	0
depressive	13	6	7	0	9	4	5	0	2	0	2	0
paranoid	2	1	1	0	3	2	1	0	2	0	1	1
Psychosis	8	4	4	0	4	2	1	1	0	0	0	0
Neurosis												
hysterical	4	1	3	0	3	2	1	0	4	0	4	0
anxiety	4	2	2	0	6	2	4	0	0	0	0	0
Feeble-minded	2	0	0	2	0	0	0	0	2	0	0	2

[a] Values = no. of patients.
[b] Postoperative psychiatric ratings: X = improved; Y = unchanged; Z = deteriorated. Some patients had more than one diagnosis.
From J. Neurol. Neurosurg. Psychiat. (1963), 26:154–165.

were mainly psychiatric. Postoperatively, the findings (Falconer and Serafetinides, 1963) suggested that improvement in epilepsy was usually followed by improvement in the psychiatric disorder. However, there were patients who did not show any improvement in their psychiatric symptoms despite improvement in their seizure status, and vice versa.

The patients with psychoses were classified as follows (Serafetinides and Falconer, 1962):

(1) Patients with mainly paranoid delusions and depression. These two features alternated in these patients. A general characteristic of this group was that, in both men and women who continued to have psychiatric symptoms, delusions were much less prominent than depression.

(2) Patients with schizophrenia-like psychoses. Thought disorder and blunt affect, as well as primary delusions and hallucinations, were present and, occasionally, catatonic features. Postoperatively, the psychiatric results were not good. Simmel and Counts' (1958) pessimistic prognosis regarding the effects of temporal lobectomy on patients with psychiatric disorders is clearly most applicable in this category of epileptics.

(3) Patients with acute confusional psychotic episodes. The episodes of confusional behavior, all postictal, were characterized by florid visual and auditory hallucinations and by paranoid and other delusions. Such episodes usually lasted a few days, or, occasionally, some weeks. The preceding seizure could be either psychomotor or grand mal. These patients had experienced several such episodes during their lifetime, and complete recovery was the rule. Afterwards they were usually able to recall some, but by no means all, of their psychotic experiences. This type of psychotic disturbance appears to be the one most directly related to seizures, and if the seizures can be stopped these confusional episodes can be expected to disappear. It is possible that Green's (1967) patients who showed improvement in their psychosis after a temporal lobectomy (5 out of 14) belonged to this category, or, to be more precise, had seizure-related psychotic symptoms. An update on the follow-up of these patients was reported recently by Falconer (1973).

The association between aggressive disorder and seizures was further investigated in this series by the author (Serafetinides, 1965). The criteria for defining aggressive behavior were acts of explicit physical violence. Most of the aggressive patients were young boys with an early age of onset of seizures. In the majority of cases the epileptic focus was in the left (or dominant) temporal lobe.

The laterality of the lesion as related to aggression was a novel observation. The question may be asked, is aggressiveness in cases with a lesion of the temporal lobe in the hemisphere dominant for speech related to impaired ability of learning?

Considering the significance of the dominant temporal lobe for speech (Serafetinides and Falconer, 1963) and memory (Serafetinides, 1968), it may be that a dysfunction of these structures in childhood will make learning exceedingly difficult, if not impossible. It is not unlikely, for instance, that the ability to learn "to behave," i.e., to control one's reactions according to a set of rules that have to be learned, will be deficient in such patients. In addition, one has to consider the special learning difficulties at school or work and the obvious consequences. It is also possible that impairment of learning ability due to a variety of other reasons may lead to violence or aggression as a result of unsuccessful coping behavior. Thus, this association should not be considered as epilepsy-specific or disease-specific, nor solely as an interactive process of cerebral pathophysiology and the demands of the environment, despite the observation of impaired insight during the aggressive outburst in some of the patients, which raises the possibility of some form of abnormal cerebral activity present at the time.

In a previous study (Dominian, Serafetinides, and Dewhurst, 1963), depression was the commonest psychiatric symptom in late-onset epileptics, and the absence of aggressive symptoms in such patients was noticed. This raises the possibility that age determines the form of behavior response to frustration, since, as already mentioned, aggressive epileptics are usually young.

A comparison of interictal and ictal emotional manifestations in temporal lobe patients will illustrate the complexities between seizures and psychological states. Thus, whereas aggressive behavior is the commonest interictal psychiatric manifestation in young patients, ictal "anger" or aggressive behavior associated with an obvious—in the clinical sense—seizure, is not frequent, even in patients with episodes of interictal aggression.

To ascertain this, the emotional symptoms closely associated with seizures were classified according to their timing as prodromal, warning, "ictal," and "postictal" emotions (Serafetinides, 1968). Except for the "ictal" emotions, the rest were recalled by the patients subsequent to the event; "ictal" emotions, on the other hand, being of amnesic in nature, were inferred through observation. Among prodromal emotions, aggressiveness predominated. Fear was the commonest warning and—inferred—ictal emotion. Postictally, aggressiveness again or depression were encountered with equal frequency. Most of the patients who displayed aggressiveness, as either a prodromal or postictal state, were among those showing aggressive personality disorder. However, most of the patients who had fear as warning, or ictally, were not characterized by aggressive behavior interictally.

Most of the subjects of this study, with some additional ones, were subsequently investigated by Taylor (1972) on the basis of later follow-up data and from the point of view of social adjustment. As might have been expected, patients diagnosed as behaviorally normal had the best adjustment both pre- and postoperatively, whereas psychotics and "others" had the worst. Neurotic and psychopathic patients occupied the middle of this continuum. Taylor concluded that " 'normal' postoperative mental state was associated with good preoperative adjustment in non-family relationships and at work, with infrequent grand mal epilepsy and 'falling attacks' after the operation, and was characterized by good social adjustment postoperatively, particularly in non-family relationships."

SECOND STUDY (UCLA HOSPITAL)

Thirty-one patients who had an anterior temporal lobectomy and six with depth electrodes implanted in the temporal lobes (Table 2) were studied. In addition to the tests mentioned in the introduction (i.e., BPRS, IHI, and SDS), demographic data were collected and each patient was evaluated clinically in terms of seizure relief (Serafetinides and Cherlow, *in preparation*).

Table 3 shows the BPRS results. The preoperative patients tend to manifest more psychopathology than the postoperative ones. While there are no overall male–female differences, unemployed female patients show a greater incidence of psychopathology than employed females. The BPRS shows also that male patients who can drive show less psychopathology than those who cannot.

In terms of hostility, employed female patients with a mean IHI rating of 1.0 are less hostile than unemployed female patients ($p < 0.05$). Thus, as with the BPRS and, as will also be shown with depression, employment seems to play a significant role in the psychiatric health of the female patients in this study.

Regarding depression, there seems to be a significant postoperative improvement both in lobectomy patients and those who had implantation only (Table 4).

Patients who have had a lobectomy within 2 years of psychiatric testing tended to be less depressed than those operated on more than 2 years before testing. Also, whereas recent lobectomy patients tended to show less depression than patients selected but not as yet operated on, no difference existed in this respect between

TABLE 2. *Patient population for Brief Psychiatric Rating Scale, Iowa Hostility Inventory, and Self-Rating Depression Scale*

	Right lobectomy (22 cases)	Left lobectomy (9 cases)	Implants (6 cases)
Handedness			
right	16	7	3
left	6	2	3
Sex			
male	12	6	4
female	10	3	2

TABLE 3. *Results from the Brief Psychiatric Rating Scale*

Test populations	Significance
Preoperative vs. postoperative lobectomy	$p < 0.1$
Male vs. female lobectomy	n.s.
Employed vs. unemployed females	< 0.02
Males who drive vs. males who do not drive	< 0.05

TABLE 4. *Results from Self-Rating Depression Scale*

Test populations	Significance
Preoperative vs. postoperative lobectomy	$p < 0.1$
Dixon and Mood (1946) Sign Test	< 0.03
Preoperative lobectomy vs. implants	n.s.
All lobectomy patients vs. all implants	< 0.02
Recent vs. not recent lobectomy	< 0.05
Preoperative vs. not recent lobectomy	n.s.
Preoperative vs. recent lobectomy	< 0.1
Male vs. female lobectomy	< 0.05
Unemployed males vs. unemployed females	< 0.01
Males who drive vs. females who do not drive	< 0.01
Females who drive vs. females who do not drive	< 0.05

selected patients and lobectomy patients who were operated on more than 2 years before testing.

These findings, although not sufficient by themselves, indicate a need for regular rehabilitative and psychotherapeutic follow-up if the postoperative beneficial effects on depression are to continue. Even if this is considered merely an hypothesis, such a systematic follow-up effort would provide a much needed test.

Since male postlobectomy patients were less depressed than females, and since Zung (1967) found no male–female differences in the normal and psychiatric patient populations he studied, we further analyzed these findings in terms of marital status, employment, and the ability to drive. The only significant findings were that unemployed females were more depressed than unemployed males, and also that females who could not drive were more depressed than both females who could and males who could not. These are interesting results, since they show that epileptic men do not suffer a greater loss of self-esteem than epileptic women from inability to work or drive; indeed, if anything, even less. These observations, similar in their direction to those on the role of employment in women patients mentioned above, are especially intriguing in relation to current attitudes on sex role and identity, but no easy explanations are forthcoming.

Horowitz (1970) also made a number of observations on the psychosocial functioning of epileptic patients treated by surgery, some of them from the UCLA series mentioned here. Thus he found that, even in patients who became seizure-free after operation, psychosocial improvement did not occur at once, if indeed at all, and certainly did not occur by itself. Even when "worthwhile" results were seen, they were usually preceded by a period of difficult readjustment that often lasted a year or two after operation. Horowitz emphasized the need for rehabilitative efforts, especially in this initial postoperative period when past patterns of behavior and identity, developed in association with long-standing seizures, had to be gradually undone and replaced by something new for which the patients had no ready-made models. (For additional information regarding other aspects of the pre- and postoperative evaluation of the total UCLA series of surgically treated patients, see also the chapters by Crandall and Walter in this volume.)

COMMENT

The relative frequency of aggressive, depressive, and other psychiatric symptoms in epilepsy, as these studies show, cannot be divorced from the question of mode of patient referral. However, it is worth noting that even in psychiatrically unselected epileptic populations, as with the patients of the second study (UCLA series), depression is not unusual and whatever psychopathology exists can be usually affected favorably by successful neurosurgical treatment.

Reports have also been published of beneficial effects on both seizures and behavior (especially aggressive symptoms) by other than temporal lobectomy neurosurgical procedures, i.e., uni- or bilateral lobotomies (Turner, 1963). There are also the well-documented beneficial results on both epilepsy and behavior of hemispherectomy in children with seizures, mental retardation, and behavior disorders, but this is a subject meriting separate treatment. (For details see Rodin, 1968, p. 124.)

The reader should be perhaps reminded, though, that whatever the implications of the studies discussed here turn out to be, they will be tempered in the future by our increasing knowledge of the genetic and biochemical mechanisms of both epilepsy and mental illness. In the meantime, however, as methods of referral and public and professional awareness improve, the clinician will be confronted increasingly with the problem of management of disturbed epileptic patients. Unfortunately, as I have stated elsewhere (Serafetinides, 1970), clinicians tend to avoid such patients either because they are convinced that epileptics are using their seizures to fight therapy and therapists alike, or because they claim that these patients have no insight or interest in changing, being too preoccupied with their seizures and medication. As a consequence, a vicious circle is established with the result that such patients are not getting the support they need. Prescribing and getting pills becomes the only contact between patient and doctor, and although this is not devoid of some psychotherapeutic function, it is not adequate. Thus, it is impossible to overemphasize the role of supportive therapy in the treatment of epileptics. This can take many forms, but it should always be supplemented by social rehabilitation measures. The findings in the UCLA study regarding the role of employment are relevant here. Anticonvulsant and tranquilizing medication, or neurosurgery whenever indicated, need to be carried out in such a supportive atmosphere if they are to be of maximum benefit to the patient. Indeed, few other therapeutic areas show so clearly the need and opportunity for integration of these three approaches—the biological, psychological, and social—as well as does epilepsy. Nor can the importance of developing services that exemplify this concept in a unifying and comprehensive way be overemphasized. Research into the complex nature of the relationship between epilepsy and psychosocial functioning must also be continued. To illustrate this, we have only to quote Rodin (1968), who found that "employment problems in the epileptic patients were related mainly to lower IQ, organic mental changes and behavioral difficulties." Although his population did not consist of surgically treated epileptics, his findings are pertinent, especially since, as he wrote, "it was surprising to note that seizure frequency was not related to the patients' employment state." This is in contrast to Savard and Walker's findings (1965) of overall psychosocial improvement as a result of decrease of seizure frequency or severity following temporal lobectomy, and raises questions that can be answered only through further research. Finally, to further compound a complicated issue, it is well to remember the well-documented observation (Gibbs, 1951) that, in some cases, seizure control by nonsurgical methods, i.e., by anticonvulsant medication alone, can lead to behavior abnormalities that can be corrected only by reducing such medication and thus allowing seizures to reappear.

SUMMARY AND CONCLUSION

A report on the psychosocial profile of epileptic patients treated neurosurgically obviously will vary in its details according to the source of patient referral (psychiatric or nonpsychiatric), hospital staffing patterns (availability of psychiatrists, psychologists, social workers), and philosophy of personnel (emphasis on—and capabilities for—long-term follow-up and rehabilitation). Keeping this in mind, if we contrast the two different populations of this report, some interesting points do emerge. Thus, it is safe to say that practically all epileptic patients undergoing neurosurgery display emotional problems in relation to their seizures and the way seizures and treatment interfere with their intra- and interpersonal psychic economy, regardless of mode of referral. The latter is important in relation to the form in which such emotional problems are encountered. Thus, it is likely that in psychiatric referrals aggression will be often met, but it should be remembered that aggression is not epilepsy-specific and rather might reflect a pathophysiologic disorder depending on a host of other factors necessary for its triggering. In the nonpsychiatrically referred patients depression is usual, but, since it is associated with a host of environmental factors, it is of the reactive rather than endogenous variety.

The postoperative results are in accord with this formulation. Thus, whenever neurosurgery is successful in reducing or eliminating seizures, aggressiveness is usually abolished and, if generous psychosocial support is available postoperatively, depression or other emotional symptoms are easier to handle. Unfortunately, providing such support is easier said than done. In fact, it has become fashionable and respectable to repeat it, pay lip service to it, or conclude with it, but the sad truth remains that there is a woeful lack of services and facilities in this area. Unless the acknowledgment of this reality is translated to firm and practical support, valuable and hard-won empirical knowledge will, by necessity, remain unutilized. Already, treatment strategies are capitalizing on such findings by applying them, for example, prognostically, thus excluding from useless neurosurgery patients with schizophrenia-like psychoses, or, conversely, considering confusional syndromes or aggressive symptoms as being potentially curable through successful neurosurgical treatment of the underlying seizures. What remains is the funding of well-staffed comprehensive programs of clinical research. This will permit further refinement of prognostic criteria such as those mentioned above, and, equally important, will provide a better understanding of the factors leading to a good postoperative adjustment, thus facilitating such an adjustment. That research—and its applications—in this area has been hampered by methodologic problems is true enough. However, such difficulties as not having "proper controls," being unable to "isolate the various variables involved," and others that could be easily added, should not obscure the fact that the greatest block to progress so far has been the lack of truly equipped systems for the study, treatment, and subsequent follow-up of patients. The present state of affairs is characterized by well-meaning declarations of needs, accompanied by the stark certainty that lack of funds, staff shortages, and lack of continuity will make it impossible to meet these needs. The answer is the creation of reliable, long-term follow-up and rehabilitative services, comprised of interdisciplinary teams that will consider and act upon all of these interconnected matters of patient evaluation and treatment on a continuing basis.

REFERENCES

Buss, Arnold H., Durkee, Ann, and Baer, Marc B. (1956): The measurement of hostility in clinical situations. *J. Abnorm. Soc. Psychol.*, 52:84–86.

Dixon, W. J., and Mood, A. M. (1946): The Statistical Sign Test. *J. Am. Stat. Assoc.*, 51:557–566.

Dominian, J., Serafetinides, E. A., and Dewhurst, M. (1963): A follow-up study of late onset epilepsy. II. Psychiatric and social findings. *Brit. Med. J.*, 1:431–435.

Falconer, M. A. (1973): Reversibility by temporal-lobe resection of the behavioral abnormalities of temporal lobe epilepsy. *N. Engl. J. Med.*, 289:451–455.

Falconer, M. A., and Serafetinides, E. A. (1963): A follow-up study of surgery in temporal lobe epilepsy. *J. Neurol. Neurosurg. Psychiat.*, 26:154–165.

Flor-Henry, P. (1972): Ictal and interictal psychiatric manifestations in epilepsy. Specific or non-specific? A critical review of some of the evidence. *Epilepsia*, 13:773–783.

Gibbs, F. A. (1951): Ictal and non-ictal psychiatric disturbances in temporal lobe epilepsy. *J. Nerv. Ment. Dis.*, 113:522–528.

Green, J. R. (1967): Temporal lobectomy with special reference to selection of epileptic patients. *J. Neurosurg.*, 26:589–591.

Horowitz, M. J. (1970): *Psychosocial Function in Epilepsy.* Charles C Thomas, Springfield, Ill.

Mignone, R. J., Donnelly, E. F., and D. Sadowsky (1970): Psychological and neurological comparisons of psychomotor epileptic patients. *Epilepsia*, 11:345–359.

Overall, J. E., and Gorham, D. R. (1962): The brief psychiatric rating scale. *Psychol. Rep.*, 10:799–812.

Rodin, E. A. (1968): *The Prognosis of Patients with Epilepsy.* Charles C Thomas, Springfield, Ill.

Savard, R. H., and Walker, E. (1965): Changes in social functioning after surgical treatment for temporal lobe epilepsy. *Soc. Work*, 10:86–97.

Serafetinides, E. A. (1965): Aggressiveness in temporal lobe epileptics and its relation to cerebral dysfunction and environmental factors. *Epilepsia*, 6:33–42.

Serafetinides, E. A. (1968): Brain laterality: New functional aspects. In: *Main Droite et Main Gauche,* edited by R. Kourilsky and P. Crapin, pp. 56–82. Presses Universitaires de France, Paris.

Serafetinides, E. A. (1970): Psychiatric aspects of temporal lobe epilepsy. In: *Epilepsy. Modern Problems of Pharmacopsychiatry,* edited by E. Niedermeyer, pp. 155–169. Karger, Basel.

Serafetinides, E. A., and Falconer, M. A. (1962): The effects of temporal lobectomy in epileptic patients with psychosis. *J. Ment. Sci.*, 108:584–593.

Serafetinides, E. A., and Falconer, M. A. (1963): Speech disturbances in temporal lobe seizures. *Brain,* 86:333–346.

Simmel, M. L., and Counts, S. (1958): Clinical and psychological results of anterior temporal lobec-
tomy in patients with psychomotor epilepsy. In: *Temporal Lobe Epilepsy: A Colloquium,* edited
by M. Baldwin and P. Bailey. Charles C Thomas, Springfield, Ill.
Taylor, D. C. (1972): Mental state and temporal lobe epilepsy. A correlative account of 100 patients
treated surgically. *Epilepsia,* 13:727–765.
Turner, E. (1963): A new approach to unilateral and bilateral lobotomies for psychomotor epilepsy.
J. Neurol. Neurosurg. Psychiat., 26:285–299.
Zung, William W. K. (1965): A self-rating depression scale. *Arch. Gen. Psychiat.,* 12:63–70.
Zung, William W. K. (1967): Factors influencing the self-rating depression scale. *Arch. Gen. Psychiat.,*
16:543–547.

Advances in Neurology, Vol. 8, edited by D. P.
Purpura, J. K. Penry, and R. D. Walter. Raven
Press, New York © 1975.

17
Critique and Perspectives

A. Earl Walker

The aim of this chapter is to show how the various aspects of the surgical
treatment of epilepsy fit together in a compatible whole, and to identify the
incompatible parts (problem areas) for future clarification. Little or no attempt
will be made to indicate solutions to these problems.

INDICATIONS FOR SURGERY

As one reads the present volume there is a recurring thought that a "basic
criterion for . . . surgical treatment is failure of an adequate trial of antiseizure
medical treatment to keep the attacks under control to a point where the patient
can live a reasonably normal life" (McNaughton and Rasmussen, *this volume,*
Ch. 3). Yet with each attack the risk of recurrent attacks increases and the
possibility of irreparable neuronal damage is heightened. Are these not adequate
reasons for reappraising this criterion? Although in the United States it is generally stated that medicinal therapy should be given an adequate trial before surgical intervention is advised, such a sequence may be inadvisable in some parts of
the world. In countries where essential antiepileptic medications are not available
or, if obtainable by devious means, are extremely expensive, the surgeon's scalpel
may be less costly and perhaps even less lethal than the physician's pills.[1] Now
that the dangers encountered in the operating theater are little, if at all, greater
than the risks of taking multiple anticonvulsant drugs, especially if these drugs
are administered in toxic or near-toxic doses for long periods of time, some
thought should be given to which is the more appropriate primary treatment.
No series of patients firmly diagnosed as having a type of focal epilepsy known
to respond somewhat to anticonvulsant drugs and/or to excision of the focus,
e.g., temporal lobe epilepsy, has ever been initially treated on a random basis by
medical and surgical therapies. If, as reported, patients may be relieved of their
attacks by cortical excisions in more than 85% of cases (Crandall, 1973)[2] or even

---

[1] McNaughton and Rasmussen *(this volume)* state that "Admittedly, drug therapy has many drawbacks. It is a tedious and troublesome form of treatment which usually must be continued for an
indefinite period; it can have unpleasant side effects, and it is a form of control, *not* a cure. Apart
from drug idiosyncrasies (such as rashes and hematological changes), side effects such as drowsiness
and irritability may be bothersome." Moreover, Rodin (1968) computes that 1.3% of patients under
medical treatment die each year—a figure five times the age-adjusted national death rate. He concludes that "operative results for temporal lobe epilepsy seem to be definitely superior to medical
treatment" (p. 124).
[2] This figure attributed to Crandall may require adjusting, since the results reported in the present
volume are much more in line with those given by other surgeons.

in 50% of cases (Falconer, 1965), primary surgical interventions may be less expensive in terms of loss of time from work, emotional and social adjustments, and even financially when compared with prolonged and sometimes toxic periods of costly anticonvulsive treatment. A single, well-controlled trial of this type should be considered seriously. If the 5-year results show surgical intervention to be superior to therapy with anticonvulsant drugs, a scientific basis would have been established for early operative therapy for at least one type of focal epilepsy.

At this time, however, few neurologists would admit that even the focal epilepsies should be considered surgical. Many physicians would point to the fact that the prognosis in focal epilepsies, particularly those due to trauma, is relatively good, and that with or without medication many of these patients live without significant handicap (Walker, 1957). Moreover, epilepsy clinic personnel may not think in organic terms, since the work in the clinic is often delegated to pediatricians, internists, or house staff, whose interest is in eliminating the seizure rather than ascertaining its physiologic mechanism.

PREVALENCE

Many "guesstimates" have been made of the size of the epileptic population which might benefit from surgical intervention. Robb (*this volume,* Ch. 1) calculates that 10% of epileptics are surgical candidates. These are considered to be patients with focal epilepsy. Between 65 and 75% of these focal epileptics had onset of seizures before the age of 20. Mathieson (*this volume,* Ch. 6) gives similar figures for the operated cases. However, only 40% of patients had surgical intervention before the age of 20. In fact, 67% of the cases are reached only at age 30, so that one may conclude that, on the average, medical management was tried for 10 years. In the series reported by Van Buren et al. (*this volume,* Ch. 8) the average was 16 years. Does this long period of futile therapy lessen the chances of a surgical success? This difficult question is not answered in this extensive review. Data derived from certain types of focal epilepsy, particularly post-traumatic, indicate that, in approximately 90% of cases, the epilepsy is stabilized by 5 years after the initial seizure. In temporal lobe cases this may not be the case, for after an initial series of seizures the patient may have a free interval of many years. In general, however, the status is usually established by 5 years. Further studies on this point are needed since early excision of foci seems to be desirable (Falconer, 1970).

DIAGNOSTIC PROCEDURES

Much has been written in this volume on what diagnostic procedures are appropriate for an individual who has had an epileptic attack. Usually only a few such procedures (well outlined by McNaughton and Rasmussen, and Walter, *this volume,* Ch. 3 and 4) are recommended for a patient just beginning his epileptic career, and it is only after the condition has failed to respond to anticonvulsive medical therapy that the attending physician considers carrying out more complicated procedures (angiography, pneumoencephalography, activated EEG) which might permit a precise diagnosis. Perhaps computerized axial tomography (EMI scan) will reveal significant alterations related to morphologic changes within the brain with no significant inconvenience to the patient and at relatively low cost and thus eliminate the need for some of the more disagreeable diagnostic aids. Further elaborations of the EMI scanner, using the principles of computerized axial tomography but with penetrating agents such as the proton beam, laser, or even ultrasonic waves, may make it possible to demonstrate morphologic or chemical changes in the brain.

The diagnostic examination of the patient being considered for surgical intervention is not universally agreed on. The clinical studies outlined in the present volume by McNaughton and Rasmussen (Ch. 3) and by Walter (Ch. 4) are essential. With the current emphasis on possible damage to the patient from surgical or diagnostic procedures, a very careful and precise description of the individual's preoperative physical and mental status is essential. Some of the many psychological tests used to define mental capacity and mentation are quite specific for certain mental functions, but unfortunately, a battery of these tests covering all the higher cerebral activities with the indications and limitations of each has not been developed. In the future, a high priority should be given to devising a set of practical clinical psychophysiologic tests for evaluation of patients about to undergo brain surgery. Such function-specific batteries would be particularly desirable for patients on whom a cortical resection for epilepsy is planned. They not only would provide standardized basal psychophysiologic data which could be used for comparisons of results in different clinics, but also would be invaluable for serial evaluation of the patient's postoperative state. They would also provide a means of testing the suspicion that some deterioration does occur in patients after cerebral lesions—morbid or surgical—especially in the later years of life (Walker, 1972).

If a surgeon is going to perform a procedure for epilepsy that has some risk, he should verify the clinical pattern of the seizures in terms of their manifestations, variations, and frequency. This may require induction of a seizure by an analeptic agent as outlined by Gloor (*this volume,* Ch. 5). This is best done in collaboration with the electroencephalographer a short time before the operation when the patient or parents have agreed to surgery. At that time, if it has not been done previously, a coded timetable of each type of seizure should be made, noting severity and frequency. In the future, a uniform plan such as used by Van Buren et al. (*this volume,* Ch. 8), should be developed for the accurate recording of seizures.

ELECTROENCEPHALOGRAPHY

Scalp electroencephalography has been pushed almost to its limits in diagnosising and localizing epileptic lesions, and it seems unlikely that, even with refinements in recording techniques, a great deal more can be obtained from visual readings of EEG tracings. However, several adjuncts to electroencephalography have not been fully explored. Computerized analyses of frequency, power, and time may compress events into readily recognized patterns of EEG complexes which are difficult to perceive by visual inspection. A compressed spectral analysis, even when carried out on only a few leads from the scalp, often provides significant data not previously suspected. A multiple toposcopic survey of DC potentials produces maps which may be of great localizing value. The changing pattern of these charges, thus far little explored, may give some insight into the propagation of epileptic activity. Certainly, future studies of these factors should bring forth very interesting dynamic patterns. Physical (e.g. hyperventilation, heat, cold) and neuropharmacologic activation using these recording techniques may be productive.

Depth recording may be carried out acutely or chronically. The acute studies carried out in the course of a craniotomy and cortical exploration which some surgeons refer to as depth recording are subject to a number of objections. Not infrequently, records made from recently implanted electrodes contain artifactual material which persists for a day or two after insertion of the electrodes. This may take the form of injury potentials or suppression of activity. Consequently, the significance of spiking in these records, especially fast spikes, is sometimes questionable. In addition, the short sample obtained, usually under some type of anesthesia, may not be representative of the waking activity of the anatomic structure being recorded. Chronic depth recording from electrodes inserted stereotactically or by hand under X-ray control, and left in place for days or weeks, not only allows artifactual material to resolve but also gives time for multiple recording sessions under many natural or artificial conditions. Records made with the patient awake and in different stages of sleep may be studied and correlated with states of consciousness and behavior. Various activation procedures may be used to induce electrical or clinical seizures. Each electrode may be stimulated electrically while the patient is being controlled clinically or by psychological testing. If portions of each of these records are put on tape, a subsequent analysis may be made for various factors.

Depth recording has been slow in gaining acceptance. Because of ethical considerations, the neurosurgeon has hesitated to insert a foreign and potentially destructive instrument into what may be normal tissue. The material of which the electrodes are made is an important consideration,[3] and where the electrodes should be inserted is a question which has been debated for years and even at this time is far from settled. Whether they should be confined to suspect areas— for example, the amygdala or hippocampus—or whether they should be placed in other areas that may be on the borderline of the epileptic focus so that the limits of the firing zone may be ascertained is a moot point. Some investigators have favored random placement of the electrodes in the approximate site of a

---

[3] This problem has been recently discussed in detail by McFadden (1969).

focus, and others have equally strongly advocated precise stereotactic implantation of electrodes within a nuclear structure. When such depth electrode studies should be made, is another unanswered question. Should they be done early in the course of diagnostic studies of a patient with focal seizures or should they be deferred until the patient has been selected as a candidate for surgical intervention? Again, how long should the electrodes be left in place, and what would be considered an adequate electrographic study to determine the preciseness of a focus? Most surgeons working with epileptics have hesitated to leave their electrodes implanted for more than a few weeks. Yet Heath (1964) has followed depth activity for months in some of his psychotic patients. There is no doubt that the activity in the depths of the brain does change over time, and that in order to obtain an adequate profile the recording should be obtained for much longer periods than is currently the practice.

In the future, one would certainly wish to telemeter the EEG to permit the patient to move around freely as the recording is being taped. At the same time, some means should be developed for videotaping the activity of the individual during the telemonitored record.

HEREDITY

Heredity, so prominently featured as a cause of epilepsy a century ago, has come full circle: with new support from electroencephalography, it has regained its prime place among the etiologic factors. Lennox's demonstration (1951) of greater familial tendencies to epilepsy in patients with generalized epilepsy than in those with focal epilepsy confirmed Foerster's (1925) concept of "Krampf-bereitschaft." The evidence for a genetic factor was most clearly presented for the spike-wave epilepsies by Metrakos and Metrakos (1961), who showed that approximately 37% of the siblings of probands with spike-wave epilepsy have this EEG trait, compared with 5% of controls. Perhaps more pertinent to the subject of this monograph was Bray and Wiser's (1965) demonstration that EEG abnormalities occurred in a high proportion of siblings of certain cases of temporal-central focal epilepsy. Further evidence came from Anderman et al. (1972), who studied the families of epileptics operated on for focal epilepsy. She found a significantly higher prevalence of EEG abnormalities among the siblings, parents, and offspring of the operated epileptics than among the same class of relatives of a control group.

With this mounting mass of evidence, the question is not whether hereditary factors play a role, but rather what genes are involved and what are the genetic mechanisms?

The neurosurgeon of the future may well depend on knowledge of his patient's heredity as one of the criteria in selection of cases. The presence of an autosomal dominant genetic factor in the family and probably in the patient may indicate an unsatisfactory surgical result. Certainly this is a promising avenue to explore.

PREOPERATIVE MEDICAL MANAGEMENT

With the introduction of more drugs and methods for determining their blood levels, the medical management of epilepsy has become quite complex. Although theoretically such pharmacologic control is quite desirable, in practice it has been rather difficult to obtain with each of these drugs. This is particularly true in children, in whom blood levels tend to fluctuate rather rapidly. Little reliable evidence defines the time a patient must maintain a therapeutic blood level in order to have an adequate trial of the drug. Obviously, some balance must be established between the desirability of an optimal test of medical management and the risk of epileptic disruption of neurons if medical therapy is carried on ineffectively for long periods of time.

THE SURGERY FOR EPILEPSY

Development of Surgical Intervention for Focal Epilepsy

It is natural that surgeons base their operative procedures on their concepts of the mechanisms involved in the epileptic attack. Since these concepts have varied considerably in the last half-century, they are worth reviewing briefly.

Sir Victor Horsley (1886), who is credited with introducing modern surgery for focal epilepsy, had seen the limbs of animals convulse upon stimulation of the cerebral cortex. As a result, he considered the epileptic area in man to be a spasmic center which, when excited, would cause twitchings of the appropriate parts of the opposite side of the body. Horsley, having no diagnostic instrumentation other than stimulating electrodes that delivered a very crude form of electrical excitation, was limited in his surgical endeavors to patients who had obvious, usually traumatic, lesions of the brain. Accordingly, with the patient under general anesthesia, he exposed the cerebral scar, stimulated it in the hope of finding an area from which he could reproduce the spontaneous convulsive manifestations, and then excised the responsive area and associated scar to white matter.

It required the use of pneumoencephalography, introduced a quarter of a century later by Dandy (1918), for Foerster (1925) to conceive of the ventricle distorted by the craniocerebral scar as wandering and inducing seizures by its tug on the cortex. Penfield's observation (1927) that a core resection of tissue to the ventricle produced a lesser scar than a simple incision of the cortex seemed to confirm Foerster's hypothesis. Accordingly, when Penfield went to Breslau to study with Foerster, he brought evidence that the tug on the cortex was epileptogenic and that resection of the epileptic scar to the ventricle would prevent the reformation of a cicatrix. Their experiences were reported in a paper in *Brain* (Foerster and Penfield, 1930). It was another decade before Penfield, based on Jasper's cortical electrical recording (electrocorticography) in the operating theater, concluded that the abnormal neuronal population about the scar was responsible for the seizure manifestation and not the cicatrix itself. Accordingly, he sucked away this abnormal cortex without resecting the scar to the ventricle.

Just after World War II, Fuster, Gibbs, and Gibbs (1948) showed abnormal spiking activity in the anterior temporal region in many cases of temporal lobe epilepsy. Accordingly, Frederick Gibbs persuaded Bailey (Bailey and Gibbs, 1951) to resect the lateral aspect of the temporal lobe in these cases. The resection was mainly confined to the cortex and white matter and only rarely compromised the anterior part of the temporal horn. There was fear that should the medial-temporal structures be damaged, serious side effects such as those seen after temporal lobectomy in the monkey might ensue (Klüver and Bucy, 1939). At about the same time, from South Africa, came a report by Krynaur (1950) of successful hemispherectomy for infantile hemiplegia and intractable seizures. This remarkable feat challenged and stimulated neurosurgeons throughout the world to perform a relatively large number of hemispherectomies.

With better localization of the seizure activity through surface electroencephalography and electrocorticography, it became apparent that not only the lateral surface of the temporal lobe but the medial-temporal structures were responsible for many of the psychomotor attacks. Accordingly, Bailey's operation was embellished by removing the anterior half of the temporal lobe including the amygdala and anterior part of the hippocampus. A number of neurosurgeons advocated this procedure and attested to its value. These included Morris (1956) in Washington, Green et al. (1951) in Phoenix, Falconer (1965) in England, and Walker (1967) in Baltimore.

It was in 1947 that Spiegel, Wycis, and co-workers (1947) introduced human stereotactic surgery, a technique which was enthusiastically pursued by neurosurgeons in many parts of the world. About that time Williams (1953) reported that with depth electrodes he was able to pick up spikes in the medial thalamic nuclei in patients suffering from petit mal. On the assumption that destruction of a center intimately concerned with the composition of the spike-wave complex might interfere with the epileptic process, Spiegel and Wycis made lesions in the medial thalamic nucleus with the aid of their stereotactic instrument.

The demonstration of preferential pathways of the seizure spread from cortical epileptogenic foci stimulated a number of European surgeons who had considerable experience in stereotactic surgery to destroy a subcortical focus, or relay nucleus or pathway. Subsequently, stereotactic operations for epilepsy have involved almost all structures of the brain including those suspected of being the focus and those suspected of participating in the propagation of the seizure. The destructive agent varies greatly from a mechanical leucotome to wax, thermocoagulation, or cryothermic techniques, to mention but a few.

Current Concepts

The papers in this volume cover admirably the general concepts, particularly those of the Montreal school, of the surgery for epilepsy. The consideration given to defining the surgical population may be unnecessary at this time since there are surgical procedures for almost every type of intractable epilepsy. The problem may be more in deciding which procedure offers the greatest prospect of relief with the least risk. The new types of surgical therapy based on ablation or stimulation of the inhibitory systems so as to decrease the general epileptogenicity of the cortex offer succor even for the so-called generalized epilepsy. For this reason, the surgeon might well be called in to see every epileptic who is not responding well to adequate doses of medication. This is particularly true for younger individuals in whom it now seems fairly well established that repeated attacks will cause deterioration of mental capacity. Although it is logical to assume that if one could eliminate or decrease the attacks the deterioration could be prevented, long-term studies are needed to determine which of the current surgical procedures will give the best results in children.

The pathologic state may prove to be the most important factor in determining the type of surgical intervention. If the pathology is extensive, a wide surgical extirpation may be necessary, for example, the hemispherectomies for intractable seizures in infantile hemiplegics which greatly benefited these young children from the standpoint of both the epilepsy and the behavioral alterations. In these infantile hemiplegics the contralateral hemisphere was found to be diffusely scarred.

In considering the types of surgery that may be used, certainly one has to acknowledge the marked technical advances in stereoencephalotomy in recent years. This technique has become so well standardized that it may be used in temporal lobe epilepsy as a preliminary therapeutic test to determine whether a stereotactic lesion is satisfactory or whether the excision of the lobe is necessary to give a good result. There is still a question as to whether a partial resection such as that achieved by a stereotactic procedure is as satisfactory as the complete removal of a lobe. Rasmussen (*this volume*, Ch. 7), discussing this problem in his excellent survey, states that the mass of tissue is related to the result. However, his cases are based on a particular type of cortical resection and he had no significant group of cases with partial resections. Van Buren et al. (*this volume,* Ch. 8) conclude that larger resections of the temporal lobe give somewhat better results. Yet his partial resections of a lobe were a motley group; his complete resections, which included the superior temporal gyrus, were more extensive than many neurosurgeons believe necessary: they remove the medial temporal structures but leave the first temporal gyrus, and their results in terms of alleviation of seizures are as satisfactory as those reported here by Van Buren et al. with more extensive resections.

Anesthesia for Epilepsy Surgery

The introduction of new anesthetic agents has greatly lightened the load of the neurosurgeon, not only in his diagnostic procedures, but also in his cortical resections for epilepsy (Michenfelder et al., 1969). The neuroleptanesthetic drugs have given the anesthesiologist agents capable of producing a satisfactory neurosurgical anesthesia. These agents may be used as a sedative or analgesic to provide adequate narcosis for the infiltration of an area with a local anesthetic, as a total anesthetic yet with the patient awake and alert, or as a component of a general combined anesthetic.

For cerebral operations, the neuroleptic agent of choice is droperidol, which blocks spontaneous and acquired movements and produces a transient state of cataplexy (Marshall, 1973). Of the analgesic agents, synthetic morphine-like substances, fentanyl is the most effective. It acts on the thalamus, hypothalamus, and reticular system producing analgesia, respiratory depression, suppression of cough reflexes, and cholinergic symptoms. These agents provide protection from traumatic and neurogenic shock by reason of the blocking effect of droperidol and the strong analgesic action of fentanyl. For neurosurgery, they give a remarkable circulatory stability. When vocal cooperation is desired during the operation, they are indispensable.

For excision of a cortical focus, a combination of these drugs and local infiltration of the incision provides a suitable state not only for electrocorticography but also for mapping motor, sensory, or psychic fields with the patient's cooperation. The disadvantages which led many neurosurgeons to abandon local anesthesia are eliminated by the neuroleptic agents, which allow the surgeon to work with an alert and cooperative patient. These drugs elevate intracranial pressure little, if at all, and have very minimal effects on the electroencephalographic pattern.

Control of Intracranial Pressure

A significant advance in neurosurgery is the ready control of intracranial pressure, both before and during operation. The use of corticosteroids (Decadron®), neuroleptic agents for induction and intubation, a free airway, adequate oxygenation, elimination of coughing, and correct positioning of the patient all lessen the risk of hypertensive episodes. In addition, the availability of agents and techniques to control increased intracranial pressure should it develop make it possible to maintain a suitable operating environment. Induced chemical hypotension, hypothermia, intravenous administration of hypertonic agents, drainage of cerebrospinal fluid, and controlled passive hyperventilation provide a variety of means of reducing hypertension. During operations, hyperventilation, probably the most effective, is used routinely.

The postoperative control of intracranial pressure relies to a considerable extent on proper fluid balance and the prevention of complications such as local cerebral edema or hemorrhage. In most cases, after a cortical resection for epilepsy, a slight restriction of fluids is desirable, but within 2 or 3 days, if the patient is taking fluids by mouth, no limitation is necessary. The patient who recovers from anesthesia and then in 24 or 36 hr becomes drowsy and unresponsive poses a problem. The possibility of a bleed in the extra- or subdural space haunts the surgeon. The repeated use of echoencephalography beginning as soon as the patient returns from the operating room is a simple means of determining any displacement of temporal or midline structures (Walker and Uematsu, 1973). It is even simpler than the dural clip which many neurosurgeons apply so that antero-posterior skull roentgenograms may demonstrate its displacement from the inner table should a hematoma develop.

Surgical Technique

The techniques employed in the resection of the lesion are mentioned by Feindel (*this volume,* Ch. 14). Improved instrumentation for operating has increased the dexterity of the surgeon. The use of optical magnification has made precision surgery possible in a bloodless operative field. Better methods of hemostasis, such as those afforded by the bipolar coagulating forceps, and hypotension have lessened the need for massive transfusions, so common yesteryear. Perhaps one of the most important of the questions raised relates to whether or not one must stimulate and record from the cortex in the case of a temporal or frontal lobe epilepsy. Is it sufficient to resect the damaged area? A number of surgeons have stated that electrocorticography did not give them much information. Falconer (1965) places relatively little reliance on the electroencephalographic findings. In more recent years we, too, have relied less on electrocorticography than some years ago.

Postoperative Anticonvulsive Medication

The question of length of postoperative anticonvulsive therapy was raised by a number of authors. Four problems are at issue: pretreatment of an epilepsy, prevention of the development of another epileptic focus after operation, prevention or eradication of a secondary focus some distance from the primary site, and treatment of the original epilepsy if the focus is not removed.

With respect to pretreatment, administration of anticonvulsant drugs over a period of 6 months to 2 years should reduce the probability of seizures to 8 and 4%, respectively. However, therapy to prevent the development of an epileptic focus poses a more difficult problem which relates to the tissue involved (amygdala, hippocampus, temporal cortex, etc.), the extent of the pathology, and the type of lesion (ischemia, thrombotic, or hemorrhagic). A relatively small lesion might have its epileptic potentialities eliminated by anticonvulsive therapy for a short period of time—say 3 to 6 months—whereas a more extensive scar might require a much longer period of time.

PSYCHOSOCIAL ASPECTS

There is no doubt that the well-being of the patient depends to a very considerable extent on his or her reintegration in family, vocational, and community life. Whether or not the seizures are all eliminated, the operative experience and the cerebral readjustment to the loss of some brain tissue require counseling and guidance for some time after operation. The patient must rely on his or her medical attendants for this, because the family is usually not well informed of the eventualities. Serafetinides (*this volume,* Ch. 16) states that in Falconer's first 100 cases preoperatively, only four were psychiatrically normal. Postoperatively, with lessening of the epileptic diathesis, the mental disorders were improved. However, in other series taken from a more general population, fewer patients had abnormal reactions.

In our experience, the postoperative psychosocial adjustments related to acute postoperative confusion—usually mild and of short duration, personality changes with lessening of aggression and mental rigidity, depression, sexual alterations, and work adjustment.

Acute Postoperative Confusion

Following operation, disorientation, hallucinations, delusions, changes in mood, and confusion are rare. When they occur, the patient has usually had such disturbances associated with the epileptic attacks. Occasionally they are a manifestation of a postoperative hematoma or subarachnoid hemorrhage. Severe headaches are a common complaint. Rarely have these disturbances required transfer to a closed psychiatric ward. They usually recede in a few days with good nursing care and, occasionally, tranquilizers.

Personality Changes

Even a few days after operation, relatives and nursing attendants will comment that the preoperative aggressiveness which made life difficult or unbearable for the patient's associates has changed to a more pleasant placidity. This is manifested by a lessened irritability and a more outgoing personality. On returning home, the patient's easier reaction to life and his associates is combined with a lessening of his mental rigidity. He has both a greater interest in and a warmer feeling toward his family. In general, he is a much nicer person.

Depression

Some months after the cortical resection, regardless of the clinical result, a reactive depression may occur related to difficulties in assuming responsibilities and obtaining a suitable job in an environment which is somewhat prejudiced because of the previous seizure state. Psychological and vocational counseling may prevent catastrophic reactions such as suicide.

Sexual Alterations

The previously hyposexual individual may find, about 6 weeks after a successful operation, that he is having a sexual awakening. This is of a global type, and is not solely related to increased libido and a craving for copulation. It occurs in both men and women and may increase over a period of months. Rarely does it assume maniacal states; perhaps it is epitomized by the request of a nice, quiet housewife who stated she was bringing in her husband at the next clinical visit so I "could tell him it was all right to do it twice a night."

However, the occurrence of this sexual awakening in young people who have previously had no interest in sexuality is alarming to patients and associates. Counseling as to what might be expected and the administration of sedatives may tide the patient over until an adjustment is made.

Work Adjustment

Not a few patients who have had good surgical results fail to make an adequate work adjustment. Some cannot obtain a suitable job and others find it difficult to maintain their occupation. Considerable and constant counseling is necessary in the first 2 years after operation.

REPORTING OF RESULTS

The results of surgical therapy for epilepsy have been critically received from the beginning of the modern era. Harken to the words of Victor Horsley, written in 1890: "Personally, I do not think that a final answer can be given on the permanency of the freedom from epilepsy until each case has been observed for five years." A number of authors (Meyers, 1954; Thomas, 1974) state that a patient should be off medication for a year or more before the epilepsy is considered arrested. Although many patients stop their medication on their own after freedom from seizures for a year or two, others do not wish to discontinue medication, asserting that they get nervous, apprehensive, and irritable without some sedative. I have patients, free of all seizure manifestations for more than 20 years, who refuse to eliminate their anticonvulsant drugs. In all other respects these patients are leading a normal life. It would seem that the personality rather than the convulsive state is being treated, and that the epilepsy should be considered arrested. Perhaps these individuals have developed a dependency akin to narcotic addiction. However, rather than attempt to force their withdrawal, it seems wiser to allow them to take minimal, often homeopathic, amounts of the medication. This is one of the problems for future resolution.

Not only is the duration of the desired follow-up questioned, but also the basis of "freedom from epilepsy."[4] While minor paroxysmal phenomena resembling

---

[4] In this book, seizure control is variously defined.

Rasmussen (Ch. 7): "A patient who has only auras" (defined as a sensory phenomenon that is without a motor manifestation, that does not interrupt the patient's mental activity or contact with the environment, and that cannot be detected by an observer) ". . . is considered seizure-free. . . ." He also classifies the attacks as minor and major, although, in his tables, the latter classification is not followed.

Van Buren et al.: A single rating of 1 (no seizures), 2 (seizure incidence significantly decreased),

the aura of the patient's preoperative seizures, but without loss of consciousness, may not be significant from the patient's point of view, nevertheless they are probably larval seizures. Yet most authors discount such attacks and omit consideration of them in follow-up analyses (Rasmussen and Jasper, 1958; Rasmussen, *this volume*, Ch. 7). One might agree with Rasmussen that a "patient who has only auras . . . is considered seizure-free in this follow-up analysis, since the social impact of these brief sensory episodes is not significantly greater than the presence of persistent spiking in the EEG." By the same logic, shouldn't the occasional twitching of the thumb, the flash of light in a visual field, and similar minor evidences of paroxysmal localized cerebral excitation also be excluded?

The classification of a "success group" as "completely free of seizures after the first year or almost so, i.e., having not more than two or three seizures in any one year" (Crandall, *this volume*) is misleading, for readers and reporters are apt to omit the qualifying phrase. A patient who has one seizure a year suffers from all the fears, stigmas, and limitations of any epileptic, but those who have not had an attack for years are neither epileptic nor so stigmatized. I would make a plea that the term "freedom from seizures" or "seizure-free" be applied on a pragmatic basis only to those patients who have no manifestations of epilepsy that render them unable to take care of themselves. This would provide a definition which could be applied medically, vocationally, socially, and on the road. An individual who, every year, has one or two attacks which disable him even momentarily should not be engaged in certain types of industry and should not drive a car. But the person who has had no such episodes in the first 2 years after operation has approximately two chances out of three of having no further attacks over a 5- to 10-year period (Van Buren et al., *this volume*, Ch. 8, Table 8). Such individuals, because they take better care of themselves than the average person, constitute no greater risks at work, play, or on the road than comparable persons in the general population (Walker, 1957).

THE FUTURE

In the future, the neurosurgeon might adopt the philosophy that he should perfect the current approaches to epileptic surgery so that his results are 100% cures. But the data presented in this monograph, as Van Buren et al. state, suggest that regardless of better selection of patients and improved surgical techniques and postoperative care, the end results may not be perfect. On the other hand,

---

3 (seizures unchanged), and 4 (seizure incidence increased). However, seizure is not defined nor is "significantly decreased."

Crandall: Group A (success group)—either completely free of seizures after the first year or almost so, i.e., having not more than two or three seizures in any one year; Group B (worthwhile improvement)—improved by at least 50% in frequency of attacks; Group C (unimproved group)—frequency of seizures is the same or worse. This classification has been used by a number of authors including Rasmussen and Jasper (1958) and Falconer (1965). Rodin's (1968) comment, after reviewing the surgical results of anterior temporal lobectomy, that "different criteria must have been applied by various authors in regard to seizure freedom" is quite appropriate.

the surgeon may seek new methods of attacking the problem that may widen the scope and effectiveness of his endeavors. The future may be gauged to some extent by the past. For what it may be worth, the current state of epilepsy surgery as indicated by a review of the world literature for the past 5 years is given in Tables 1 and 2.

It seems that the target for epilepsy surgery will continue to be the temporal lobe. Not only are more hospitals doing this type of surgery, but many more temporal lobectomies are carried out than any other procedure. Although some surgeons advocate the trial of a simple stereotactic operation on the amygdala before excising the whole lobe, this policy is not being widely accepted. The number of hemispherectomies will probably level off as fewer cases become available.

In the United States, surgery for epilepsy—cortical resections, lobectomies, and hemispherectomies—has been performed only in a few large clinics. This reflects,

TABLE 1. *Operations on the cerebral hemispheres for epilepsy (world literature in the past 5 years)*

Targets	No. of reports	No. of cases
Temporal lobe	15	583
Hemisphere	10	161
Corpus callosum	2	3
Fornix	1	1
Cortical foci	1	916[a]
Miscellaneous	4	1191[a]

[a] The majority are probably temporal lobectomies but the numbers are not given.

TABLE 2. *Types of stereotactic surgery for epilepsy (world literature in the past 5 years)*

Targets	No. of reports	No. of cases
Amygdala	10	159
Thalamus	4	24
Forel—H	3	54
Fornix	2	33
Internal capsule	1	7
Putamen	1	69
Miscellaneous	3	576[a]

[a] Mainly thalamotomies and amygdalatomies but the numbers are not given.

in part, the busy surgeon's reluctance to spend long hours in the clinic working up an epileptic case and in the operating room searching for an elusive epileptogenic focus; in part, the neurologist's desire to exhaust all medical therapy; and in part, the prejudices of some physicians who refuse to admit a therapeutic failure and boast that they never refer a case for surgery. Hence, the amount of epilepsy surgery performed in the U.S. has not increased appreciably in the past few decades. Even stereotactic surgery for epilepsy, introduced by Spiegel et al. (1947), never gained the popularity in the U.S. that it has attained in some other countries.

The recent success in pacemaker instrumentation has led to a resurgence of interest in stimulation of inhibitory mechanisms as a means of relieving seizures. Initial reports of cerebellar stimulation are promising, but more cases must be studied over a 5-year period to assess the value of this technique. Chronic intermittent stimulation of the intralaminar system, another inhibitory center, has been tried for pain and will unquestionably also be used for intractable epilepsy. Great caution must be used in interpreting the results, for the dice of the Gods are loaded. A year ago, I inserted a stimulating device in the midline cerebellar nuclei of a 16-year old girl who was having many psychomotor seizures daily and occasional major attacks. After a few months, the generalized seizures stopped and the automatisms were reduced to an occasional episode. The patient and her parents were delighted at the result—a result that was not due to the cerebellar excitation, for the connecting wire to the electrodes broke 2 weeks after insertion!

A number of problems seem likely to beset the neurosurgeon operating to treat epilepsy in the future. One of these relates to the medico-legal aspects of his procedure. Although most adults are intelligent and able to understand the nature of the operation and give informed consent, this is not the case with some deteriorated adults and with children. The question must be raised as to how such individuals may be protected from unnecessary, risky, or experimental procedures and yet have the benefits of modern surgical intervention for incapacitating seizures. The current policy of the Department of Health, Education, and Welfare (Brown et al., 1973) recognizes three cardinal principles: that the rights and welfare of the subjects involved are adequately protected, that the risks to the individual are outweighed by the potential benefit to him, and that informed consent is obtained in an adequate and appropriate manner.

The basic elements of an informed consent are as follows:

(1) a fair explanation of the procedures to be followed, including identification of those which are experimental;

(2) a description of the attendant discomforts and risks;

(3) a description of the benefits to be expected;

(4) a disclosure of appropriate alternative procedures that would be advantageous for the subject;

(5) an offer to answer any inquiries concerning the procedures; and

(6) an instruction that the subject is free to withdraw from the project at any time.

This assumes that the subject is himself capable of giving an informed consent. Who may consent for the patient when he is incapacitated? Under what circumstances can a substitute or agent consent instead of the parent? May parents ever consent to a risky procedure on behalf of a child when the benefit is primarily for science and the benefits for the child are minimal? Such questions may best be resolved by local hospital committees composed of physicians in the specialty of the case, social workers, and other medical personnel as seem desirable, meeting for the express purpose of protecting the subject's rights. If this group approves the procedure, it is presented to the subject's personal physician, personal lawyer, and immediate kin with periods of time being allocated for reflection, questioning, and debate before consent is given.

Surgery for epilepsy seems likely to be involved in the current controversy regarding psychosurgery. Strong sentiments in some quarters favor outlawing all psychosurgery. While epilepsy surgery, which treats an organic brain disease, is not now under attack, depth recording, which some consider essential for the accurate localization of an epileptogenic focus, is common to many psychosurgical procedures. To prevent the surgeon, operating for epilepsy, from becoming embroiled in this controversy, the indications, contraindications, and limitations of depth recording in each case should be critically identified. The surgeon must weigh the risks against the probable benefits to the patient. Unquestionably, one of the most difficult problems in the diagnostic examination of an epileptic relates to the bilateral phenomena, usually spiking, that are present to a greater or lesser extent in the EEG in most cases. Depth recording offers a means of differentiating primary and secondary bilateral synchrony from multiple independent foci.

There are many other long-term effects of operative removal of the cortex which have not been sufficiently studied. These relate to changes in personality, alterations in global sexuality, decreased life expectancy, and suicide in the first few years after operation. Further, studies on the effect of temporal lobectomy on sleep and dreams may show a change in the ratio of the different stages of sleep, especially rapid eye movement sleep. Finally, the psychosocial changes following a temporal lobe resection may play an important role in the decrease of epileptic attacks.

It is thus apparent that the surgery for epilepsy requires a team effort, with each highly skilled member cooperating in the initial examination, operative procedure, convalescence, and familial, social, and vocational rehabilitation. Even with this collaborative effort, the results of the surgical interventions are not always successful for reasons as yet poorly understood. However, the outlook for the future with better methods of case selection, improved diagnostic techniques, new and promising surgical procedures carried out under ideal analgesics, and means of providing comprehensive counseling, brings hope for the epileptic patient.

ACKNOWLEDGMENT

This chapter is based in part on work done under grant NB-03392 from the National Institutes of Health.

REFERENCES

Anderman, E., Metrakos, J. D., and Rasmussen, T. B. (1972): The relationships of genetic factors to surgical outcome in patients operated for focal epilepsy. *Electroencephalogr. Clin. Neurophysiol.,* 33:452.

Bailey, P., and Gibbs, F. A. (1951): The surgical treatment of psychomotor epilepsy. *JAMA,* 145:365–370.

Bray, P. E., and Wiser, W. C. (1965): Hereditary characteristics of familial temporal-central focal epilepsy. *Pediatrics,* 36:207–211.

Brown, B. S., Wienckowski, L. A., and Bivens, L. W. (1973): *Psychosurgery, perspective on a current problem.* National Institute of Mental Health, Department of Health, Education, and Welfare Publication No. (HSM) 73–9119, Washington, D. C., 17 pp.

Crandall, P. H. (1973): NINDS research project: Stereotaxic surgery stops some seizures, adds to scientists' knowledge of the brain [by Joanna Fulmer]. *National Spokesman,* 6:4.

Dandy, W. E. (1918): Ventriculography following the injection of air into the cerebral ventricles. *Ann. Surg.,* 68:5–11.

Falconer, M. A. (1965): The surgical treatment of temporal lobe epilepsy. *Neurochirurgica,* 8:161-172.

Falconer, M. A. (1970): Significance of surgery for temporal lobe epilepsy in childhood and adolescence. *J. Neurosurg.,* 33:233–252.

Foerster, O. (1925): Zur Pathogenese und chirurgischen Behandlung der Epilepsie. *Zentralbl. Chir.,* 52:531–549.

Foerster, O., and Penfield, W. (1930): The structural basis of traumatic epilepsy and results of radical operation. *Brain,* 53:99–119.

Fuster, B., Gibbs, E. L., and Gibbs, F. A. (1948): Pentothal sleep as an aid to the diagnosis and localization of seizure discharges of the psychomotor type. *Dis. Nerv. Syst.,* 9:199–202.

Green, J. R., Duisberg, R. E. H., and McGrath, W. B. (1951): Focal epilepsy of psychomotor type: A preliminary report of observations on effects of surgical therapy. *J. Neurosurg.,* 8:157.

Heath, R. G. (1964): *The Role of Pleasure in Behavior.* Harper and Row, New York.

Horsley, V. (1886): Brain surgery. *Brit. Med. J.,* 2:670–675.

Horsley, V. (1890): Surgery of the central nervous system. *Brit. Med. J.,* 2:1286.

Klüver, H., and Bucy, P. C. (1939): Preliminary analysis of functions of the temporal lobe in monkeys. *Arch. Neurol. Psychiat.,* 42:979–1000.

Krynaur, R. A. (1950): Infantile paraplegia treated by removing one cerebral hemisphere. *J. Neurol. Neurosurg. Psychiat.,* 13:243–267.

Lennox, W. G. (1951): The heredity of epilepsy as told by relatives and twins. *JAMA,* 146:529–536.

Marshall, B. M. (1973): Neuroleptanesthesia in neurosurgery. *Int. Anesthesiol. Clin.,* 11:103–124.

McFadden, J. T. (1969): Metallurgical principles in neurosurgery. *J. Neurosurg.,* 31:373–385.

Metrakos, K., and Metrakos, J. D. (1961): Genetics of convulsive disorders. II. Genetic and electroencephalographic studies in centrencephalic epilepsy. *Neurology,* 11:474–483.

Meyers, R. (1954): The surgical treatment of "focal" epilepsy: An inquiry into current premises, their implementation and the criteria employed in reporting results. *Epilepsia,* 3:9–36.

Michenfelder, J. D., Granert, G. A., and Rehder, K. (1969): Neuroanesthesia. *Anesthesiol.,* 30:65–100.

Morris, A. A. (1956): Temporal lobectomy with removal of uncus, hippocampus, and amygdala: Results for psychomotor epilpesy three to nine years after operation. *Arch. Neurol. Psychiat.,* 76:479–496.

Penfield, W. (1927): The mechanism of cicatricial contraction in the brain. *Brain,* 50:499–517.

Rasmussen, T., and Jasper, H. (1958): Temporal lobe epilepsy, indication for operation and surgical technique. In: *Temporal Lobe Epilepsy,* edited by M. Baldwin and P. Bailey. Charles C Thomas, Springfield, Ill., pp. 440–460.

Rodin, E. A. (1968): *The Prognosis of Patients with Epilepsy.* Charles C Thomas, Springfield, Ill., 455 pp.

Thomas, M. H. (1974): Levels of progress in prevention of seizures and restoration of the person with epilepsy. Presented at the Western Institute for Epilepsy, March 19, 1974.

Spiegel, E. A., Wycis, H. T., Marks, M., and Lee, A. J. (1947): Stereotaxic apparatus for operations on the human brain. *Science,* 106:349–350.

Walker, A. E. (1957): Prognosis in post-traumatic epilepsy, a ten-year follow-up of craniocerebral injuries of World War II. *JAMA,* 164:1636–1641.

Walker, A. E. (1967): Temporal lobectomy. *J. Neurosurg.,* 26:641–649.

Walker, A. E. (1972) Long term evaluation of the social and family adjustment to head injuries. *Scand. J. Rehab. Med.,* 4:5–8.

Walker, A. E., Leuchs, H. K., Lechtape-Grüter, H., Caveness, W. F., and Kretschmann, C. (1971): Life expectancy of head injured men with and without epilepsy. *Arch. Neurol.,* 24:95–100.

Walker, A. E., and Marshall, C. (1961): Stimulation and depth recording in man. In: *Electrical Stimulation of the Brain,* edited by D. E. Sheer. University of Texas Press, Austin.

Walker, A. E., and Uematsu, S. (1973): Echoencephalography. *Curr. Med. Digest,* 913–927.

Williams, D. (1953): A study of thalamic and cortical rhythms in petit mal. *Brain,* 76:50–69.

SUBJECT INDEX

A

Activation of seizures
  for diagnostic studies, 68-69, 71-74
    bemegride in, 72-74
    in electrocorticography, 96
    hyperventilation in, 71, 96
    methohexital in, 72, 96
    pentylenetetrazol in, 72-74
      diazepam with, 73-74
    photic stimulation in, 71
    in sleep, 72
    by withdrawal of medication, 71
Adolescents, social rehabilitation of, 278
Afterdischarge, in electrocorticography, 97-98
Age
  and onset of seizures, 17-18, 109, 113, 115
    in temporal lobe epilepsy, 158
  at operation, 268-269
    in frontal lobe epilepsy, 200
    and pathologic categories, 116
  and selection of patients for surgery, 44, 55
Ammon's horn. *See* Hippocampus
Amnesia. *See* Memory
Amobarbital, intracarotid
  in preoperative studies of speech and
    memory, 314-318
  in secondary bilateral synchrony diagnosis,
    77-83, 201
Amygdala
  extent of excision of, 289-290
  stereotactic lesions in, 31, 251-255
Amytal. *See* Amobarbital
Anesthesia, 141-142, 340-341
  in temporal resection, 186-189
Angiography, cerebral, 41, 53-54
  microangiography, 294
  in temporal lobe epilepsy, 162
  in tumors with epilepsy, 230-231
Anticonvulsants. *See* Medical therapy
Arteriovenous malformations, with epilepsy,
    232
  surgery in, 234
    results of, 237
Astrocytomas, 231
  results of surgery in, 234-235
Auditory function tests, 303-304
Auras, clinical patterns of, 269-270
  in temporal lobe epilepsy, 159
Automatism, 6-8

B

Behavior disorders. *See* Psychiatric disorders

Behavioral therapy, effects of, 25, 27
Bemegride, for activation of seizures, 72-74
Biofeedback therapy, 27
Bombardment, and spread of seizures, 5, 6, 8
Brain scanning, value of, 41, 52, 230

C

Capsular lesions, stereotactic, 242-243
Carbamazepine therapy, 43, 50
Card-sorting, after frontal lobe excision,
    310-312
Carotid arteries
  injection with amobarbital or pentylene-
    tetrazol, for secondary bilateral
    synchrony diagnosis, 77-83, 201
  preoperative intracarotid amytal studies of
    speech and memory, 314-318
Case reports of surgical results, 285-289, 295-
    296
Celontin therapy, 43
Central region epilepsy
  attack patterns in, 208
  electroencephalography in, 208-209
  etiology of, 207
  surgery in, 209-211
    psychological aspects of, 312-313
    results of, 211
Central region turmors
  incidence of, 232
  surgery in, 233
Centrencephalic integration, 7
Cerebellum, role in epilepsy development,
    28-29
Cerebral maturation, and onset of seizures,
    17-18
Cerebral pathology, and epilepsy development,
    19-20
Cerebrospinal fluid, after cortical resection,
    150-151
Children
  anesthesia for, 142
  psychological testing of, 304
Chlorpromazine, in temporal resection, 187
Cingulum, stereotactic lesions in, 30, 251
Circuits of spread, in seizures, 5, 31-34
Clonazepam therapy, 50
Clorazepate dipotassium, 50
Cognitive function. *See* Intelligence
Commissurotomy, cerebral, 259-260
Complications of surgery, 149-151, 273
  in frontal lobe epilepsy, 203-204